TAO TANTRIC ARTS
for WOMEN

Cultivating Sexual Energy,
Love, and Spirit

Minke de Vos

Destiny Books
Rochester, Vermont • Toronto, Canada

Destiny Books
One Park Street
Rochester, Vermont 05767
www.DestinyBooks.com

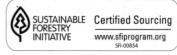

Text stock is SFI certified

Destiny Books is a division of Inner Traditions International

Library of Congress Cataloging-in-Publication Data
Names: Vos, Minke de, 1955– author.
Title: Tao tantric arts for women : cultivating sexual energy, love, and
  spirit / Minke de Vos ; foreword by Mantak Chia.
Description: Rochester, Vermont : Destiny Books, 2016. | Includes
  bibliographical references and index.
Identifiers: LCCN 2015042842 (print) | LCCN 2015048396 (e-book) |
  ISBN 9781620555163 (paperback) | ISBN 9781620555170 (e-book)
Subjects: LCSH: Sex—Religious aspects—Taoism. | Sex—Religious
  aspects—Tantrism. | Sex instruction—Religious aspects—Taoism. | Sex
  instruction—Religious aspects—Tantrism. | BISAC: HEALTH & FITNESS /
  Sexuality. | SELF-HELP / Sexual Instruction.
Classification: LCC HQ61 .V67 2016 (print) | LCC HQ61 (e-book) |
  DDC 306.7—dc23
LC record available at http://lccn.loc.gov/2015042842

Printed and bound in the United States by Lake Book Manufacturing, Inc.
The text stock is SFI certified. The Sustainable Forestry Initiative® program promotes sustainable forest management.

10 9 8 7 6 5 4 3 2 1

Text design and layout by Virginia Scott Bowman
This book was typeset in Garamond Premier Pro and Gill Sans with Jensen Pro and Futura used as display typefaces

Drawings by Minke de Vos (unless specifically attributed)
Minke's drawings inked by Gary Wildeman
Photo art on page 245 by David Gyurkovics
Poems and lyrics by the author (unless specifically attributed)

To send correspondence to the author of this book, mail a first-class letter to the author c/o Inner Traditions • Bear & Company, One Park Street, Rochester, VT 05767, and we will forward the communication, or contact the author directly at
www.femininetreasures.com.

Contents

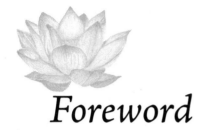

Foreword

In my thirty years of teaching the Universal Healing Tao, I have worked with many dedicated practitioners, and Minke de Vos is one of those bright guiding lights. I met her in 1983 and was impressed by her spontaneous, powerful awakening of the energy channels and subtle states of being, which demonstrated her deep roots in the Tao.

Minke has taught with me in the Darkroom retreat, Healing Love workshops, and other international trainings. It was a pleasure experiencing her creative and harmonious way of teaching. Her joy and passion for practice is contagious. After she facilitated the women in the workshop, they returned glowing!

Sexual alchemy is a core Taoist practice, as sexual energy is the fuel for our development on all levels. The ancient roots for cultivating sexual energy are now taking root all over the world and instructors like Minke and her partner, David Gyurkovics, are making it available for people to learn these valuable practices internationally. Their retreats are seeding grounds for training skilled certified instructors to bring the energy arts into their communities.

The Taoist sexual arts are a growing field of interest for men and women. Through the integration of internal research and Western science, our understanding of the importance of creative life force is expanding. I am happy to introduce Minke's teachings to a growing body of women and men, who will greatly benefit from the practices.

Remember: "When you practice, you get it!" I hope that Minke's beautiful playbook will inspire your practice.

Mantak Chia

～◯

MANTAK CHIA, world-famous Inner Alchemy and Qigong master, founded the Universal Healing Tao system in 1979 and has taught and certified tens of thousands of students and instructors all over the world. The director of the Tao Garden Health Spa and Resort in northern Thailand, he is the author of more than fifty books, including *Healing Love through the Tao* and *Chi Kung for Women's Health and Sexual Vitality*.

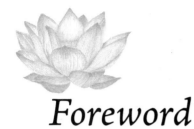

Foreword

There is an overabundance of new age and self-help books on how to improve one's sex life. But few of these books offer genuine wisdom and skill in managing sexuality at all levels of one's life. Minke de Vos's *Tao Tantric Arts for Women* is about achieving total integrity with one's sexual energy. It is packed with cream-of-the-crop methods and insights that only someone who has lived her life and relationships to the hilt could share.

Minke's approach is much deeper than that of ordinary psychologists, Western sexologists, or weekend tantra workshop experts. It's because she has done the hard work of cultivating herself for decades following a very deep path that integrates Qigong (Chi Kung), Taoist Inner Alchemy meditation, sacred dance and song, and traditional tantric principles.

She uses a very sophisticated and elegant model of the human energy body that allows for a much higher-level skill set. Most of the "neo-tantrics" I've encountered have their hearts in the right place but simply lack the high-level internal energy skills needed to take their students to a deep spiritual reawakening.

I have cotaught with Minke at our Healing Tao USA summer retreats (currently in Asheville, North Carolina) over the last ten years. This has given me a chance to witness firsthand how she uses her feminine energy cultivation methods to quickly touch people and empower them to change their own lives. She teaches with her whole being, focusing her strong feminine presence in creating safe and satisfying pathways for transformation.

I've watched her countless times become a natural magnet for women seeking clarity and strength in their sexuality. The women who emerge from her jade egg and breast massage breakout sessions are glowing and radiant. But in our coed sessions, she is equally inspiring to men. She helps them grasp the elusive feminine sensitivities within themselves needed to harmonize their relationships with women. She helps get them in touch with their often-suppressed inner female. Finding and balancing both the male and female soul polarity within a single-sexed body is both the challenge and the secret of Minke's success.

Minke is able to share the Taoist truth that sexuality is a special frequency of highly volatile energy connected to the soul of every human. In this approach, sexual energy cultivation doesn't have to involve sexual activity. Sexual Qi, called Jing Qi, can be directed outward for romance or inward for spiritual cultivation, or it can be focused within our body for medical and emotional healing. This is the core secret of Taoist inner sexual alchemy, known as the Enlightenment of Kan and Li (water and fire).

Minke ran a retreat center called Silent Ground on an island off the coast of Canada for twenty years in which students would come for months at a time to do serious practice with Taoist Inner Alchemy and Qigong. This was not a place for weekend workshop junkies hoping to find a new Band-Aid for their suffering. She required her students to develop energetic skills that allow one to progress from the personality's physical body consciousness to the soul's energy body to our collective spirit body, also known as awakening our Oversoul.

It was the deep work she did on herself at Silent Ground that gives Minke an edge over other teachers of the Tao and Tantric Arts. She has fully lived what she teaches; she has walked her talk for a very long time. She dances with the litheness of a young girl and when she laughs you know her inner child is alive and well. She wears a deep wisdom with humbleness and grace. She has trained deeply in the spiritual sciences needed to speed up both self-healing and self-realization.

Minke knows how to guide women to open up their energy channels using the Tao Microcosmic Orbit, movement, Qigong or sacred dance, emotional alchemy of the Fusion of the Five Elements, and inner soul integration of water-and-fire sexual alchemy. These methods allow the highest level of sexual healing, sexual integration of shadow side of the soul, and sexual illumination that overflows into the spirit level.

That might seem scary to some; it is a lot to commit to. But Minke has a talent for making the journey fun and easy. So it is natural that she often starts her students with a single method, such as the Inner Smile, or the Six Healing Sounds combined with jade egg, before they feel safe in progressing to deeper levels. It's not necessary to jump in with our whole body and soul onto this path. That is part of the beauty of Minke's book—it offers a smorgasbord of feminine treasures that people can pick and choose from, to creatively shape their own sexual path.

This book is thus a resource for women of many different paths. Whether you seek healing from exhaustion and trauma, want to enhance romance in the bedroom, or are attracted to using your soul's sexual polarity to supercharge your spiritual path, this book has much to offer you. It is a cornucopia overflowing with jewels of wisdom and practical advice. It is distillation of a highly talented woman who has spent her entire lifetime in assembling and refining these jewels.

If you want to improve your life and the life of those you love, please take the time to practice what she so generously offers in her book. This will keep the flow of sexual energy moving in ever-expanding cosmic spirals of love and harmony.

In gratitude for Minke's open-hearted offering,

MICHAEL WINN

Michael Winn cowrote with Mantak Chia the classic *Taoist Secrets of Love: Cultivating Male Sexual Energy* and was chief editor and writer of Mantak Chia's *Healing Love through the Tao: Cultivating Female Sexual Energy*. Michael Winn is founder of Healing Tao USA. His forthcoming book is *Primordial Tai Chi: Way of Enlightened Love.*

Invocation and Intention

Humbly I thank my many teachers,
All beings who help me cultivate my life
and realize my higher consciousness.

May life-force energy flow through my being,
and Divine Presence penetrate my body and soul.
May my love be free and graceful!

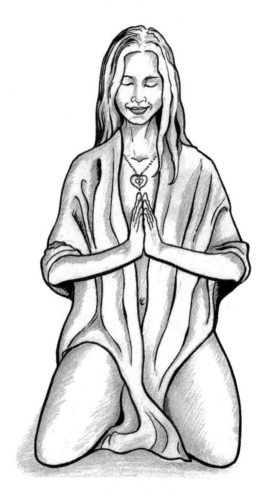

The Divine in me bows to the Divine in you.

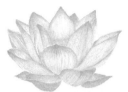

Acknowledgments

I dedicate this book to the Tao,
the Divine Feminine,
and infinite creative possibilities.

I feel we urgently need these practices to awaken our natural healing energy. As we heal and love ourselves, we heal and love the world. The cultivation of energy has been a strong thread in my life, which continues to pull me through challenges and weave the manifestation of my life purpose.

I feel so inspired by the Divine Feminine and so supported by the Divine Masculine in this co-creation. Gratitude wells up in my heart for all those who gave their kind attention to making this book accessible to a broader community.

- I am deeply grateful to Mantak Chia and all the Universal Healing Tao instructors who have contributed to bringing the Oriental Inner Alchemy secrets to the world.
- I appreciate all the joy and wisdom from teaching with Michael Winn of Healing Tao USA. Great thanks for his big perspective in his brilliant foreword.
- Thanks to my mother, Janke van der Kooi, for her belief in my unique gifts. Thanks to my father, Antoon de Vos, for his loving understanding of nature and for teaching me to draw.
- Thanks to Christer Ekstrom, my ex-partner, for building up with me

Silent Ground, a unique center that held long-term retreats dedicated to meditation, healing, and art.

✍ The sacred union with my partner, Dave Gyurkovics, is a continual source of unconditional love, support, and joy, for which I am deeply grateful.

✍ Thanks to Wendy Lang for teaching the Medical Qigong Training. This training has deepened my connection to the Divine for guidance and healing. The books by Professor Jerry Alan Johnson, about Chinese Medical Qigong therapy, have been a profound resource in my research of the esoteric meaning of ancient healing methods.

✍ Thanks to Shashi Solluna for coteaching Tao Tantric Arts Teacher Training for Women with me. Her passion for deep exploration and the evolution of tantra has been very inspiring.

✍ Thanks to Darshan Yoriko Takui for making some of the original illustrations, which inspired me to draw and create visual transmissions.

✍ Thanks to Gary Wildeman, a comic book artist and drummer, who brought playfulness and precision to inking the illustrations and drawings. And to Dave Gyurkovics, whose skill of observation and touchup refined the final presentation.

✍ I am so grateful to Stephanie Lafazanos for her eloquence and coherence in helping me to write the book. We enjoyed drawing on our internal research as teachers of Tao Tantric Arts. In our creative space, channeling of the Divine opened up and came through with ease and grace.

✍ Thanks to Kenneth Wapner for his expert help with my book proposal and Jacob Larmour for prepping the manuscript. Great thanks to all those at Inner Traditions/Destiny Books for making this book as successful as it can be.

✍ I would like to thank all the participants in our classes, workshops, and retreats over the years. I have learned so much from you! Everyone's questions and enthusiasm have contributed to the momentum of this book's emergence.

✍ Thank you all for reading and practicing, as your loving attention keeps this book's creative energy alive!

Introduction to Oriental Terminology

Terms in parentheses are alternate spellings.

Bells of Love: The breasts, which resound the feelings of the heart

Cauldron: A pot of transformation in our core, between the navel and the spine, about two finger-widths below the navel

Crystal Palace: The center of the brain, and the location of the master endocrine glands

Dantian (tan tien): An elixir field for brewing qi—an area like a ball of energy. There are three dantians: the upper dantian is located in the head; the middle dantian is in the chest; and the lower dantian is in the lower abdomen.

Jade Fountain: Female sexual organs; our fountain of youth and spring of life

Jade Stalk: Penis

Qi (chi): pronounced "*chee*"; energy, life force, the breath of life that nourishes us

Qigong (Chi Kung): Energy cultivation, mastery of subtle energy; an Oriental breath therapy that may include meditation, breath work, and movement

Sexual Palace: In women, the Sexual Palace is the Ovarian Palace—the uterus. In men, it is the Sperm Palace, in the area of the prostate gland.

Tantra: A weaving of opposites, a transformation of spirit into matter, matter into spirit, or fear into love

Tao (Dao): The path of living in harmony with nature

Yoni: A Sanskrit word from the Yogic tradition that means "womb," "symbol of life," or "sacred place" (*Vagina* means "sheath for a sword.")

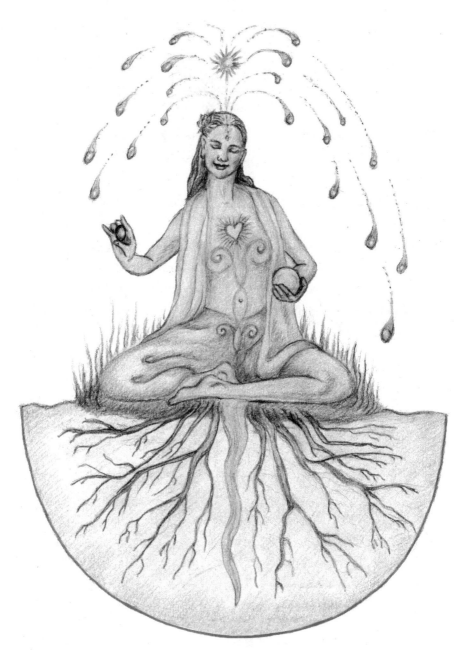

Feminine transmission

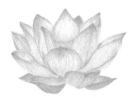

Introduction

*Cultivating a relationship with your feminine essence
makes fragrant the river of love
between you, your loved ones, and life itself.*

The purpose of this book is to inspire you to nurture and evolve yourself through regular practice. I believe the Sacred Feminine is reemerging at this time. Women are naturally drawn to empower themselves as the Goddesses that they are. The refined practices as presented in this book are a portal for individuals and groups of women to create a new reality for ourselves.

The book is intended to help you build an energetic foundation for cultivating your sexual creative energy in a safe way. The purpose of the practices is to take you on a journey of progressive dimensions of exploration:

- ⚹ Your journey begins by opening the channels and healing yourself.
- ⚹ The second dimension focuses on empowerment and strengthening yourself.
- ⚹ The third dimension focuses on manifesting your creativity and harmony.
- ⚹ The fourth dimension is the development of conscious relationships with your loved ones.
- ⚹ The fifth dimension is spiritual alchemy of your inner male and inner female and giving birth to your inner sage.

1

By progressing through these dimensions you will build a solid foundation for self-cultivation. The Universal Healing Tao offers an excellent system to enhance self-mastery. It builds the foundation from rooting in the earth and being in the body. It is a "down and through" path, which incarnates your spirit into the body with awareness: the deeper you go, the higher you rise. You create a safe channel for transferring energy through your being and avoid the dangers of striving for ascension without sufficient grounding. If a tree does not grow deep enough roots, it can get top heavy, topple over, and crash.

If you do not embrace yourself as a raw sexual being and are just fascinated by spiritual light, you can get caught in "spiritual bypassing"—cutting yourself off from your true power and the juice of life. Making the physical reality transparent to the light of the spirit is spiritual work. It is the sexual energy that weaves all these dimensions together.

You might think sexual energy is just about sex, but it is actually about how alive you feel! You can cultivate this essential vitality for your life as a whole. Tantra actually involves the heightening of your awareness in all aspects of your life, including not just sex but how you drink tea, walk, or sleep. It weaves the sacred into your daily life.

Keys to Cultivating Qi

- Be relaxed, loving, and playful!
- Circulate your sexual energy from your genitals to the rest of your body.
- Conserve, generate, and transform your sexual energy for longer-lasting pleasure, health, and spiritual awakening.
- Stay wild!

The practices included in this book were designed to help you tune your own instrument. When you play with your beloved, you make music, make love, and make life harmonious. You are prepared for grace, harmony, and bliss to happen! Be patient, beginning your own personal practice with single cultivation (solo practice). Much satisfaction will come when you apply the energetic gestures with your partner, although this is not the end goal. The nurturing of self-love is meaningful and fulfilling within itself.

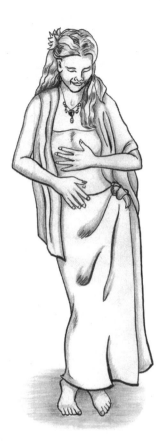

Loving your instrument

By applying the practices and principles in this book you can open a treasure chest of creative opportunities for growth. Along the way you may stir up challenges and issues that want to be liberated. Through mindfulness, self-understanding, and compassion, you can embrace these issues and resolve them at a gentle pace that is organic for you. You are not alone when you connect with your creative essence and higher guidance. Your intuition and heart's knowing will lead you, as well as pave the way for others around you.

How to read this book? After you read a practice it's good to close your eyes and visualize yourself doing it; in this way, you can accomplish the practice in your kinesthetic imagination. Apply the principle "Where the mind goes, qi flows." You will reap the benefit as if you were doing the practice with movement of your physical body. This is a convenient way to practice internally if you are reading this book on an airplane or in a coffee shop, for instance, and don't want to draw attention to yourself.

When you are in a safe space, practice with your whole being. Take the time to embody these practices by gently nurturing yourself on all levels.

You will bring more joy, love, and compassion into your life.

I recommend that you read and practice with this book like you would a cookbook: when you feel tantalized by the description of a practice, cook it up and eat it right away! For those of you who do not use recipes, let it be an inspiration. Once you understand the essence of qi cultivation and transformation you can create your own Qigong forms and delicious dishes!

Pillars for Practice

There is such an abundance of treasures in this book, you may wonder which are the main practices that you should focus on.

These are the practices that best support this energetic path:

Tao Energy Fundamentals

Inner Smile

Six Healing Sounds

Microcosmic Orbit

Qi Self-Massage

Sexual Energy Cultivation

Three Fires

Breast massage

Yoni Breathing

Jade egg practices

Triple Purification

Tao Tantric Qigong

Lotus Sublimation

Belt Channels

Thrusting Channels and Fountains

Kidney Breathing

Embracing the Tree

Bone Breathing

Moon and Sun practices

Alchemy of Love

Harmonious Exchange

Water Wheels

Divine Union

PRINCIPLES FOR SELF-CULTIVATION

The practices in this book are drawn from ancient Taoist principles of energy flow in the universe and in our bodies.

To follow the Tao is to live in accordance with the natural way. Nature goes through the cycles of the seasons, and the ancient Taoists created formulas for practice based on these cycles. The five-element cycle that underlies much of Taoist thought also forms the underpinning of many of the practices in this book.

The creation cycle is used to cultivate energy, while the control cycle is used to counterbalance opposite elements. (See chapter 2 for more information on these five-element cycles.)

The stages of a woman's life cycle can also be viewed as the seasons: maiden (spring), wild woman (summer), mother (fall), and crone (winter). Spring and summer are yang seasons, and fall and winter are yin seasons, so we are conscious of balancing active yang with restful yin practice.

The Medicine Wheel acknowledges the cycles of the moon phases in understanding the menstrual cycle: ovulation is likened to the full moon, the premenstrual period corresponds to the waning moon, menstruation is like the dark moon, and the postmenstrual period corresponds to the waxing moon, with the still point in the center of the wheel.

We also apply the principles of Medical Qigong, which include purging, tonifying, and regulating. When we move into a new house or state of being we first need to clean the house, repair it, fortify its structure, and create a balanced atmosphere in which to live.

The golden triangle or sacred trinity of body, soul, and spirit is applied continuously in these teachings. You are always addressing bodily awareness, emotional transformation, and creative intention.

PRACTICAL NOTES AND CAUTIONS

Sexual energy is like fire.
It can warm your house or cook your food.
If you don't treat it wisely with respect,
it can burn your house down.

These practices are powerful and require your loving attention. If you have a medical condition, please consult a physician or doctor of traditional

Chinese medicine. Listen to the needs of your body. If you have any questions, please contact a Universal Healing Tao instructor or Tao Tantric Arts Facilitator.

In general, the practices included in this book are a safe way to work with Kundalini—the powerful sexual energy currents—as they are well grounded and well founded. Throughout the book, we will identify contraindications for specific practices and conditions.

When the sexual energy is awakened it will start to clean up the body and emotions to prepare for the rebirth of your subtle bodies. You might experience detoxification symptoms as well as a release of psychic toxins. Rest, get bodywork, be in nature, move, dance, and give yourself time to integrate.

Special Cautions

- Pregnant women should avoid drawing sexual energy away from the growing fetus. Instead, channel earth energy up and into the body to support growth.
- Women with IUDs should avoid weight resistance training, as the IUD could cause tears in the uterus.
- Those who have mental and emotional challenges should practice Inner Smile, Six Healing Sounds, and Microcosmic Orbit to harmonize the inner life before actively cultivating sexual energy. Because sexual energy amplifies our emotions and thought patterns, it is important to avoid putting gasoline on a fire that may be self-destructive or imbalanced.

Through self-observation you can read the warning signals of your body and emotions when they are in the bud formation, rather than remaining unaware until your body screams at you through disease. These practices are really the art of preventive medicine. Through self-awareness and self-care you can prevent some pain and suffering arising from negligence.

These practices can be very energizing! If you practice this at night without balancing and centering, you might end up cleaning the whole house or writing a book! At the end of every session, absorb excess energy and heat into the bone marrow via Bone Breathing, and balance hot and cold energy by running the Microcosmic Orbit. Center and store energy in the navel center to finish. If there is still excess energy, cool down with the triple warmer healing sound.

If your body is shaking and moving spontaneously, allow the energy to move you and unwind blockages. Please see the description of Unwinding in chapter 8. If the energy gets too high, a venting point is the Mingmen, the Door of Life, behind the navel on the spine. Breathe into this First Aid point to reset yourself with source energy. The other First Aid point is the Bubbling Spring on the soles of the feet. (See Self-Acupressure in chapter 2 for these point locations.)

You can trust the innate wisdom of your natural sexual energy. Resistance and suppression of this powerful life force can create mental, emotional, and physical imbalances. Cooperate with this energy, as it is always working to heal and balance you!

PROGRESSION OF PRACTICES

It is important to understand why we do practices in a certain order. Cultivating sexual energy requires the preparation of your body-mind, just as the process of cultivating a garden requires that we weed, till the soil, nourish with fertilizer, and plant the seeds before we can harvest and store the fruits. Part of the preparation of your body-mind is emotional transformation. We open channels to circulate the qi. We store the energy to build a reserve.

The structure allows us to be spontaneous and creative; discipline breeds freedom.

- Warm-ups, Qigong, and Tao Tantric Yoga loosen tension, open the body, and ground our energy in the earth.
- Healing work transforms the emotions and clears obstructions to free expression of your sexuality.
- The Inner Smile and breast massage open the heart, activate the hormones, and fuse the virtues of the organs into compassion. When the heart opens, the yoni opens.
- Belly and ovarian massage improve the qi and blood circulation and release energetic knots around the navel.
- Cleansing the uterus from negative emotions allows us to fill our creative center with compassionate vibrations.

⚔ Practicing Yoni Articulation and Yoni Breathing awakens and circulates the sexual energy. Yoni Toning connects our throat and sexual chakras, freeing our creative voice.

⚔ Jade egg practice strengthens the pelvic floor; warms up, circulates, and activates the sexual energy; articulates the vagina as an instrument of love; stimulates the reflexology zones inside the vagina; and opens portals for endless dimensions of orgasm. Tao Yoni Yoga uses various postures and movements to channel the sexual energy.

⚔ Tao Tantric Qigong and Qi Weight Lifting enliven your movement and strengthen your internal powers.

⚔ Kidney and Bone Breathing build up your reservoirs of energy.

⚔ Circulation of sexual energy moves and refines the energy in the major channels.

⚔ Harmonious Exchange enhances the conscious exchange of energies with your partner.

⚔ Inner Alchemy balances and transforms fire and water into unconditional love and marries your inner masculine and feminine energies into conscious wholeness.

Ultimately, developing compassion and inner beauty is our best protection and a gift to the universe. What we radiate comes back to us. Let us support and encourage each other to be creative and healthy. Practice with other women for a powerful exploration of your essential energy. The tools you learn will help you transform your life and support your healing journey into radiant wellness. Enjoy these expressions of love!

These practices are based on an ancient tradition and applied in creative ways. Once you get the essence, please add your creativity to your practice! When you do it, you will start to reap the countless benefits.

🕊 Minke's Journey of Rebirth

My youth was full of wonder! As a teenager I had a deep respect for sex and felt this act was truly sacred. It could create a child and profoundly change one's life. The other girls in my high school seemed more casual in their exploration of sex; it was entrenched in the drug, alcohol, and rock-and-roll scene.

I loved kissing and playing but as for full intercourse I wanted to make sure the guy was "right" for me. My first serious boyfriend felt an amazing energy coursing through me and described it as champagne bubbles! In uni-

versity my boyfriend and I went all the way. Delightful sensations arose but I felt something was missing. I recognized that his hands were not the hands of my long-term lover.

I choreographed a dance of the five elements, intuiting all the colors and movements of the elements from dream states, and later read about them in a Tibetan Buddhist book. In a rainbow costume my movements were like stirring a cauldron. The other five dancers poured their negative emotions into this cauldron to be fused into compassion. All at once I popped out of my body and saw myself dancing from above in the auditorium. I realized that I was more than a physical body; I was a microcosm of the vast universe. Little did I know that I would one day be teaching Fusion of the Five Elements and Microcosmic Orbit, which are central to the practice of Inner Alchemy.

During this very creative time in my life, my menstruation stopped. I felt very healthy, vibrant, and inspired. I felt that I was channeling sexual and emotional energy into my dance. It wasn't because of hormonal imbalance or weakness, but due to the raising of the creative force into expression, known as "slaying the red dragon" in Taoist classical texts.

After university I left Canada and the possibilities of homesteading and children for another adventure. I went to Germany to study Eurythmy, an ethereal dance also called "visible speech and song." My body was becoming transparent and open. I could feel energy flowing through me, carrying me like an angel through space.

My body moved spontaneously every time I meditated, as the qi circulated around and through me like fountains and whirlpools. These patterns of qi, I later discovered, were embraced in the Universal Healing Tao system and cultivated in practices like the Microcosmic Orbit. Many other rhythmical patterns pulsed and circulated in different centers, which I counted and recorded in my journal.

On my holidays I went to Switzerland, where I met my future husband. I fell in love with his voice before I saw him. He was a meditator, and I accompanied him on retreats in the Swiss Alps. My meditation was simply following the breath. When I started to meditate, a surge of energy moved through my Core Channel like a volcano and overflowed through all my channels. Many awakenings proceeded as I went through a birth of my energy body over nine months.

I felt sometimes like a flaming ice cube: crystal clear and frozen in stillness with a glowing auric field. The steaming reversal of fire and water inside *made me sweat, in a cold chalet, where you could see your breath! The bliss of "cosmic orgasm" made my body feel buoyant and light-filled. The boundaries between the universe and myself often dissolved, leaving vast spaciousness.*

My soul body spontaneously extended above me. I felt a strong pull on my crown like someone was pulling my hair. Then I felt about fifteen feet high, giving me a grander view of the present moment. A bright light in my core developed, which I called a "diamond." I felt like a Madonna, giving my "diamond" devoted attention with unconditional love and compassion. For about nine months it was like a fetus stirring inside of me.

Currents were so strong that they moved my body involuntarily. I trusted the process like a woman giving birth. Carefully I observed the awesome wisdom of the energy. The process of freely flowing energetic openings continued. Through voice and gesture the immortal body, or higher self, communicates directly. It became more and more vivid how the Divine lives within me and manifests through me. The energy was often blissful and loving and I would describe it now as a spiritual orgasm. Waves of compassion would move me to tears beyond the pain of my present personal life.

We did many meditation retreats together, and on one moonlit night, we came together as a couple. After four years of Eurythmy dance training, we moved to an isolated island in Desolation Sound, British Columbia. My partner was familiar with the yogic tradition of tantra and was skilled in moving sexual energy and seminal retention. Our energy bodies exchanged bliss in a very vivid way beyond our physical bodies. This subtle-body lovemaking was seamless with the exploration of our energy bodies and was revealed more and more as we dedicated ourselves to Taiji, dance, and singing.

In 1983, my husband experienced a powerful Kundalini awakening that shook his world. I felt like a midwife for his energetic birth. Fortunately, we learned of the Taoist master Mantak Chia when my friend and Taiji teacher gave us his first book, Awakening Healing Energy through the Tao. *Upon learning about this Taoist map for our experiences, we urgently flew to San Francisco to meet Mantak Chia and other Healing Tao instructors. He was impressed by our stories of spontaneous awakening. It showed how the ancient teachings are universal in nature. He then invited us to become instructors of the Healing Tao system (whose international branch was renamed twenty years later as Universal Healing Tao).*

For twenty years we devotedly ran Silent Ground Retreat Center on Read Island, British Columbia. It was a spiritual home for the cultivation of medi-

tation, healing, and creative arts. My training with the Healing Tao community clarified safe and effective ways to work with energy and Inner Alchemy. It was fulfilling to see the development of those who applied their teacher training, backed by substantial practice.

Our lifestyle at the retreat was a very special opportunity for inner research. We worked consciously with the sexual energy, and the students at the retreat could feel this profound energy in their meditations and Qigong practices. We also channeled this energy into the singing voice. This connection of my sexual center and throat chakra allowed many poems to be channeled through me.

For a second time my menstrual cycle stopped for nine months. The energy was channeled into meditative states and spontaneous poetry. Again I felt full of life, very blissful and lucid. It was a gift of the Spirit. I felt how sexual essence can profoundly be transformed into energy and spiritual presence. Many female students had lighter menstrual cycles with less discomfort. I made a conscious decision not to be a mother in this lifetime, but rather to be a "spirit mother" for many, in service of their spiritual development at the retreats. My shamanic name is Mingka, White Crane Woman. Mingka means "bright soul."

After a long marriage of about twenty years, there came a time when my husband and I grew apart. I needed more affection. My heart's flower was withering. The divorce was very stressful emotionally. I was leaving my home and my life's work as well as my relationship.

I was vulnerable and developed a severe heart condition, which the doctors say was caused by a virus. I was increasingly ill and dying for about nine months. I tried to heal this condition with Western and alternative medicine but the damage called for a heart transplant on April 6, 2004.

I was close to death's door and was given a second chance. I called this, "new heart, new start." My sense of life purpose was enlivened. I watched my body regrow itself from skin and bones into new muscle and new hair. This was the miraculous work of sexual energy! The jing knew the original blueprint and put me back together again beautifully.

I practiced Microcosmic Orbit, Inner Smile, and Kidney and Yoni Breathing throughout my illness and recovery to restore my physical body and energy. The Inner Smile of loving acceptance never left me. My remarkable recovery was living proof of the effectiveness of the Taoist practices.

Four months after the operation, my dear friend Dave and I taught

Healing Love at Hollyhock Retreat Center. I was still limping a bit as I had a drop foot. I used my intention to encourage the nerves to grow together, to dance and kiss each other. It worked! I was so grateful to be able to walk and dance again!

The Divine kicked me out of the monastic lifestyle. Now living in the marketplace, my vision is to help others cultivate their connection with the great universal spirit, to become peaceful with their soul's experiences, and to manifest wisdom and compassion through their bodies.

Not everyone has such a dramatic story, but we all have ups and downs in life. I believe these fundamental practices are very supportive in the healing process of conscious living and thriving! Now I am living my passion teaching body, mind, spirit, and energy arts internationally. My "baby" is Feminine Treasures, which emerged through working on myself and with other women in classes and retreats. Many women contacted me asking to learn these practices from a woman rather than from a man. Up until now, many of these practices have been taught by men.

Songs and poems have poured through me out of my connection with divine love and creative energy. A lot of these creative impulses I have integrated into the Feminine Treasures training and the Sacred Femininity one-month teacher training in Tao Tantric Arts. In co-creating this training with Shashi Solluna, I have been fortunate to experience women from all over the world blossoming into their full potential.

My present partner, Dave, has played a vital role in supporting my growth. His love makes my inner flower blossom! His wisdom casts light where I need more awareness, to transform the past and live even more fully in the present. I am most grateful to the power of love to heal and the power of conscious sexual exchange to open each other to the Divine.

My newly liberated self is exploring the full spectrum of the feminine and enjoying being sexy, sweet, wise, or motherly as the moment calls for. Living and dancing my passion is a counterbalance for the more masculine, ambitious aspects of modern life, like being on the computer, texting, and other verbal and writing-based communication.

My friend Wendy Lang, who did an eight-month retreat with us over twenty years ago, asked if I would organize Medical Qigong training for her in Vancouver. I have completed this training to the master's level and am certified by the International Institute of Medical Qigong. It opened doors to the psychic, psychological, and spiritual dimensions of energy healing.

The Medical Qigong sessions have also been an important step in awakening and healing from my heart transplant. Five years after the operation, Wendy gave me a session that helped reset the rhythms of my heart, which still had the sporty, athletic rhythm of the donor, into the rhythms of my inner dancer.

Ten years after my heart transplant a primal fear reared its head and I found myself in another crisis wondering when, where, and why I would die. I cried to the Divine that I might live and do the creative work I came here for. This anxiety was creating high blood pressure and I lost my natural self-confidence. The fear felt like black dense metal in my back, which pushed me from behind and made me feel like running away from the darkness in my heart. This fear manifested in my life as a robot-like, habitual way of distracting myself through work.

Wendy facilitated me through a soul retrieval journey, where I faced my worst fear of dying. I found myself crossing the street and suddenly I fell to my death but something lifted me to the edge of the street. I was not ready to die; there was still so much creative will in me. Dave rushed to my side and I got to look into my partner's loving blue eyes for the last time. It was very hard to leave him and all the loved ones in my life. I felt the shock at their hearing of my death and felt the love behind their tears.

I passed through the veil and was greeted by a circle of angels. They opened a portal for me to review my life, which appeared as sunny or stormy weather conditions passing through my world. I went higher on a beam of rainbow light and became a star. It was peaceful and I felt supported by a grid, the Divine Masculine safety net. There was no touching and yet I felt I was touching everything through this network of light. I could play, spin, spiral, and sparkle. Floating in a grid, I was supported yet free. My "eternal soul star" reincarnated in my heart center. My physical heart received light transmissions from the star, which brought into balance the beating of my heart's wings. It felt like this internal bird could fly over the entire ocean. The twelve angels formed a halo above my head, which felt like a wedding ring that married me to the Divine.

As in near-death experiences, when I reentered my body the healing light spread into every cell and created a deep trust in love that penetrated right into my bones. What was once the heavy metal of fear transformed into diamonds of mirrors, which reflected light, suspended from Divine sources. What was once worry transformed into wonder. I could see the bright stars in my eyes!

Life was no longer a burden but an opportunity to play! I believe creative or Kundalini energy has been playing an essential role in my personal evolution. I am confident that this will ripple and continue to inspire many women on their path of unifying their primal creative life force with their spirituality.

Thank you for the opportunity to share this story. I encourage you all to write your sexual and spiritual adventures. Blessings of love and bliss to you all! I offer my joy and love for practice!

Alchemy of Opposites

When I curl over and cry
and you roll over and run,
Distant, yet love draws near.

With a sigh of passion
I long to open to you,
You long to penetrate me.

Pushing, pulling, faster and faster,
Vibrating like a sperm's tail
Swimming into the egg.

Born under one sky again and again,
Our splits and our tiffs
Arise and resolve in the Tao.

With a sigh of compassion
I dissolve into you,
You merge into me.

Love is the alchemical agent
Fusing opposites into harmony.
Our longing returns to the Source.

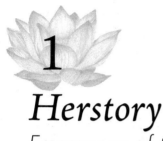

1

Herstory
Emergence of the Divine Feminine

Kuan Yin is the goddess of compassion. Her name means "she who hears the cries of the world." When I channel Kuan Yin, internally I say, "Kuan Yin and I are one." Then I allow her wisdom to come through me.

The message from Kuan Yin is that we are not alone. At this point in time the Divine is helping us to lift suffocating veils of suppression from the Feminine so that we can breathe in the power we need to rise again. At the same time, the divine being of the earth is bubbling up fountains of life force in dry and barren places. These fountains are found within our own feminine sexual organs, giving us the potential to emerge with renewed life force and purpose.

The playful dance of the Tao is like a cosmic seesaw: when the yin rises, the yang recedes, and when the yang rises, the yin recedes. We are coming to a time of equilibrium when the seesaw is even and the masculine and feminine can look into each other's eyes and see the Divine in each other. This is a profound opportunity for love that opens us to higher consciousness.

Humanity's Core Channel, expressed through our upright spine, connects the Divine Masculine—heavenly energy—with the Divine Feminine—earthy energy. This Core Channel has an opportunity now to connect deeper into the earth, a process that in turn invites the life force to come up as a fountain of renewal. In this way, each individual becomes a shining source of love, compassion, and creativity. This incarnation process of bringing heaven down to earth is feminine, like a baby spirit incarnating through the mother's body. It is the process of involution—divine light or spiritual potency birthing into matter—and is the necessary prerequisite of evolution.

Our common mother nourishes all of us and in turn we should also nourish her. This increasing wave of life force, like the power of water, will gently soften and wash away the roughness of old structures. The pain and suffering of the past era is old energy; our energy is freer now to be invested into a new and more harmonious epoch.

SAPPHISM AND SISTERHOOD

Women are like fingers of the same divine goddess,
moving with emotion, intuition, and sensitivity,
nurturing each other as the divine Mother,
upholding and cherishing our one blessed earth.

Entering through the portal of time, visualize yourself in nature: playing and harvesting with other women; massaging, bathing, and soothing each other's pain and sorrow; dancing for the pure joy of it! Let us not forget the roots of our sisterhood that go way, way back and that carry our evolution forward.

Our feminine nature longs to touch and be touched. Touch is the earth element. It is very nurturing for the body, which is the feminine aspect of ourselves. In modern life there is a lot of taboo around women touching each other, although this is gradually softening through the "free love" hugging culture. Sapphism is a feminine form of connection, intimacy, and bonding. Sensual intimacy between women was once common in the Orient and an accepted way for women to nurture themselves. Yin and yin nourish each other (fig. 1.1).

The "tend and befriend" response is natural for females in times of stress. When women come together to heal, share their stories, and celebrate, something magical happens. The entrainment of feminine essence when we are together increases oxytocin production, which gives us that good feeling. Through sharing the emotional ups and downs of life through stories, the pressure of anxiety and stress is released, allowing sexual energy to move freely through the body. Women dancing together generate joy and ecstasy!

Feminine energy is contagious; it rubs off on others. The cascading laughing, giggling, and heart-opening connection multiplies our sexual, orgasmic energy. When we go back to our partners or husbands, the polarity between masculine and feminine is increased.

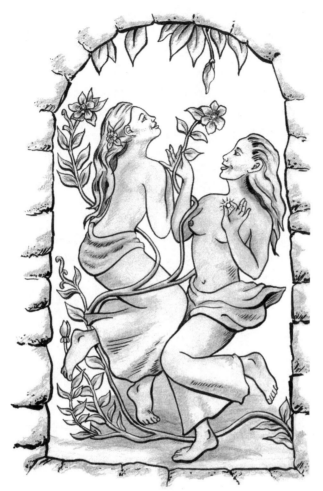

Fig. 1.1. Sisterhood celebrating nature!

❋ Women's Circle Practice

When women get together to laugh and cry, it makes them softer and more beautiful. We all love to be heard, seen, and understood. I invite you to sit with a girlfriend and allow her to share her fears, desires, and needs, witnessing with no judgment and loving acceptance. Create an equal opportunity for both of you to share and witness.

As a group practice, sit in a circle of women. Pass around two crystals, one light and one dark. Each woman can place the light crystal in one hand and the dark crystal in the other. Look into the deep, dark stone in your right hand as if you were looking into a crystal ball, and speak from that shadow part of yourself. What is holding you back in this moment? Look into the light-colored stone in your left hand and share from your heart all that you are grateful for and joyous about in your life. When everyone has had a chance to reveal the light and dark within, bring your hands together in prayer position as if fusing the opposites into love and compassion in the heart. All bow to the support of sisterhood.

The Goddess Rejoices

Woman of all ages form a cauldron,
Luscious, sweet, and wise,

Gathering together to embrace our essence,
Gathering our energy to grow our beauty.

Stories of separation drift into the distance
As the moment of connection draws near.

We are the women on the edge,
Pressing through the walls of time.

Being embraced by the angels,
our future births are blessed.

Beloved Mother of All welcomes us home
And the Goddess within rejoices.

FEMININE ROOTS
OF TAOIST SEXUAL PRACTICE

Taoist sexual practices evolved in ancient China from a combination of elements, including the ancient, deeply feminine shamanic tradition, medical practice, and scholarly philosophy.

Wu Yi Taoist Shamans

The Wu Yi were shamanic Qigong healers in ancient China. The ancient Chinese character *wu*, which means "magician," depicts a person standing between heaven and earth. The Wu Yi lived in deep connection with nature, celebrating their interrelationship with everything. This communion with Mother Earth is fundamentally feminine, and indeed, the majority of the Wu Yi were women.

The inner explorations of the Wu Yi revealed the inner workings of energy. These magicians were highly respected in their communities and consulted for various occult practices, including healing and clearing spiritual disharmony in relationships. In times of drought the Wu priestesses would dance and offer prayers to invoke rain. In times of disaster they would wail and chant, pleading with celestial immortals to soothe the people's grief.

The Wu Yi consulted tortoise shells for divination and dream interpretation and studied the energetic changes of the sun and moon, of the planets and stars. They were aware of the changes of the mist and dew—sometimes called "honey dew" or "celestial wine"—as they represented luxurious growth and abundance. Rainbows, composed of yin and yang, were investigated as the will of the Tao (Divine). Qigong grew out of these ancient roots and is the "grandmother" or spiritual basis of traditional Chinese medicine, acupuncture, Taiji, and Feng Shui.

Do you relate to the healing and intuitive abilities of the Wu Yi? In recent times there has been a resurgence of women who relate to being a goddess or priestess, as if we are remembering our ancient shamanic roots and finding renewed empowerment.

The Yellow Emperor's Classic

> *The Yellow Emperor asks, "How can I tell if a woman is*
> *experiencing pleasure?" The Plain Woman replies, "There*
> *are five signs, five desires, and ten movements by which*
> *you can observe her transformation and understand her*
> *reactions."*
>
> Su Nu Ching

The roots of the Taoist sexual arts go back to the oldest sex manuals in the world, the Chinese *Handbooks of Sex* and *Tao of Love Coupling*, written five thousand years ago by the legendary Yellow Emperor, Huang-Ti (2697–2598 BC). Under his rule, the Chinese nation developed and refined many practices, including agriculture, herbal medicine, and silk cloth industry. The Yellow Emperor is said to have had three female sex advisors and one male sex doctor. Their conversations were compiled into a book titled *Su Nu Ching,* or "Classic of the White Madam."

This legendary text became part of *The Yellow Emperor's Classic.* The *Suwen,* or "Basic Questions," is generally thought to have been created between the Warring States period (475–221 BC) and the early Han period (206 BCE–220 CE). It is the most important ancient text in Chinese medicine as well as a major book of Taoist theory and lifestyle. It brought together three different modes of practice: the shamanic magical world of the Wu Yi; the body-based methods of the Skill Masters, who were versed in healing exercises and sexual cultivation; and the Scholar-Physicians, who used medical methods and theories. Out of this hybrid combination, Oriental medicine was born.

The ancient texts of the *Suwen* contain detailed descriptions of postures and timing for lovemaking in order to optimize its healing effects. For men, this involves the practice of seminal retention to preserve jing and enhance health, longevity, and spiritual development. Although semen is retained, the mystical energetic practice of pulling up and circulating sexual essence allows for the potential of long-lasting, full-body orgasm. For women, there are ways to support and expand orgasmic fulfillment. The Yellow Emperor's secrets tell us how he enjoyed one wife of the first rank, the Queen of Heaven; three precious consorts of creativity, preservation, and immortality; nine wives of the second rank, embodying the energy of the nine planets; and twenty-seven wives of the third rank, who symbolized the twenty-seven constellations in the sky. Eighty-one concubines were for playful lovemaking. It was said that the Emperor should make love with nine chosen consorts every night and satisfy them fully so the planets were pleased. By retaining his semen through the arts of love, the Emperor concentrated his internal power, then offered his seed to the Queen of Heaven at the full moon.

The Yellow Emperor's Classic expressed the importance of sexuality in a variety of applications in our lives:

- ⚔ The arts of the bedchamber such as "entering and penetrating"
- ⚔ Invocations of the cosmic forces of yin and yang
- ⚔ Physical behavior such as "using, doing, and sleeping"
- ⚔ The potential energy drain of sexual activity
- ⚔ Specific medical conditions and possible symptoms or diseases

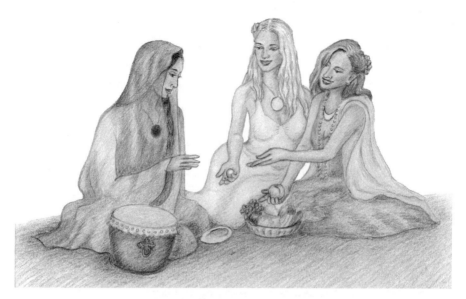

Fig. 1.2. White Madam reveals the jade egg
to Mystery Girl and Harvest Girl.

The Three Female Advisors of the Yellow Emperor

Let me introduce you to the female mystics behind Oriental medicine and sexual arts (fig. 1.2).

Su Nu, the Plain Girl, the Queen of the White River, is earth's embodiment of all creativity. The Yellow Emperor named his sex manual *Su Nu Ching*—"Classic of the White Madam"—after her. Her yoni was said to be like a beautiful conch shell, and her naked body soft as silk.

Ts'ai-Nu, the Harvest (or Elected) Girl, the Goddess of Many Colors, is earth's natural narcissism, which honors the natural beauty of our bodies. She is also the eroticism of all preservation and teaches us about conserving our sexual essence through the erotic channeling of sexual energy.

Hsuan-Nu (Shuen-Nui), the Dark Girl or Mystery Girl, is called the Peach of Immortality or Transcendence. She bears the sweetening fruits of the earth and lasting transcendence through the arts of sexual cultivation. She made magic drums for the Yellow Emperor and helped him slay the Monster of Time—the debilities of aging due to stress.

❦ A Visit with the Yellow Emperor

Entering into the beautiful palace garden of the Yellow Emperor, we greet him
on his dragon bed and hear the sweet voices of his female advisors. Delight-
ful melodies are played on the zither. The aromas of wine, fragrant orchids,
and lotus flowers fill the air. Under the moonlight the three female advisors
initiate the Yellow Emperor—the Son of Heaven—to the supreme truths
concerning sexuality and harmonization with his queen and concubines.

Elixir of Life

The forces of the three female advisors—creativity, preservation, and
transcendence—form a precious tripod of immortality and refine the
Elixir of Life. They are three, yet they are one, like the bright white full
moon, the half-moon, and the dark new moon are all phases of the moon.

The Elixir of Life was made potent, and obstacles of stagnation and
death were overcome, through cultivating the sexual essence. The sexual
essence is the water of life that is warmed by the spirit's light. When sun
and moon make love, they create steam that rises like mist on a lake in the
warm sun. This mist is described as the celestial dragon or Kundalini serpent
power, which is refined sexual essence. This blissful essence purifies our bodies and creates a loving glow that expands into the energy field around us.

These sexual and longevity secrets were lost over time, but now the
wisdom of the three mystical female advisors is again beginning to inform
our modern life.

> *Then the bliss of the Celestial Dragon rose from the lake*
> *with the sun and moon in eclipse,*
> *the Divine Union illuminated the mountains.*
>
> SU NU CHING

Arts of the Bedchamber

The Importance of Conserving Essence

> *At the beginning we speak of Essence;*
> *when the two essences of male and female mix*
> *we speak of spirit.*
>
> SU NU CHING

Essence or jing is the quintessential matter that gives life. When masculine
and female essences unite, the creation of a new human being with spirit

consciousness is born. Essence is the fundamental material, creative matrix, and reproductive force that determines the constitution of all things.

Our essence is the potent energy that makes life possible. Essence is condensation of qi in its yin aspect. Jing Qi is a yin/yang pairing in which the yang qi transforms and transports the yin essence. The best essential energy goes into procreation to further our evolutionary survival. Even if parents are unwell their children can be born well. Conserving jing is important as "it takes money to make money." A sufficient reserve of essence is needed to build vitality.

Men often feel depleted after ejaculation. One ejaculation is said to be a loss or investment equivalent to about thirty-six hours of mental work or seventy-two hours of physical work. Sperm is also full of protein and nutrition. This is why it is important for women to understand how to support a man's vitality through his practice of recycling his essence by lifting it up to higher centers and circulating it in the Microcosmic Orbit. Then, even if he does ultimately ejaculate, he has absorbed the essence into his body and/or his partner's body.

You might be surprised at how many concubines and wives the Yellow Emperor had around him—at least 120! How could he please them all without being drained of his vitality? Apparently there were previous emperors who had died at early ages due to sexual energy drain (but what a way to go!). Thanks to his female advisors, the Yellow Emperor found ways to have orgasmic experiences without draining his energy. He even improved his health at the same time! The same methods would rejuvenate the women, keeping them beautiful and vital for a long time. How did they do this?

The Female Initiatresses

The three female advisors initiated the Emperor into ways of the cosmos, including the energetic differences between heaven and earth. They taught that heaven has a solitary role of emptiness while earth embodies the fullness and multiplicity of life. Heaven rules with universal laws and the earth flourishes through the continuous creation of life in many forms. Through this understanding one can live in harmony with the polarities of masculine and feminine.

The Emperor's advisors had a deep intuitive understanding of the true nature of masculine and feminine polarities; they understood the masculine as consciousness and the feminine as the body and the flow of life. They taught that on the sixteenth day of the fifth month of every year (midsummer), the roles of heaven and earth are reversed. On this day the three advisors would determine the order of events and the Yellow Emperor would comply, thereby ruling his empire well. This shows that the three female advisors had an influence on the important events of the empire.

The Secret of the Jade Egg Practice

The secret of the jade egg practice was developed by the three female advisors to make the vagina articulate and sensitive, so that a woman could play with the Emperor's Jade Stalk and give him an orgasmic experience while he was withholding ejaculation. The advisors impressed on him the importance of circulating the sexual energy throughout his whole body, providing full-body orgasm, thus preventing genital orgasm and losing his vital essence. The jade egg was placed inside the vagina and moved in such a way that it would massage the reflexology zones of the vital organs. The jade egg practices have the result of lessening blood loss and discomfort during menstruation because the blood is transformed into qi and circulated through the body to nourish the soul and spirit.

The wisdom of these feminine mystics still exists within the Taoist Healing Love practices and is continually developed by modern women who are neither concubines nor nuns. The Tao Tantric Arts training offers women and men these sacred practices adapted to support the needs of modern life.*

Taoist Secrets Come to the West

In the 1950s and '60s, yogic and tantric practices from the Hindu traditions were being discovered in Europe and eventually came to North America. Many of these yogic traditions emphasized celibacy as a way to conserve sexual energy for yogic development.

In 1980, Mantak Chia came to New York and began to teach Chinese people there how to open the Microcosmic Orbit. His teacher in China had stressed to him the importance of teaching Chinese people. Westerners then heard of Master Chia's teachings and asked him to

---

*I am grateful to the lineage of mystical and wise women for bringing these life-enhancing practices to us and influencing Oriental medicine with their profound ways of embodying source energy.

teach them. He developed workshops and began to teach in the United States and Europe.

Prior to this, sexual practices had been held secret in China. Taoist masters kept them secret, and also made a business of teaching them. These masters felt that sexual energy was too powerful and that most people's moral development wasn't sufficient to deal with it. In the Universal Healing Tao system that Master Chia founded, however, the issue of moral development was integrated into the system: the safety valve for working with volatile sexual energy is to cultivate emotional harmony through the Inner Smile and Six Healing Sounds, to integrate and harmonize it with the Microcosmic Orbit, and to ground it with Iron Shirt Qigong.

Through his teachings, Mantak Chia stressed that the Taoist practices are a science for health and longevity. They are food for developing the soul and spirit. He saw that these practices were badly needed in the Western world to free up our repressed sexual energy and to transform our world. Other pioneers, like Dr. Stephen Chang, also shared Eastern methods of cultivating sexual energy.

At about the same time, the meditative practices of Tibetan Buddhist tantra came to the West. These teachings helped prepare people morally for practices like the Microcosmic Orbit by requiring them to do thousands of prostrations.

We are so fortunate today that we can go to a bookstore and discover how different spiritual traditions dealt with sexuality. The secrets are now open secrets that we can apply in our lives!

FEMININE AND MASCULINE TREASURES
The Dance of Yin and Yang

Hold your male side with your female side,
Hold your bright side with your dull side,
Hold your high side with your low side,
Then you will be able to hold the whole world.
When the opposing forces unite within
there comes a power abundant in its giving
and unerring in its effect.

LAO-TZU
TAO TE CHING (TAO OF VIRTUE), VERSE 28

Wuji (Wu Chi) is ultimate emptiness—the pregnant void with potential for everything to arise. The heart of Taoist cosmology is the cycling between the unmanifest Wuji and the manifest Taiji (Tai Chi)—between Tao-in-stillness and Tao-in-movement with its continuous dance of yin and yang.

Yin and yang refer to the light and dark sides of the mountain. The universe can be seen as a dance of polarity between these two energies. One is not better or worse than the other. We need both for the world to go around. The table below describes the core essence of these polar but complementary opposites.

ATTRIBUTES OF YIN AND YANG, MASCULINE AND FEMININE

ESSENTIAL YIN	ESSENTIAL YANG
Earth	Heaven
Moon	Sun
Water	Fire
Stillness	Movement
Life force, Shakti	Consciousness, Shiva
Flow	Form
Cool	Warm
Passive	Active
Inward and deep	Outward and surface
Contracting	Expanding
Dark and night	Light and day
Descending	Ascending
Slow	Fast
ESSENTIAL FEMININE	**ESSENTIAL MASCULINE**
Fullness	Emptiness
Sensual	Mental
Body	Mind
Everything	Nothing
Being	Purpose
Receptive	Penetrative
Nurturing	Protective
Chaos and spontaneity	Order and focus
Subtle	Direct
Surrender	Control

ESSENTIAL FEMININE	ESSENTIAL MASCULINE
Sustains	Initiates
Radiant	Integrity
Cooperative	Competitive
Emotional	Rational
Expressive	Witness
Colorful	Simple
Inviting	Directing
Social	Solitude
Communing with nature	Conquering nature
Thrives on praise	Thrives on challenge
Process oriented	Goal oriented
Vagina	Penis
Soft and curvy	Hard and angular

Feminine and Masculine Essence

Within each of us are the gems of both feminine and masculine energy. In every movement, the flow itself is the feminine aspect, while your awareness of the flow and the way you direct it are masculine aspects. These are different yet inseparable.

What makes you feel happy? What qualities would you call a good day? A man or woman with a feminine essence would delight in activities like cooking or dancing. If we have a developed masculine capacity, we might feel proud at accomplishing a goal.

Rather than seeing this as stereotyping, I'd like to see this as a palette of human expression that we can artistically play with to bring more polarity and spice into our relationships. We need polarity for sexual attraction!

The second part of the table above shows how yin and yang are expressed within each of us as our masculine and feminine aspects. The chart also shows what the masculine and feminine thrive on in our relationships. Often yin craves yang: the deep, dark part of our feminine self longs for fullness, color, and radiance. In a similar way, the masculine part of our self, which is light, craves the deep, inward meditative stillness needed to nurture itself.

You can also use this understanding to recognize qualities that you may have lost along the way. As children, many of us covered up qualities that the adults around us disapproved of. As we peel off the shells of our conditioning we can reclaim feminine or masculine aspects of ourselves that we might have rejected long ago.

For example, have you ever heard, "Be still, be quiet, be a good girl"? You may have become a rebel girl in reaction! As you mature, you start to become your authentic self, who can respond spontaneously with any of the qualities on this chart. Your gifts are unlimited and multifaceted. I hope this will help you recognize and appreciate the ways that your masculine and feminine gifts play out in the world.

Playing with Sexual Polarity

Many women cultivate their masculine capabilities of planning, ambition, and getting things done. It is crucial that they remain able to switch polarities consciously in order to maintain their own health, well-being, and relationships. If you live a concrete, rushed lifestyle, for instance, and find yourself being bossy, pushy, and sharp-tongued, you will benefit from being able to shift at will into a feminine polarity. You can imagine, for example, that you are on a tropical island like Hawaii—warm and luscious. Perhaps play some flowing music, relax, and move your hips like the ocean. You will feel sexy by enjoying your own body and movement. The feminine brings us out of our head and into our body.

Receptivity and Presence

There is a corresponding tension for every thought. Simple ways to become more receptive are relaxing your jaw, muscles, and joints. Soften your eyes. Unclench the base of your body. Become a listening vessel and breathe in that which you are receptive to.

Presence requires relaxation along with structure; aligning yourself with heaven and earth allows you to be totally there. Witness the other without judgment. Be conscious of your breathing and your heart.

True and False Yin, True and False Yang

"False" is a limited or contracted expression of our unlimited true nature. Both true yin and true yang are heart-centered; the heart center is their balance point. False yang is head-centered: the head becomes overheated and the heart becomes cool. False yin is belly-centered: the heart becomes overheated and emotional as the belly and sexual waters become cool or frozen with fear. When women live primarily in the emotional heart, rather than the inner soul heart, they are led by emotions that are partial, rather than by unconditional love and compassion.

It's important to understand that every male body and every female body has within it the challenge of balancing the yin and yang forces flowing within. Some women may have an extremely yang nature and some men may have an extremely yin nature. The important issue is whether a person's energy flow is dominated by true yin or yang or false yin or yang. False yang manifests as personal will and control, while false yin leads to submission and victimhood.

Under the dominance of the patriarchal grip, the water/yin becomes frozen. At this time in history, women are becoming liberated, and with this emergence new qi is awakening! The true water wants to flow and be warmed by the true fire! The spiritual journey is from the personal to the transpersonal level, moving from false masculine and false feminine qi toward the Divine Masculine (divine will) and Divine Feminine (divine surrender).

Feminine and Masculine Spiritual Practices

Feminine spiritual practices are devotional, embodied, and celebratory. They may include singing, dancing, chanting, celebration, sensual feasts, healing others, circles for sharing, compassionate service, and communion with nature.

In contrast, the masculine spiritual practices are focused on higher consciousness, awareness, witnessing, and mindfulness. They may include self-observation, stillness meditation, emptying the mind, no distractions, mountain meditation, Zen-like austerity, discipline, and inquiry.

Self-Expression through the Five Elements

Out of yin and yang are born the five elements, the five tendencies of energy: fire rises, water sinks, wood expands, metal solidifies, and earth is stabilizing and centering.

How are the five elements expressed in your life? You might express fire with your creative flair and flaming enthusiasm for life; water with your deep feeling and sensuality; wood with your enjoyment of walking in the forest and dancing; metal with your sharp, discriminating mind and self-reflection; and earth with cooking a delicious meal or gardening.

FEMININE ARCHETYPES

I honor the maiden, wild woman,
mother/ healer, and wise woman within me.

Many different feminine qualities exist within the feminine essence. By exploring various archetypes of the feminine, we can experience a fuller range of our divine essence.

Archetypes of the Seasons

The cycle of a woman's life turns with the wheel of yin and yang. As we pass through the seasons of our life, we pass through four archetypes.

Spring: We emerge into our maiden aspect. The virgin or maiden is associated with innocence, youthfulness, birth of new life, and finding boundaries. Her qi is uprising and buoyant.

Summer: As energy builds into full yang we step into the wild woman aspect—our full and blossoming nature. The wild woman dances with wild, spontaneous energy! The lover or wild woman is associated with expansive experiences, adventure, romance, and ecstasy.

Autumn: After the wildness we may choose to channel energy into motherhood, creating, or healing. We become the archetype of the Mother, Healer, and the Creatrix, who is associated with channeling energy into manifestation, healing, and transformation.

Winter: Drawing our energy into our core, we become the Wise Woman or crone, who is associated with extracting the essential out of all experience in the form of wisdom. The blood stops flowing out, stays within, and returns to the heart in order to nourish spiritual development. The Wise Woman holds the inner secrets and mysteries. The ultimate dissolving into the yin is to pass through the space between worlds—to leave the physical body and enter the spirit world. The Wise Woman knows the way, supporting the eternal cycles of life and the immortal seed of life within.

Individual women may embody one archetype more than the others; on the journey to greater wholeness we can play with stepping into the shoes of other archetypes. Men are natural "hunters" and they hunt, or at least

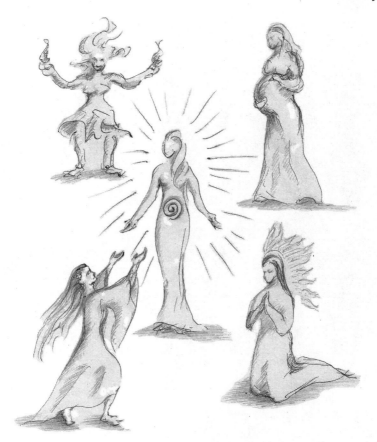

Fig. 1.3. Weaver of the women's web

notice, different flavors of the feminine. If you embody these different flavors yourself, this nourishes the men in your life. It also adds spice to a possibly flat, boring life.

Full-Spectrum Goddess

Chorus of the song:
Yes, I'm a full-spectrum goddess
So many flavors
That no man can guess

Verses:
I've got a wise woman in my bones
Her ancient roots stem beyond the known

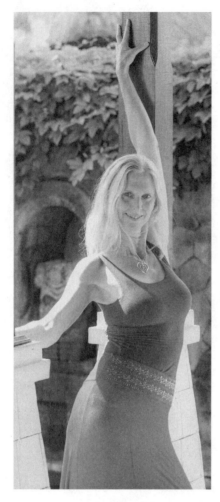

Fig. 1.4. Full-spectrum goddess
(Photo by Michael Julian Berz)

I've got a sweet girl in my smile
Her joyful heart shines for miles and miles

I've got a warm mother in my womb
Creating life from moon to moon

I've got a sexy lover in my blood
Her passion swells in blissful floods

Ending:
So many flavors (3x)
Only goddess can guess!

Women's Roles Dance Drama

This dance drama is a wonderful way to embody some of the many feminine archetypes. You could approach the gestures in the same way you would try on a dress that pushes your edge. Notice which roles feel undeveloped or out of your comfort zone. Great expressive energy builds when a group of women move in a circle together!

When feminine arts stem from virtues like love, compassion, strength, and authenticity, the positive response is profound. When they arise from a shadowy, distorted energy they will have the opposite effect from the desired result. When a woman flaunts her flirtatious talent to manipulate or her neediness to demand attention, she will only repulse her partner. If she is nagging, he will not listen. When out of balance with self-love, devotion can become suffocating to a partner.

Devotional, Longing

"I long for your presence.
I bow to my Beloved
And fill my heart."

Reach up with alternating hands, showing yearning with your whole body for all the qualities you long to connect with. Bow with devotion. Gather qi from the earth to replenish the heart.

Flirtatious, Inviting

"Come, just come. Come, just come."
"Catch me if you can, Catch me if you can."
(But remember that if there is neediness in your flirting—
"I need you. Give me attention!"—you will only repulse men!)

Call with your arms and hips, then move away like a mermaid from a sailor, waving your tail behind you.

Romantic, Loving

"I'm in love with you. You're in love with me.
Living life in tune, we dance in harmony."

Hold one hand to your heart and the other hand to your (imaginary) partner's heart. Dance a waltz, looking into each other's eyes. Swivel and spin around, becoming dizzy with love!

Independent, Adventurer

Cowgirl, galloping, slaps her behind with one hand while the other hand swings a lasso. "Yeehaw!"

She rides after him and gets too close . . .

Challenging, Seductive

"Give me space. Take me if you dare!"

The right hand pushes away and the left hand sexily strokes over your body. Have you ever said, "Give me space"? When you get too much distance the challenge becomes how to bring back passionate attraction. The art is to feel free and also open to being ravished.

Initiatress, Awakening

Express your heart-felt concern for your partner when his/her path wobbles. *"It kills me to see you like this."* Support your partner's highest destiny.

Scene: the cowboy is drinking in the saloon and gets into a fight.

"Wake up! I love you!" Stamp and raise your arms into the center of the circle, then turn to the left and open your arms from your heart. Speak out to your past lovers, present lovers, warriors, world leaders, and your inner masculine.

Supportive, Strong Woman behind the Man

*"I support you to follow your path.
I support you to get on track."*

Speak with an uplifting gesture and then a pushing forward, as if behind his middle back. Feel the support of the women behind you. Turn and bow with gratitude to all those beings who are supporting your path.

Compassionate, Forgiving

Embody the compassionate qualities of Kuan Yin with this dance: Hold a pot in your left arm; with your right hand scoop soothing, healing waters out of the pot and onto the earth. Offer the water to parts of the world and yourself that are suffering.

Face inward and scoop the healing waters from the cauldron, washing yourself and soothing what may ail you

Chant: *"Kuan Yin Pu Sa . . . Kuan Yin, goddess of compassion and mercy."* Her name means "she who hears the cries of the world."

Pu Sa means Boddhisattva, and Kuan Yin is the ultimate Bodhisattva who comes to help those in suffering.

Lover, Surrendering

"I am the cup, I am the wine,
I am the lover, in sweet surrende

Open your arms, with a soft receptive chest.

Press your hands and chest forward. Ripple the pa
ing the pelvis and chest. Wash blissful qi over your crc
of the body with a soft chest and arms flowing down lil
the love, the lover, and the beloved merge.

Lover of Life, Beauty Path

"I see the beauty in all beings.
I feel the grace in everything."

Seeing the beauty in everyone and every being, gesture and step to the right,
then left, then circle to the right.

Gesture and step to the left, then right, then circle to the left, with a soft
hand like a whirling Sufi dancer.

Gratitude

Bow in gratitude to these attributes within yourself.

STAGES OF WOMANHOOD

Each of us moves through multiple stages of development from childhood to adulthood and beyond. While the times of transition can be
difficult, the essence within us seeks to evolve and can help us move
from each stage to the next. That essence, in the form of sexual energy,
exists in the body from the time of conception and is cultivated throughout our lives.

- In the fetus, sexual energy is creating a body.
- In childhood, sexual energy prepares the body for puberty.
- During the teen years, its natural desire is hunting for a mate.
- During adulthood, it is creating family, service, and tribe.
- In elder time, sexual energy moves more inward into wisdom.

We can help ourselves and those around us move through the stages
of womanhood with grace by supporting the appropriate expressions of

...gy at each stage. The supportive practices mentioned in this ...will be explained further in following chapters.

...een Development

The teen years are an exceptional time of physical, emotional, and sexual development. Supporting young girls as they approach these tumultuous changes will help them become the strong, multifaceted women they are meant to be.

Physical Development

It is important for young women to prepare their bodies to be strong enough to carry another being inside of them. A pregnant woman must produce sufficient blood to nourish the growing fetus. Her physical body needs to be strong enough to carry a child. For this she needs a good diet and exercise.

In most schools, competitive sports are the basis of physical education. This can be very invigorating and develops the masculine edge, which thrives on challenge. To create wholeness within young women, inclusive and expressive activities like creative dance will bring out the feminine qualities of grace, flow, and connection. Qigong, which plays with archetypal animal movements and powers, encourages a range of expression, such as the strength of the tiger and the magic of the dragon. The emergence of the Divine Feminine begins with the education of the girls!

Emotional Development

It's important to give teens an opportunity to be teens. Although learning to be responsible and caring for their family and environment is good practice, too much responsibility can be a burden. Be mindful that your teens do not play parental roles for their siblings or even their parents.

Teens need to act out their rebellious qi without harming anyone. Rebellious qi will create new revolutions for all of us.

Body Image

Teenage girls should be encouraged to accept their bodies just as they are, whatever their shape, size, and fitness level. Through this acceptance they will love and take care of themselves.

Through praise and encouragement, parents play an important role in helping young men and women to see their unique beauty. Teens should be encouraged to practice the Inner Smile by smiling lovingly to themselves in the mirror. Perhaps gentle reminders like "I love myself" can be posted on the mirror. This self-love will show as an unmistakable inner glow.

Girls should be encouraged not to wear underwire bras as they can disturb breast development by cutting off the flow of qi. Breasts need room to grow! A plant in a small pot will not grow to its full potential. Girls can be taught to massage their breasts, which will encourage them to grow firm, full, vibrant, and just the right size for them.

Initiation

Becoming a Woman

In the past, communities would celebrate the day when a girl became a woman. Through song, dance, challenging games, and feasts, a young woman's entry into adulthood has traditionally been marked by community-wide celebration. Many modern people are now developing ways to bring this sense of ritual initiation back into our lives. Parents and communities around the world are rediscovering and creating opportunities for coming-of-age celebrations.

Creating Rites of Passage

First, create safety and a heightened respectful atmosphere by setting "sacred space" for your right-of-passage ceremony. Invoke the powers of the directions and nature spirits, since our feminine cycle is a part of nature.

Invocation

We call on the spirit of the west and the metal element
to empower our lives with courage and integrity.
We call on the spirit of the north and the water element
to pervade our lives with wisdom and peace.
We call on the spirit of the east and the wood element
to fill our lives with kindness and abundance.
We call on the spirit of the south and the fire element
to infuse our lives with love and compassion.
We call on the spirit of the center and the earth element
to support our lives with openness and trust.

We call on the spirit of the heaven and earth
to guide and nourish our highest destiny.

- ♦ Invite people to share from their hearts through a ritual like passing around the talking stick or offering a blessing of flowers.
- ♦ Create a unified field through chanting words of spiritual power, dancing, and drumming. A beautiful way to animate the passage into a new phase of life is to create a tunnel of people with their arms making an archway. The young "Moon Goddess" walks through the tunnel after her first moon blood, where she is blessed with words and gentle touch and is welcomed into a women's circle.
- ♦ Invite the elders and the spirits of the young woman's ancestors into the circle and acknowledge them with gratitude, asking them to support her growth and development.
- ♦ Honor the uniqueness of each young woman by creating an opportunity for her to shine and offer a gift of her own creative expression.

In addition to initiation rituals, there are regular habits and practices that can help bring a sense of honor and celebration to a girl's relationship with her body.

Fertility Celebrations

Menstrual blood is not just discarded material from the uterus but is sacred essence, vital for life! We highly recommend watching the movies *The Moon inside You* and *Monthlies,* by Diana Fabianova. Both films are about young girls coming into puberty and menstruation. Families can have a welcoming attitude to menstruation, as with every cycle a teen's body is preparing a feast for a child to grow. By honoring the fertility within each teenager, they will promote abundance in their own lives and the earth around them.

There are many traditions where teenagers can be taught to honor the earth each month as they pour their menstrual blood into the earth with a prayer. If using a menstrual cup, the blood can be collected and poured into the ground or beneath a plant in a meaningful way. The blood can be used to "paint" a medicine wheel symbol, for instance—a cross within a circle—to signify the root chakra and honor the forces of all four directions, above and below.

Normal Self-Care

When mothers are practicing breast and yoni massage as part of their regular self-care, by example, their daughters sense that this is natural and normal.

Movement

Transforming emotion with movement frees emotion.

Bodily disciplines like martial arts, gymnastics, and dance will help young people feel their power and boost their self-esteem. Enjoying these activities without self-criticism and competition or comparison is important. These kinds of physical activities, which channel sexual desire and emotional states, give young people a sense of self-control and self-mastery.

Dancing is a way that young people express their fertility. Folk dances are a safe way for young men and women to meet within a community setting. During folk dances they are in a space of celebration and joy; they can express themselves through movement and feel who they are energetically attracted to beyond external appearance or status. Dancing helps release inhibitions and shyness around the body and helps young people open their hearts to one another.

Pagan fertility rites like the Maypole dance portray the sexual alchemy mythologies with the spiraling of the colorful flowing feminine ribbons that weave around the masculine erect pole.

The Turtle and Buffalo Qigong practice in chapter 7 will get the fire awakened in the Sexual Palace. Awakened energy is moved up the spine to the brain and down the front of the body to the dantian. When teenagers practice this they are more alert in their mind and can get their homework done and have more time to play!

Menstrual Health

The ancients called menstruation "heavenly water": *heavenly* indicates the True Qi descending from the heavens and *water* indicates heavenly clouds generating water. The kidneys store our essence and are responsible for our growth. The kidneys need to be strong enough to ensure that there is an abundant supply of blood in the Core Channel—"Sea of Blood"—to overflow from the uterus.

Menstruation marks a healthy purification stage, during which the body can discharge excess fats, proteins, and impurities. The body will also discharge psychic toxins, imbalances, or suppressed emotions during this time. Cooperate with this natural process by breathing out impurities and excesses into the earth.

Lunar Alignment—Cycles of Menstruation and Ovulation

In the past, when we were more in touch with the natural light of the moon, we could receive its effect on ourselves. With electric and city lights, we tend to be distracted from natural light and less aware of its effects on us. The ancient Taoists considered ovulation to be a powerful time and called the day a woman ovulated her "full moon." When the moon is full, energy naturally ascends in the body. During ovulation, about fourteen days before menstruation, large amounts of hormones circulate in a woman's body, increasing her emotions and passionate, magical powers.

During the new moon the energy in the body is naturally descending. When a woman menstruates during new moon she is influenced by her instinctual center, the sexual organs, which are tied to the moon and nature cycles. When a woman menstruates around the full moon, her cycle is influenced more by her erotic center (the brain). Generally, when a woman is more yang she will menstruate during the full moon. When she is more yin she menstruates during the new moon.

These two traditional feminine patterns are known as the Red Moon cycle—when a woman menstruates around the full moon and ovulates at the new moon—and the White Moon cycle—when she ovulates around the full moon and menstruates at the new. The medicine women, midwives, and wisdom keepers were following the Red Moon cycle. They channeled their sexual energy into healing and the empowerment of others rather than giving birth to children. The White Moon cycle represents the fertile power of earth and the motherly nature of women menstruating around this time.

In the past, many women would go into the red tent together. You might find yourself connecting to a tribal rhythm with women close to you. Have you ever consciously shifted your menstruation time? Did it feel empowering? Our moon cycle tends to change with life circumstances and our longings for raising a family or serving a career, creative expression, or spiritual path.

Lunar Alignment at Birth

Aligning with your innate cycle gets you in touch with the anchor that was imprinted in your body-mind when you were born. Your lunar alignment at birth is the exact phase of the moon in which you were born. You can find your exact lunar date and percentage of moon phase by entering the birthdate and location/hemisphere you were born in at www.stardate.org.

How much of the sun's light was the moon reflecting at your first breath? The cosmos is a reflection of spirit's message to us. What was the particular cosmic charge that you were born with? The moon reflects your emotional karma and what your soul lessons may be. Why did your higher self choose this particular astrological imprint and moon phase? The sun-moon imprint at birth is akin to micro solar systems in everyone's bodies. Apparently your innate ovulation date is the phase of the moon at which you were born. So special attention can be given to the phases of the moon for both contraception and fertility.

Premenstrual Syndrome (PMS)

PMS is a time when the truth or the darker sides of the emotional spectrum come to the surface of a woman's feelings. Often women feel sensitive, irritable, emotional, or sad. It is good to observe if there is a pattern from month or month: are you irritable because your body would like to rest and you are forcing yourself to keep working?

By going into the red tent with friends or by yourself, you can reflect on the emotions that are arising. Here you can ask the emotions what is their message or spiritual goal for you. Use journaling and the Inner Smile practice to embrace these difficult emotions internally. Practice the Six Healing Sounds (see chapter 2) instead of throwing emotional garbage into your environment, which affects those around you.

Menstrual Cramps

Menstrual cramps are a sign of cold, damp, contracted, and stagnant energy in the lower abdomen. Just as you hug yourself and shiver when you're cold, cold energy in the lower abdomen causes contraction and spasms of the muscles. To relieve these contractions, we recommend abdominal massage with warming oils like sesame and stimulating essential oils like geranium, rosemary, and ginger. Traditionally, the hot water bottle is a girl's best friend and will relax the lower abdomen so the blood flows naturally. You can also relieve menstrual cramps by rubbing and tapping the sacrum.

Postures that are helpful for cramps open the kidneys and pelvis and encourage deep groin and pelvis breathing. Child's Pose, for example, or hugging the knees to the chest, or squatting like a frog are all helpful positions. Breathe slowly and deeply while widening the kidneys and groin with each inhalation. As you exhale, internally blow warmth down from your heart, melting the excess coldness and cramps.

Breast massage, ovarian massage, and jade egg practices on a regular basis will relieve menstrual cramps and discomfort. Unfortunately, doctors these days are prescribing pills to artificially control menstruation, but with this they are stopping a natural cycle of life and young women are not feeling the connection to nature and their body.

Diet for Reducing Painful Periods

When women bleed, their bodies are discharging excess fats and proteins. It makes sense not to eat excesses of these foods just before you menstruate, but to wait until after your period when you crave these foods to build up your blood again. To reduce pain and discomfort during menstruation, eat heavier foods like animal protein for two weeks after your period.

Internal dampness stagnates like a swamp in the lower body and can cause menstrual cramps. To prevent cramps, avoid eating damp-producing foods like dairy, sugar, peanuts, and bananas for two weeks before your period.

Avoid Overexertion

Avoid straining and compression during menstruation, as increased qi flow can increase blood flow. Qigong postures like Embracing the Tree can be practiced on a structural alignment level. Bone Breathing is excellent to restore the blood in the bone marrow. Avoid the fast bellows breathing, which will increase the blood flow, and avoid pulling the energy up the spine at this time as there is a natural flow down to the earth. Rather, during bleeding time, pull up earth energy by pumping with the anal sphincter muscles to direct earth energy up to the kidneys and the spine. Wait for a few days after menstruation to do the jade egg exercises.

❋ Menstrual Practices

We can become allergic to our sexual energy if it is suppressed; the creative force then becomes self-destructive. Liberate this energy for positive change! Make friends with your sexual energy.

● Warm Up Your Ovarian Palace

Channel smiling, loving energy from your heart into the sexual organs and kidneys. Put your right hand on your heart and left hand on your Ovarian Palace and breathe. Warm up internal "coldness" that can cause cramps.

● Womb Wrapping

During menstruation you can gently wrap the uterus with qi to heal the "inner wound" more quickly, preventing unnecessary loss of blood and qi. Spiral the earth energy counterclockwise, from the front to the left, penetrating into your vagina and uterus. This practice is also healing after a miscarriage.

● Womb Breathing

Cooperate with the cleansing, building, and regulating aspects of the menstrual cycle.

Place your hands in front of your hip bones. Feel the breath expand like a beach ball into the Sexual Palace, hips, and sacrum. Relax on the exhalation. Breathe out wounded, dissatisfied, frustrated, resentful feelings like cloudy, gray smoke. Breathe out impurities, excesses, and suppressed feelings into the earth, which acts like a compost pit below you. Transform the energy into forgiveness and unconditional love. Breathe in golden light and loving, healing energy.

● Red Spiral

During your menses you can pour some of your physical or energetic blood back into the earth. Squat and place your hands in prayer position in front of your heart. Rotate your hips and imagine a red spiral going into the earth in a clockwise direction (moving forward and to the right). Pray that your blood essence makes life fertile and abundant. Be grateful for all the lessons and gifts this month has given you.

Conception

The Power to Choose

The instinct to become a mother is a powerful drive. Every month there is a reminder of the potential muffin that could grow in your oven. It is very special at this time to be able to make the free and conscious choice whether or not to conceive a child. It is important to look at where that choice comes from.

The choice to not conceive could come out of fear of committing yourself to this devotional lifestyle. On the other hand, some women would rather be free to study, travel, or work on their careers. And some women may face challenges such as not having met the right guy or health issues or conflicting desires.

One way to make the conscious choice is through using the practices of the jade egg and Inner Smile to ask the womb if it desires a child. In meditation, smile to your heart and all your organs with the inquiry about having a child. Does the whole body say "YES!"? Or does it say "I'm not ready yet" or "This feels like it is not meant to be"?

It's also good to inquire with permission about whether your partner is ready, willing, and able to be the father of a child. This can be done by meditating together with soul gazing. It is possible that a baby's spirit has, like Cupid, brought a couple together to be its mother and father. You can ask this little Cupid questions that are in your heart. Preparing the field of unconditional love will attract a baby spirit as it is the optimal environment to grow in.

Natural Methods of Birth Control

If the time is not right for you to conceive a child, there are several natural ways of supporting your choice. One source of natural birth control is a clear intention that becoming a mother is not your path at this time, for the sake of all beings. Many women I know have a big event coming up and they tell their body, "Please don't menstruate until this event has passed," because they want their full strength for it. Intention is very powerful!

DUAL CULTIVATION

Working on dual cultivation as a couple is a powerful form of conscious birth control. The man has an opportunity to practice pulling out or pulling the energy up before the point of no return, preventing pregnancy. A man really needs to know himself and the woman also needs to know him, to not draw the ejaculation out of him. Like musicians they both need to pay sensitive attention to energetically building into an orgasmic crescendo without dropping their instruments!

The man needs to be curious and responsible enough to know where his partner is in her cycle and adjust accordingly, either by avoiding penetration or by being very careful to not ejaculate within her. That means the woman needs to be in touch with her cycle and open enough to express it to her partner.

OBSERVING CERVICAL MUCUS

A popular natural birth control method is based on self-observation of cervical mucus, which produces a wet or slippery vaginal sensation leading up to ovulation. You'll be able to follow a pattern of cervical mucus changes over the course of each menstrual cycle.

Cervical mucus is affected by estrogen six days before ovulation, when it starts to become clear and elastic like stretchy egg white. This mucus stretches between your thumb and index finger and is sometimes called "spin." Sperm can thrive and survive in this cervical mucus and be viable when the egg arrives—so this is not a good time to have your partner ejaculate within you if you wish to avoid pregnancy. Ovulation is likely to occur the last day your mucus is in this phase.

After ovulation, when cervical mucus is affected by the production of progesterone, it becomes tacky between your thumb and index finger— sticky and opaque white. As the mucus changes, it becomes less hospitable to the sperm. Be aware of of lubricative sensations in the vagina. After you ovulate your vaginal sensation will go back to feeling more dry.

To avoid conception it is best to prevent ejaculation inside the woman's body for about three days before and about three days after ovulation. If you have irregular cycles and it is hard for you to track your natural rhythm, it is very important for you to track your temperature as well as the cervical mucus. You will be taking your basal body temperature upon waking up, before getting out of bed in the morning. There is a slight rise in temperature when you are ovulating. This is a sign that you are in "heat."

As you record the story of changes in vaginal sensations and cervical mucus, you can put them in the context of the cycles of the moon. With daily tracking, cervical mucus methods of birth control can be 78 to 97 percent effective. However, research has shown that this effectiveness can be increased to 98.5 percent by integrating lunar biorhythmic calculations into your mucus and temperature tracking. Proven by comprehensive research on over ten thousand women, lunar biorhythm tracking accounts for the likelihood of spontaneous ovulation that may occur due to your lunar alignment, no matter where in the cycle you are.*

Four Easy Steps to Natural Fertility/Contraception

1. Keep track of the first day of your period and count from there.
2. Be aware of mucous secretions: clear and stretchy (ovulation); white, creamy, and tacky (farther from ovulation).
3. Be aware that there is a slight temperature rise or spike at ovulation.
4. Be aware of your innate lunar date (exact phase of the moon on the day you were born).

Becoming a Mother

*This is a time for nurturing and stabilizing yourself
and receiving the support you need.*

If you feel that you are ready to have a child, spiritual practice can support you through each stage of this marvelous journey.

Preparing the Womb for Conception

You can invite conception by preparing your body, mind, and spirit.

⚔ **Prepare a succulent home** for your child if you want to become pregnant. You can use your innate lunar anchor to nourish your essence at that time by taking blood tonics and eating food that nourishes the blood.

⚔ **Ovarian Breathing.** While this practice is usually used for harvesting potent qi from the developing egg to nourish the body, you want to do the opposite of this when you are trying to get pregnant or are

*See http://nfmcontraception.com.

pregnant. Use Ovarian Breathing to charge the egg or embryo with as much good qi as possible.

⚹ **Qigong.** The Fountain of Yin and Shower of Yang practice detailed in chapter 7 is a good practice for gathering qi in the womb.

⚹ **Fertility meditation.** Practice the following meditation to ready your womb for conception.

✳ Preparing the Fertile Ground

Consciously breathe in the fertile Mother Earth energy, which builds the substance of the body and gives us support.

- Sit or stand with your palms down to the earth.
- Turn your palms to the sky and breathe in heaven's qi to energize your body.
- Let heaven and earth couple at your navel center and form a ball of balanced Yuan Qi. Breathe into the qi ball with your palms facing each other.
- Place your charged-up hands on your Ovarian Palace and absorb the energy into your womb.
- Talk to the life force: "Please make my body fertile ground to grow a healthy baby. My yoni is fertile and ready to grow a healthy baby."

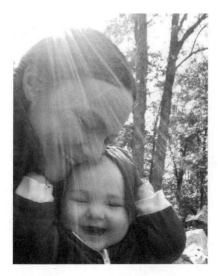

Fig. 1.5. Mother and child bathed in the light (Photo by Michael Winn)

Conception

At conception, the yin and yang energies of the parents merge with the divine potential of the Tao—with the primordial, true, unified generative energy of creation. The Taoist classics described the act of creation and the formation of a spiritual embryo in this way: "formless produces form, immaterial produces substance." The mother's womb is a container for the primordial energy of creation (Yuan Qi), which nourishes the embryo.

Through meditation, you can talk to the growing cells and the life force. Breathe and smile and say affirmations inwardly such as, "May the natural order of cell growth make this baby vital, strong, and healthy." Tell all the cells, "I love you. I thank the Divine, the universe, for supporting the natural growth of my baby." Imagine your Inner Smile as golden loving sunlight shining on the ocean of your womb.

Pregnancy—Ripening the Fruit

Pregnancy is a time of female empowerment and inner growth. This yang process needs the balance of yin, calm, peace, gentleness. Recall the Taiji symbol—yang within the yin in one lobe and yin within the yang in the other lobe. Nesting time allows the mother to build her energy for the birth, like calm before the storm. The child grows well in a peaceful, meditative space like a seed grows in the quiet earth.

A harmonious internal atmosphere is very important, as the fetus feels all the mother's emotions. Furthermore, a positive environment allows for healthy growth of the cells and immune system. Relax and let go of stress and negativity, which can be toxic for the fetus. The Inner Smile and Healing Sounds meditations can release stress and increase positive virtues.

During this time, the mother's priorities should be aligned to being a mother. If being a mother conflicts with her career goals, the fetus will feel this.

Practices during Pregnancy and Childbirth

Pregnancy is an opportunity to deeply connect with your body, heart, and spirit, to surrender to all the changes and prepare for the great letting go. General ways you can support yourself and your baby during this time include the following:

⚔ **Diet.** Avoid cooling foods like excess raw, dairy, damp, or frozen foods. Mild and balanced foods are beneficial, as are foods with high iron levels. Listen to your body's needs!

⚔ **Voice programming.** It was discovered that pheasant's sounds preprogram their chicks in the egg to function when they are hatched. Sing or speak to your baby pleasant messages like, "My princess you are growing beautifully. You are welcomed into this world with love." Sing the baby's name if you already know it.

⚔ **Music.** Many researchers over the years have demonstrated the benefits of music to the growth and development of living things. For instance, it was found that plants grow better when exposed to harmonious music, like Mozart.* And the energetic field of even a simple object, such as a cotton ball, expands with sound prayer.†

⚔ **Lovemaking.** Massage and cuddling are comforting and can ease back discomfort. Intercourse will cause gentle contractions of the uterus and will massage the baby with love. Avoid intercourse, however, if there is a danger of premature labor. If you need to induce labor, intercourse can be a good way to move the baby into the world with dynamic love.

⚔ **Qigong** is moving, breathing meditation that is low impact. It cultivates calm focus and free movement of qi. Movements that gather qi from nature are very supportive, like Ocean Breathing (see chapter 7). Avoid pressing and tapping acupressure points as many points are contraindicated during pregnancy.

⚔ **Dance.** Hula dancing, or any movement that activates the Belt Channels, will spiral qi around the hips and keep the back and pelvis flexible and relaxed. These movements also contain and protect the energy field. The mother can hold a jade egg in her vagina as she dances spontaneously like the ocean or the wind.

❋ Specific Practices for Pregnancy

In addition to the activities above, there are several practices that are specific to the gestational period, or that have specific modifications for pregnancy.

---

*Peter Tompkins, *The Secret Life of Plants* (Cambridge, UK: Cambridge University Press, 1973).
†Fabien Maman, *The Tao of Sound* (self-published by Tama-Do Academy in the Czech Republic, 2011).

● Prenatal Breathing

The Microcosmic Orbit, also called Prenatal Breathing, refers to the flow of energy that balances the flow of yin and yang meridians and supports the growth of the fetus.

The Orbit contains the energy and protects the mother's energy field. It holds in the baby and in this way helps prevent miscarriage. The Microcosmic Orbit also reels in qi from the universe. As you meditate, intend the Orbit to pull in whatever elements are needed to nourish you and your baby.

● Dual Orbits

Sense the Microcosmic Orbit in your body and in the fetus. The qi in the growing fetus flows in the fire cycle—up the spine and down the front of the body. When the child is born, qi flows in the water cycle—up the front and down the back—until puberty. In adulthood, qi can flow in either the fire or the water cycle.

Allow both of your Orbits to harmonize, even though their speeds and directions may be very different. Avoid manipulating the qi as the qi is very wise!

● Water Wheels

Invite and scoop ocean or earth's water power into your Orbit to nourish the kidneys and then wash over the fetus. Circle around your heart and wash love over the fetus. Circle over the head and then wash wisdom around the fetus. (See chapter 7 for a detailed description of the Water Wheels practice.)

● Building Earth Energy

The energy of the earth element is very important during pregnancy as it builds blood and the physical body. Use earth energy for Upward Draws and avoid drawing energy away from the growing fetus. It is not recommended to practice with the jade egg while pregnant. Do not interfere with the energy field as nature is very wise. A pregnant woman should not unusually overexert herself. Practice noticing all the various pelvic muscles and tightening and relaxing them (mostly relaxing). Practice ejecting the yoni egg a few times and notice the inner gesture. Hugging trees is a great way to absorb earth energy, as is Kidney Breathing.

● Breast Massage

The Stomach meridian, whose energy has a lot to do with nourishment and trust, flows through the nipples. Worry and anxiety can therefore cause blockages to the natural flow of qi in the stomach, the spleen, and their meridians. Breast massage is helpful for releasing such blockages and for relieving painful and engorged breasts. It softens and opens the heart, helping the mother to accept the changes in her life. If the breasts are very sensitive, an ethereal massage with the intent of soothing can be practiced.

Harvest the virtue energies from the organs and fuse them into compassion. Send this high-frequency energy down to the uterus to nourish the unborn child. Nipple massage will prepare the glands for whatever changes are needed. It can also help relieve anxiety when combined with the Inner Smile and full breathing. (See chapter 4 for detailed breast massage practices.)

● Tao Yoga

Several Tao Yoga exercises are also good during pregnancy.

- **The Cat:** Arching and curling the back while kneeling on all fours eases back pain.
- **Spinal Pelvic Rock** frees up the circulation of the Microcosmic Orbit.
- **Kidney Breathing:** Lying on your back and hugging your knees against your chest, breathe earth energy into the spine and kidneys. Kidney Breathing is good for building up energy.

❀ Orgasmic Birthing

Open up to the possibility of having an orgasmic birth.

- Clear the fear of your own birth from your womb and vagina with Womb Breathing.
- Practice the Inner Smile and Healing Sounds meditations to transform any anxiety in your organs that you or your ancestors might have had around giving birth or being born. Balance these contracted feelings with love and openness.
- Open your body and let your hips spiral like the ocean. Rotate your hips counterclockwise to spiral up the Earth Qi to nourish the baby. Rotate your hips clockwise to spiral down Heaven Qi to facilitate giving birth.

- Be free with sound, especially orgasmic sounds. The "a" sound makes the body more receptive and deeply flowing: try the heart sounds "ah" and "mmma-a-a-a-a" and "ha-a-a-a-a-w" to keep the heart open. When the heart opens, so does the vagina.
- I highly recommend the DVDs *Birth as We Know It* (available at birthintobeing.com) and *Orgasmic Birth* (available at orgasmicbirth.com). What a way to be born!

Recovery after Childbirth

After childbirth, the pelvic floor can remain painful for some time. Place your healing hands over your yoni and breathe slowly and deeply. Soothe the area with blue, gentle light to heal inflammation.

Breast-feeding will tone the uterus. Wait until the walls of your vagina are healed before practicing with the jade egg. Start with gentle practices lying down. Wait until the tissues are strong before practicing standing practices.

> I was blessed to meet Minke de Vos two years after the birth of my first son, which was an orgasmic experience that radically expanded my capacity to feel pleasure and opened me into my inherently ecstatic nature. When she began to share some of the practices from the Feminine Treasures, I lit up with delight as I discovered that many of these ancient techniques for cultivating our feminine radiance that she was transmitting, I was already connecting to as the innate wisdom emerging through me from the inside out, guiding me into these spaces of cultivation and renewal. In receiving her embodied wisdom, the deepest core of my being was affirmed, like the Universal acknowledgment that I was on the right track to keep listening and allowing this inherent wisdom to inform my practice from my connection to what feels natural and nourishing.
>
> One of the greatest gifts she gave me in our initial meeting has given back exponentially in my life: a jade egg and the introduction to the practices. I began to work with it on a consistent basis and was astounded at what awoke within me! Within a few weeks of cultivation, the vitality of my yoni and womb came online in a way I had never before known, and I not only regained the strength and tone that had existed prior to being stretched open in birth, but far surpassed it into new realms of articulation and expansion in the subtle energies of pleasure.
>
> AMBER HARTNELL, WHO STARRED IN
> *BIRTH AS WE KNOW IT*

Breast-Feeding and Breast Care after Childbirth

Breast milk is formed from the yin blood and produced by the spleen and stomach. Before pregnancy, yin blood flows downward as menses. During pregnancy, the yin blood flows through the Conception Vessel and Thrusting Channels to nourish the fetus. After birth, the body fluid turns from red to white and moves upward to become milk. Excess stress, grief, anger, or stagnation can make the milk toxic. If the baby consumes this toxic milk it can cause malnutrition.

Gentle massage of the breasts acts like a water wheel that pumps Earth Qi up through the inside of the legs, through the pelvis, and up through the breasts. For lactating mothers breast massage relieves engorgement soreness by increasing drainage of lymph nodes and milk ducts and promoting blood circulation. Massaging the breasts can stimulate letdown and expression of milk and increase milk flow. Channel the Mother Earth energy up to the breasts and massage in the lusciousness of life force to replenish the breasts. After childbirth women can emphasize the uplift in their breast massage to prevent sagging. It is vital for a mother to smile to her breasts and be grateful to her breasts as a source of nourishment for her child and herself.

> I have noticed a resurgence in my feminine energy and an overall sense of renewal. As for the breast massage I have noticed that my breasts look and feel fuller and are improving back to their normal state after having two children; even my partner noticed! It's nice to know that a self-loving practice can enhance the tone and fullness of my breasts, almost reversing time!
>
> RACHEL, MOTHER

Menopause

Second Spring

Menopause is a second spring during which the energy that was once lost in menstruation can be channeled into the body and mind instead. This is the body's way of antiaging. Instead of the blood being used to grow a physical child, the qi in the blood is freed up to grow your inner spiritual child. Many women become very psychic and powerful in this period of life.

Practices that build kidney energy are good during the menopausal time. (See "Building Your Core Reserves" in chapter 8.)

Hot Flashes and Insomnia

During menstruation, the Core Channel and the uterus fill up with blood, which then moves downward. During menopause, this flow is reversed and moves upward to the heart, the Palace of the Spirit. The tendencies of aging—the separation of the polarities of hot and cold—can cause disturbing symptoms in menopause. Women often become yin deficient as yang speeds up, causing heat to rise in the body. Sometimes the rising energy is chaotic and overly hot, leading to symptoms like hot flashes and insomnia. The deep water reserves in the kidneys start to dry up.

It is possible, however, to alleviate these common symptoms with regular practice. To prevent this extreme polarization, we need to energetically link up our lower and upper body by replenishing our kidneys and the Qi Belt. We have a yin and a yang kidney, which are like cold and hot water taps in the body. Keeping the Mingmen—the Door of Life—open and "moving" the qi between the kidneys will help keep this balance.

Circulating energy around the Microcosmic Orbit is excellent for curbing hot flashes, insomnia, and other menopausal experiences. Channeling energy in the Microcosmic Orbit will balance rising and descending energy—the fire and water. Circulating qi in the fire cycle orbit transforms the emotions, which "burn up" inside. Circulating qi in the water cycle—the wisdom cycle of the crone—will help replenish feminine water. (See Microcosmic Orbit meditation in chapter 2.)

The Healing Sounds can also be used to release excess heat, coldness, and other imbalanced qi. The heart sound, "ha-a-a-a-a-w," calms the false fire in the heart, associated with overdoing and overgiving, which are both real dangers for women. As we let go, we can perceive our true feelings and needs more clearly. When there is too much heat that rises to the heart and head, it is difficult to sleep. Practices like the triple warmer sound will bring excess heat down from the upper body to the belly and feet.

Women in this time of life are often sandwiched between having children at home, caring for aging parents, and working at a job. With this busy schedule there is not much time to rest and replenish the blood. The kidneys need sufficient blood to circulate to keep the body at a comfortable temperature.

A practice to help replenish the blood is to rest for at least twenty minutes daily, practicing deep breathing, listening to music, meditating, or praying. This is not a time to be watching TV or reading a book, because "where your mind goes qi flows." Make time to come back to that conscious yin state of receiving life force from nature and the universe. Be still, or in subtle movement, with a quiet mind and awareness of your body. It is highly recommended that you lie down on the earth, allowing your body's magnetic field to be reset by the earth's resonance.

Taoist Practices That Promote Hormonal Balance

Taoist sexual energy practices are a way to prevent the hormone factory from shutting down. After menopause, the adrenals take over from the ovaries in hormonal functions, and therefore it's important to keep the adrenals happy and replenished. Replenish the adrenals by having enough sleep at night, particularly before midnight, and by doing Kidney Breathing. See an herbalist about taking herbal formulations to nourish yin essence. Goji berries are considered a superior tonic that can be taken on an ongoing basis to preserve youthfulness.

Kidney Breathing. This is an important practice for replenishing yin energy after menopause. Holding the breath and earth energy in the kidneys will recharge your batteries. Make sure to bring the excess warmth of the heart to the kidneys to calm the heart and warm the kidneys. For a more yin style, you can do this practice lying down with your knees up and feet flat on the earth. (See chapter 8 for a detailed look at Kidney Breathing.)

Deep Sea Turtle Breathing will open the Mingmen. (See chapter 8.)

Dragon Washes Her Face. This practice brings the heat down the Thrusting Channels to prevent hot flashes, which can dry up the deeper reserves of energy. The downward strokes of the arms calm the nervous system, preventing insomnia. By stroking the left and right channels alternately, the sympathetic and parasympathetic nervous systems are balanced. This will calm the adrenals and destress the body. (See Triple Purification practice in chapter 6.)

Dantian Breathing centers the heat below the navel and develops core power. When you store the heat in the proper place, the heat will be less chaotic.

Bone Breathing builds the blood in the bone marrow so you have enough blood to circulate (see Bone Marrow Neigong practices in chapter 8).

Bone Packing. The bones are a great place to store excess sexual energy and heat. This practice stores energy, prevents stiffness, and builds bone mass, preventing osteoporosis.

Triple Warmer Sound—"he-e-e-e-e"—cools the body, balances the temperature, and is a great way to induce sleep. It can also be practiced to chill down a hot flash.

Microcosmic Orbit channels free up energy in a balanced, centered way. Circulating the energy balances the hot and cold in the body. It distributes qi evenly throughout the glands, promoting hormonal balance. Starting the Microcosmic Orbit early will give you a smooth ride through this stage of your life.

Breast massage enhances the activation of female hormones, while nipple gland massage balances those hormones. Self-massage improves blood and lymph circulation, preventing stagnation and cancer. This ancient practice has helped women keep their breasts healthy for thousands of years. It also gets you in touch with your heart and feelings. It is an excellent antidepressant!

Qi Self-Massage. Self-acupressure and self-massage stimulate the anti-aging human growth hormones and help rejuvenate the body. Massage improves blood circulation. (See chapter 2.)

Jade egg practices prevent the vagina muscles from atrophying. If you don't use it, you lose it! These practices prevent vaginal dryness by stimulating the flow of creative juices and natural lubrication.

Moonlight practice will fill you with deep yin energy. It will keep you in connection with the powerful cycles of the moon. Bathing your yoni in moonlight will recharge it with the force that moves the tides of the ocean.

Flowering Women

When the flowers within us
Blossom together
The garden is fragrant
Our hearts fill with color.

When the buds of our being
Arise from the source
The palace is golden
Our bodies are glorious.

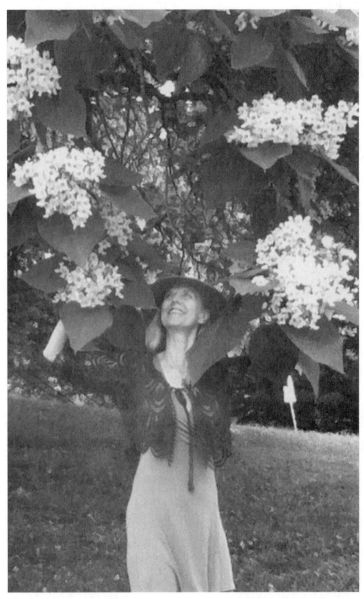

Fig. 1.6. Flowering Woman rejoices! (Photo by Marian Rose)

When the stars of the heavens
Shine light through our bodies
Our ancestors rejoice
Our cells are reborn.

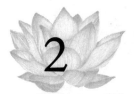

2
Tao Energy Fundamentals
The Basic Practices

In the framework of Taoist practice, the cultivation of sexual energy begins with an understanding of how energy moves through our bodies and through the universe around us. This chapter includes practices for drawing on our sources of energy to begin meditation, as well as some of the fundamental practices for cultivating that energy, including the Inner Smile, Six Healing Sounds, and Microcosmic Orbit.

The Tao is a down and through path: by going deeper into the body we realize the microcosmic wisdom within and are then able to open ourselves to the cosmic creative dance. The deeper you go the higher you rise. We work through the dense aspects, making them more transparent so the light of consciousness can shine through. We widen our inner embrace to feel and transform the dark aspects of ourselves, and this fuels our love and ecstasy.

By practicing Tao Tantric Arts to cultivate sexual energy and grow love and light, you will set into motion a natural self-healing process with benefits on all levels:

- ⚔ Physically: cleanses, balances hormones, strengthens the pelvic floor, boosts the immune system, rejuvenates, promotes longevity
- ⚔ Energetically: circulates vital qi through the body
- ⚔ Emotionally: gets us in touch with our feelings
- ⚔ Spiritually: allows us to become present with heightened consciousness

THE THREE TREASURES

Jing, Qi, and Shen

The Three Treasures are like a candle: jing is the wax and wick, qi is the flame, and shen is the light.

Jing is dense like ice, appears solid, and has a strong form.
Qi is fluid like water that moves in and out and through everything.
Shen is transparent like all-pervading vapor.

THE TAOIST CANON

The Three Treasures of jing, qi, and shen (essence, energy, and presence) are a microcosmic trinity of the primordial breath. The Taoist path of qi cultivation integrates the Three Treasures by transforming them into one another in processes of dematerialization or of materialization. In dematerialization, jing transforms into qi, and qi transforms into shen—essence into energy into presence. This is a transformation of something dense into something more transparent and light-filled. This path of evolution heightens our awareness that we are more than our physical bodies, and that we are one with all of life in the spirit.

The path of materialization, on the other hand, is a path of creation: the transformation of spirit into manifestation on a denser plane is a process of giving birth.

The Interdependence of Jing, Qi, and Shen

The soul is composed of all Three Treasures, which resonate at different frequencies like the three phases of water. They are mutually dependent on each other for maintenance and survival.

Jing—Essence

What is the nature of sexual energy?

Jing is our essence and pure potentiality. It is our tangible basic vitality, which is the denser, lower vibrational frequency of our human energy matrix. It creates and sustains the body's physical form. It has a bonding sticky quality and is like an energetic glue that holds matter together.

When we are consciously healing, we can direct the jing to multiply our cells. It is the orgasmic vibration that helps the cells multiply in a proper way, being the architect, designer, and holder of the original blueprint of our DNA and ancestral imprints. When DNA yin and yang strands wind around each other, their spiraling dance is like making love! Its nature is growth and reproduction.

The color frequency of sexual energy is pink. Pink is the mixture of the red blood building power and white of the egg/sperm building power. Pink is a warm color, which expresses the warmed up, lightly aroused energy. Visualize the colors as they appear in nature—the pink of a sunrise, cherry blossoms, or a ripe peach. Hot pink has romantic overtones and a cultural association with being sexy.

Qi—Energy

What is the nature of life-force energy?

When jing is transformed into Jing Qi, it interacts with vibrational fields of jing and shen. It has a middle vibrational frequency, which contains and sustains thoughts and emotions. Our mental and emotional energy is sourced in our vital organs, which are differentiated by the five elements: earth, metal, water, wood, and fire.

The human qi field is the bio-electro-magnetic body that consists of the energy channel system, which distributes vitality throughout the body.

Shen—Spirit

What is the nature of spirit?

Shen is the spirit and psyche, invisible and intangible. Shen maintains the body's qi. Its higher vibrational energy sustains the vibration of the mind, which is the process of awareness and consciousness. Shen exists throughout the whole body and is not limited to the brain. It is our presence and our "I am" being-ness.

The Three Treasures and Sexual Identity

If we identify with our physical body, we are limited to either our male or female body. If we identify with our qi body, however, we become aware of both masculine and feminine energies within ourselves. When we identify with our shen or spirit body, our nature is pre-gender or nondual.

Kundalini

Kundalini is the primal power of our evolution and spiritual development, sometimes called the serpent power. This metaphor of the Three Treasures corresponds to the Hindu "Sat, Cit, Ananada," meaning "existence, consciousness, and bliss."

The dormant Kundalini—the coiled snakes at the root of our body— is like our jing. The awakened Kundalini—the snake energy rising—is like our qi. The merging of the masculine and feminine snakes with our higher consciousness is like our shen.

Three Dantians

The three dantians are the energy centers in our bodies that store and transform the Three Treasures. *Dantian* means "elixir field." When the Three Treasures, or three dantians of the head, chest, and lower abdomen, work together, we live in a harmonious flow state (see fig. 2.1 on page 62). We need all three dantians for communication that is sustainable, responsible, and trustworthy.

Lower Dantian

This area or ball of energy includes the solar plexus and the perineum. The root of the lower dantian is the umbilicus, where we were nourished as a fetus. Your core power can be concentrated here, slightly below the navel. Drop an imaginary plumb line from your crown to your center. Find the pivot point that is your center of movement and practice spiraling around it. The lower dantian:

- Stabilizes and contains
- Acts like a cauldron for cooking energies
- Is the center of will, action, digestion, touch, vitality, power, and being
- Controls the transformation of jing into qi
- Is associated with the earth, stability, security, and grounding
- Stores jing in the kidneys and sexual organs
- Is the center of awareness and gut intuition that is instinctual, like sensing someone coming up from behind you
- Is connected to the first Wei Qi field, which protects the physical body

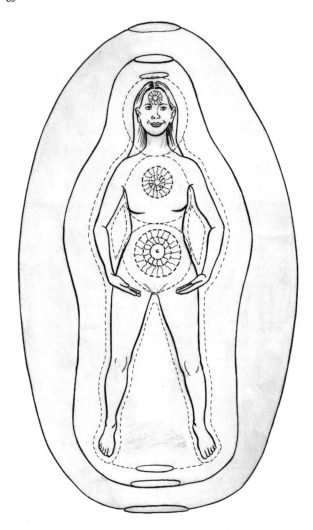

Fig. 2.1. Three dantians and three Wei Qi fields

Middle Dantian

This area or glowing ball of energy includes the heart and lungs—the rhythmical system. The heart's electromagnetic field is five thousand times more powerful than the brain's and can be felt at least twenty-three feet away. This field shrinks when we are upset and expands in the state of love.

The middle dantian:

⚔ Is the center of feeling and emotional perception
⚔ Controls the transformation of qi into shen

⚔ Is associated with the human plane, between heaven and earth
⚔ Is the center of consciousness, presence, love and compassion, passion, and flaming enthusiasm for life, which is fed by values and virtues
⚔ Is connected to the second Wei Qi field, which protects the energy body

Upper Dantian

This area or ball of energy includes the brain, master glands, senses, and throat.

The upper dantian:

⚔ Is the center of thinking, mental activities, and purpose
⚔ Guides hormones, senses, and language
⚔ Controls the transformation of shen into Wu Ji, infinite space of the Tao
⚔ Is associated with shen, presence, Heaven Qi, and light
⚔ Is the center of Observer Mind, insight, intuition, and vision
⚔ Is connected to the third Wei Qi field, which protects the soul/ spiritual body

Taiji Pole

The Taiji Pole is another name for the Core Channel that connects all three dantians. Running from the crown to the perineum, the Taiji Pole is like a tent pole that holds us up energetically between heaven and earth. Practices that cultivate energy in the body—like the Three Minds into One Mind exercise below—often focus on this Core Channel.

✸ Three Minds into One Mind

Modern life pulls our attention and energy in so many directions that many women feel too spread out. After a day of multitasking and serving others, this exercise is a fantastic way to pull yourself together.

- **Observer Mind.** Smile into your head and pull the tentacles of dispersed thoughts into your upper dantian. *The seed of thought is silence.*
- **Consciousness Mind.** Smile into your heart center and pull the tentacles of dispersed emotions into your middle dantian. *The seed of feeling is love.*
- **Awareness Mind.** Smile into the core of your belly and pull the tentacles of

dispersed actions into your lower dantian. *The seed of desire is contentment.*

- *One Mind.* Three minds become one mind, connected to the universe. Breathe between the universe within and the universe without. *In the seed is the whole universe.*

BEGINNING YOUR PRACTICE
Setting Intention and Warming Up the Qi

Visualization becomes actualization
as the qi body responds to our creative intention.

Before beginning your sexual energy practice (or any energy practice), it is important to set clear intentions so that the energy you cultivate is properly aligned.

❋ Aligning with Higher Purpose

Unconditional love powerfully transforms our lives and ripples out into the world around us. If your motivation is pure, upholding wisdom, love, and compassion both personally and globally, the transformation power is amplified. This will noticeably raise your internal power.

- Become aware of the intention in your heart. What is it you would like to heal, grow, and become? Sense a shiny star in the halo above you. Let this personal guide star resonate with your intention. Call on your higher guidance—the guides, guardians, angels, and other beings of light who are supporting your evolution.
- Affirm your intention to cultivate your sexual energy—for example, "I surrender to higher love, joy, and wisdom. I cultivate creative energy to serve the Divine."
- Broadcast your intention out into the universe. Let it multiply and come back to you. Feel your star getting brighter and stronger. The higher the motivation, the more the cosmos will help you raise your sexual energy.
- Bring the starlight down your Core Channel to the center of your head, brightening your Observer Mind; to the center of your heart, warming your Consciousness Mind; and to the center of your belly, energizing your Awareness Mind (fig. 2.2).

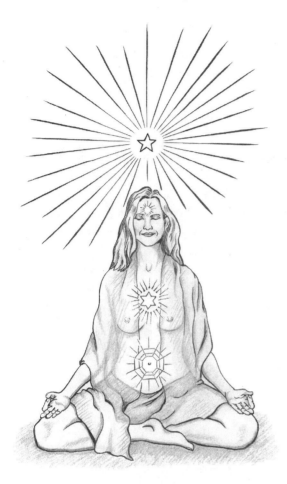

Fig. 2.2. Aligning with higher guidance

When you have aligned your body, mind, and spirit with your intention, your next preparation is to warm up the qi.

❀ Practices for Warming Up the Qi

The warm-up practices offered below open the spine, which is a super-highway for our energy system. They expand our breathing capacity, shift the focus from the mind to the body, release tension, and allow the body to relax.

● Sitting Posture

Sit comfortably on a chair with your feet flat on the floor. If you are sitting cross-legged on the floor, make sure your knees are supported with your back erect. Align yourself between heaven and earth with equal weight on both sitz bones. Lengthen the back of the neck by slightly tucking your chin. Allow the spine to lengthen as you inhale and to soften as you exhale.

● Spinal Cord Breathing

Inhale and arch your back, opening the front door to your heart (fig. 2.3). Squeeze your shoulder blades together, open your palms, and rock your tailbone back. Keep the back of your neck long and open your eyes.

Exhale and curl your back, opening the back door to your heart. Tuck in your pelvis and curl your hands, elbows, and head into a ball. Close your eyes.

Open like a flower with each inhalation and curl into a little seed with each exhalation. The heart is an organ of soul perception, like the chakras and our eyes. It is important to open these doorways at times, and also to close them at times for rest.

You can vary the speed of the rocking, which creates waves throughout your body. This movement can be applied in lovemaking, as you ride on top of your lover!

● Double Lift

Breathe in two times, sipping through your nose while lifting your shoulders toward your ears. Then drop your shoulders with an exhalation. Make the "ha-a-a-a-a-w" sound through your mouth.

● Shimmy

Shake your shoulders like a belly dancer. Release any heavy emotions from your chest. Shake off stress. Sigh with a descending heart sound, "ha-a-a-a-a-w."

● Spinal Rocking

Let the waves rock your spine from side to side from the bottom up. Start by wagging your tail, then rock the lower lumbar, then the middle thoracic, then the cervical vertebrae of the neck. Become supple like a snake, rising in a slow sensuous ripple. Smile into every vertebra, as each one is a blessing. Shift your awareness gradually back down the spine and settle into stillness. This movement will relax your nervous system.

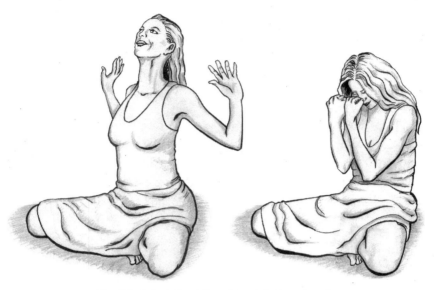

Fig. 2.3. Spinal Cord Breathing: inhale and arch,
exhale and curl

● Chest Lift and Sink

Inhale, lifting your sternum toward the sky and smiling to your thymus gland. Exhale with a "ha, ha" sound, sinking the chest two times. Let go of any heavy emotions sitting on your chest. Give your immune system a boost.

● Wind Stirring the Clouds

Hug yourself and lean to the right, dropping your head down as you exhale. Lean left and lift your heart to come up as you inhale. Change arms and circle in the other direction. This rotation opens the point between the shoulder blades and stretches the kidneys, liver, and spleen. It also relaxes the diaphragm for deeper breathing.

Let go of your jaw and the base of your skull while dropping your head. Imagine that you are sweeping the past out of your hair! End by dropping down to the earth, touching the ground with your hands. Release any stress into the earth and slowly roll up with an inhalation.

● Hinge Up

Clasp hands behind your back and then, as you exhale, hinge forward forty-five degrees. Inhale as you rise up to a vertical position and pull your hands down, stretching open the chest and fascia. This opens up the chest and aligns the sacrum. Imagine you are the woman on the bow of a ship, braving the waves and storms with grace.

ENTERING MEDITATION

Beginning each meditation with good foundations will help you move into a strong and deep practice. The following exercises establish a good sitting posture, awareness of your breath, and relationships with your sources of energy. All of these foundations are important prerequisites for directing energy in the body.

✸ Meditation Posture

Sit tall on your meditation throne. Your spine is erect yet breathing, softening a bit on the exhalation and elongating on the inhalation. Your chin is slightly tucked and the crown is lifted. Open the front and back of your heart. Widen your eyes and lips, into an effortless smile. Allow your mind to drop down into your belly. Feel the rise and fall of your breath.

✸ Preliminary Breathing Practices

Breathing practices help calm and direct your energy before, during, and after meditation.

● Internal Ocean Breathing

Feel an ocean of qi in your belly, breathing in and out with the rhythm of the waves, rippling an ocean of breath throughout your body. Allow the rise and fall of the breath to caress the inside of your body.

● Skin and Hair Breathing

Feel your skin become soft and sensitive. Feel every pore of your skin breathing like a little mouth. Sense your hair like antennae picking up frequencies from the cosmos.

● Aura Breathing

Become aware of the skin of your aura breathing and filtering energies so they're just right for you. The radiance of your aura is powerful protection.

Create a safe and sacred space within your aura so you feel comfortable to explore your inner world. If you like, you can create ambience by sensualizing soft light, fragrances, and colors.

● Centering Breath

Breathe in and out through your nose. Fill your lower abdomen like a beach ball, expanding on all four sides. Continue to inhale and fill the chest, armpits, and scapula. Fill yourself with life force. Exhale down the Core Channel/Taiji Pole. Blow the essence of the breath down into your cauldron (a pot for transforming qi), behind and just below the navel.

❇ Drawing from Three Sources

When we smile with love, gratitude, and appreciation to Mother Nature, we boost her immune system. Nature responds to our delight and gives generously of its treasures. Three satellites—power centers or chakras below and above your body—are called transpersonal points by the Taoists. Through these satellites you can tune in to different energies or octaves of earth and heaven to receive soul nourishment and insights. There is one of these outer chakras for each layer of our Wei Qi field. (See fig. 2.1.)

● Earth

Women need a lot of earth energy, which builds the blood and substance of the body. When we are in nature, tuning in to the frequency of the earth's electromagnetic field (7.8 hertz), our bodies can repair, rejuvenate, and heal more efficiently.

- Sense your core as the center of the earth in your body. Breathe from your core through your legs and feet down into the earth. Send down deep roots like a grand old tree that has withstood many, many storms. Go down through the rocks and underground waters, through the bones of our ancestors, to our common root at the center of the earth.
- Draw up earth energy—which is neutral, nourishing, stable, and gentle—through the soles of your feet and perineum. Breathe it up the body like sap rising up a tree.
- Expand your awareness below your body:
    First transpersonal point: become aware of your innate power of physical survival and belonging to the earth.

Second transpersonal point: expand your awareness to embrace the energetic grid of the earth.

Third transpersonal point: merge with the consciousness of the earth.

● Heaven

Plug yourself in to the universal sources of light to recharge yourself.

- Become aware of your crown and let it open like a flower opening to the morning light. Create a satellite or personal guide star to tune in to the planets and stars. Draw universal, heavenly energy in through this star, and penetrate your body with light. Listen to the silent wisdom of the stars and download it into your body-mind.
- Align with the three heavenly transpersonal points—energetic portals to high octaves of soul and spirit guidance—to receive insights from celestial realms.
- Expand your awareness above your body:

  First transpersonal point: become aware of your ethereal soul and a halo above your crown.

  Second transpersonal point: connect with divine unconditional love, which radiates the colors of the rainbow—the virtue and wisdom of the five pure lights.

  Third transpersonal point: embrace the sacred geometry matrix of the heavens and merge with the vast consciousness of the eternal Tao.

● Human Plane

The human plane connects us with all that lives between heaven and earth: all the human beings, animals, plants, and nature spirits.

- Become aware of a source of happiness, which could be a beautiful scene in nature. A golden sun is an image of unconditional love, shining its light on all beings equally.
- Connect with the radiant light of inter-being. Breathe in benevolent rays through the mid-eyebrow and eyes. Draw in golden light from the cosmic smile and shower it into your body with the Inner Smile meditation.

● Heaven and Earth Alignment

- Align your Core Channel with heaven and earth. Sense the force of gravity grounding you and the force of levity uplifting you. For effortless sitting, imagine a star above upholding you and roots below grounding you.

- Couple the heaven and earth energy with the Original Qi in the cauldron at your navel. This area is like a pot for storing and fusing energy into an elixir and condensing it into a pearl.

● Three Sources Qigong

- Reach your arms up to the sky and breathe in the energy of the stars, planets, sun and moon, the vastness of the Heaven Qi, and the infinite Tao.
- Bring your arms down to your heart. With your hands in prayer position, fill your heart with love, joy, and gratitude for being in this body at this time. Smile down and radiate the love into your body.
- Move down into a squat to touch the earth; feel the pulse of the earth in your palms. Breathe in the nourishing and supportive qi. Gather Earth Qi and draw it up the yin channels (inner legs) to your creative center, your yoni. Draw the qi up to your heart and bow to your Tao community with reverence for all of life.

CREATING EMOTIONAL HARMONY

The cultivation of sexual energy amplifies our emotions in the same way that gasoline feeds a fire. For this reason, it is very important to practice harmonizing your emotions as you cultivate sexual energy. Embracing the opposites of light and dark is the Taoist way to grow harmony. These opposites fuse into Yuan Qi, unconditional love.

Emotions and the Five-Element Cycle

Two fundamental practices for harmonizing emotions are the Inner Smile and the Six Healing Sounds meditations. These meditations use different aspects of the five-element cycle to structure and direct the emotions.

Creation Cycle

The creation cycle follows the seasons and grows the virtues of the organs: lungs/autumn → kidneys/winter → liver/spring → heart/summer → spleen/Indian summer.

- Lung/metal falls into the water and nourishes it. Integrity breeds serenity.

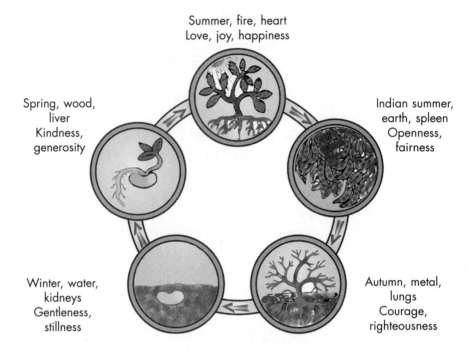

Fig. 2.4. The creation cycle in nature
(Illustration courtesy of *Cosmic Fusion* by Mantak Chia)

- ✍ Kidney/water nourishes the wood. Serenity breeds kindness.
- ✍ Liver/wood fuels the fire. Kindness gives birth to love, honor, and respect.
- ✍ Heart/fire warms the earth and nourishes it with ashes. Love gives birth to openness.
- ✍ Spleen/earth condenses into metal. Openness stimulates courage, justice, and integrity.

We use the creation cycle in the Six Healing Sounds meditation. This order can also be applied in other practices if you would like to focus on growing virtues.

Control Cycle

The control cycle is effective in balancing and controlling overactive organ energies. It is the classic order for smiling to the organs in the Inner Smile meditation.

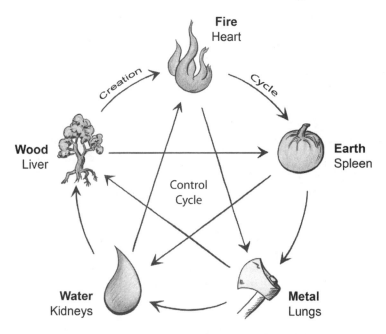

Fig. 2.5. While the creation cycle nourishes the virtues of the organs, the control cycle uses the virtues of opposite organs to balance negative emotions. For example, the warmth of love in the heart melts sadness in the lungs.

The order of the control cycle is this: fire → metal → wood → earth → water.

- ⚔ Fire (heart) melts metal (lungs).
- ⚔ Metal cuts down wood (liver).
- ⚔ Wood's roots break up the stuck earth (spleen).
- ⚔ Earth dams up water (kidneys/bladder/sexual organs).
- ⚔ Water extinguishes excess fire (heart).

The Inner Smile Meditation

The lifting of your lips uplifts your energy, like turning on a light switch (see fig. 2.6 on page 74). Frown and notice how your body dims and sinks inside. Now smile and notice how the pelvic floor lifts and creates a natural uplift in your body. An inner smile radiates powerful healing energy. Accepting your life unconditionally is the spiritual quality we cultivate with the Inner Smile practice.

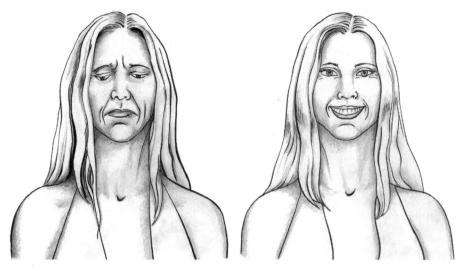

Fig. 2.6. Inner frown and inner smile

Benefits of the Inner Smile Meditation

The Inner Smile meditation has many positive effects, including the following.

SETS A POSITIVE TONE FOR THE DAY

Smile to the world and the world smiles back at you. The Inner Smile affirms the law of attraction so you can attract the synchronicity of positive events toward you. If you wake up to rainy and gloomy weather, you can set the dial of your inner mood to your inner sun. You become freer from the influence of your environment and the moods of those around you.

*The golden sun
touches our foreheads,
the day opens
with a smile.*

AWAKENS YOUR BUDDHA NATURE

The Inner Smile cultivates the spiritual quality of loving acceptance. Sense the Divinity in every cell, in all of life. An enlightened state is the lasting, eternal inner smile of our Buddha nature. This state of being calms the monkey mind and integrates mind, soul, and body.

TRANSFORMS EMOTIONAL STRESS INTO VITALITY

The magic of your inner smile melts the contraction of negative emotional energy and transforms it into expansive virtue energy. This process liberates a lot of qi that was used to suppress negativity in the body.

RELAXES AND BALANCES THE BODY

Smiling inside adjusts the alkaline balance of the body. Conditions like cancer thrive on acidity. Our DNA mirrors our whole body and emotions, such that negative emotions make your DNA contract and wind up tighter, while positive feelings make your DNA relax and lengthen into their proper shape.

GIVES RADIANCE AND BEAUTY TO YOUR EXPRESSION

There are different types of smiles, such as baby, mysterious, care-worn, wise, humorous, etc. The most important is the smile of love and acceptance. The Inner Smile is a genuine whole-body smile, not just a superficial head smile.

People who don't like themselves tend to shrink. Self-accepting people radiate their uniqueness and beauty. Lifting the corners of the lips helps create the inner smile: notice that your organs feel uplifted, and that the energy in your body rises up to create feelings of peacefulness and contentment. You can "fake it till you make it" because just the motion of the lips uplifts the energy in the body.

BRIGHTENS YOUR INTUITION AND SENSITIVITY

Smiling brings energy up to the third eye—the wisdom eye—where we can see each other's mysteries. You can sense energetic blockages in the body before they manifest. You can listen to and communicate with the soul and spirit of your organs. Your body's functions will work much better!

BOOSTS ENERGY LEVELS AND THE IMMUNE SYSTEM

Smiling plays an important role in the immune system. If someone gives you one nasty look, this can lower your white blood cell count for six to eight hours. Smiles do the opposite: they raise the white blood cell count, which in turn boosts the immune system. Muscle testing is a great way to test how smiling affects the human body. You'll notice that smiling and positive affirmations uplift your body and make your muscles strong. Frowning and negative affirmations will make the muscles weaker and the body energy will feel heavy and sinking. Negative emotions can shrink the thymus gland.

UPLIFTS SEXUAL ENERGY AND STRENGTHENS THE WHOLE BODY

When you smile, become aware of how your pelvic floor tones and smiles with you. Sexual energy is effortlessly attracted to the radiance of your open heart. How can we grow an abundance of vitality? Smiling is one way! If you show you are appreciative and grateful toward those who are working for you (your organs), they will work better!

OPENS THE HEART WITH UNCONDITIONAL LOVE

The essence of authentic connection starts with love for oneself. Love is the energy of the heart, the center of our feeling. To really open to another, our whole being needs to expand in love. Mantak Chia likes to say, "When we are orgasmic our DNA multiplies in the proper way." Imagine the strands of DNA as yin and yang lovers!

HELPS THOSE AROUND YOU FEEL MORE COMFORTABLE

When you smile to someone, notice how they smile back and feel relaxed and accepted. When you give gratitude and loving attention to people, they feel better—even when they are not present. Talking bad about another will make that person feel bad. Rather than dumping your negativity on others, recycle your emotions into vitality with the magic of your loving smile. Talking positively boosts our immune system for hours!

MAKES YOU FEEL POSITIVE ABOUT YOURSELF AND YOUR LIFE

The Inner Smile is a profound way to boost positive self-image and self-confidence. When you have negative judgments of your body, every cell of your body hears that. Feel how your body contracts when you look in the mirror with criticism and judgment. When you practice loving acceptance with how you look and feel, your natural beauty can unfold from the inside. Treat your body like a work of art that you sculpt with your positive thoughts and activities. Appreciate how the wrinkles and white hair are part of the unfolding artwork of nature.

Inner Smile Practice

Prepare for the Inner Smile practice by tuning in to the love and light that connect you to the Divine.

✸ Source of Unconditional Love

Imagine something that makes you feel happy, like the smiling face of someone you love, a beautiful place in nature, or the sun. The sun is an image of unconditional love that shines on all beings equally.

- Draw smiling energy through the third eye into the center of the head— the Crystal Palace that activates the master glands of the body. Refract/ direct the golden light from the Crystal Palace into your body.
- Lift your lips into a peaceful, effortless smile like a Madonna or Buddha.

✸ Shower of Golden Light

Spread warm, golden smiling energy to melt away tension and transform negativity. Negative emotions can also be released into the cauldron to be neutralized, balanced, and transformed by the light of your awareness, then fused with other elements.

- Smile and breathe into parts of your body-mind calling for loving attention. Smile until your whole body radiates with virtue energy and heightened awareness.
- Connect with the cosmic smile of your higher self. Watch with loving understanding and acceptance as thoughts and feelings come and go, like clouds drifting in the vast, open sky. Open inner spaciousness. Make room for growing what you want to enhance in your life.
- Connect with the golden sunny glow of unconditional love and let it flow down the front, middle, and back of your body, melting any tension and transforming any negativity.

✸ Inner Smile Meditation

In this practice, we follow the control cycle to progress through the organs.

- Draw a warm, golden light of loving acceptance in through your third eye. Light up the glands of bliss (the pituitary and pineal glands). Relax your senses and facial muscles and softly lift the corners of your lips. Melt tension in the neck, thyroid, and parathyroid glands. Smile to your thymus gland in the upper chest and affirm your body's ability to heal itself.

- Smile to your heart and feel your inner sun radiate into the whole body. Feel the warmth of unconditional love melt any contracting tension of negativity into the expansive glow of virtue energy.

    Let your whole body smile. Tell every cell, "I love you. Thank you for supporting my life."

- Smile to your lungs and let the sun's rays disperse any heavy, gray clouds of sadness or tiredness. Fill the lungs with white light and the feeling of courage and strength.

- Smile to your liver. Melt any anger and frustration with the warmth of your smile and transform it into kindness. Fill your liver with the green light of a forest or jungle and the abundance of nature.

- Shower your spleen with smiling light, transforming stress and anxiety into openness and trust. Fill your spleen with the yellow light of a sunflower at harvest time.

- Shower the warm, golden light down your back to the kidneys, melting icy cold fear into gentle, peaceful blue water. Smile to your bladder and give thanks for all that it does for you.

- Smile down to your sexual organs. Spiral and wrap them with golden light, as if they were a precious gift. Draw passion up from the sexual organs to grow compassion in the heart. Feel your heart's flower open as it drinks the sexual water.

- Draw up sexual energy and mix it with smiling energy in your saliva, then swallow. Smile down and move the golden elixir through your stomach, small intestine, large intestine, and anus/pubococcygeal/qi muscles. Breathe softly into your belly.

- Breathe golden light into your third eye and create a beam like a floodlight that shines from the Crystal Palace. Sweep the beam sideways across your forehead to clear away any mental tension. Sweep the beam forward and backward in arches through the left hemisphere of your brain to clear any old stuck thoughts. Sweep the beam in arches over the ear through the right hemisphere of your brain to make room for new inspirations to flow in. Balance the two sides of your brain by sweeping the beam sideways, which can create a light sense of bliss. Beam into the back brain (cerebellum) and allow it to relax. This calms the heart and breathing rhythms.

- Spiral the warm, liquid light down through your spine, vertebra by vertebra to the sacrum and coccyx. Relax and lengthen the spine. Breathe up the spine to above your head. Shower from your personal star a waterfall of love and appreciation down through your auric field, skin, muscles, tendons, bones, and bone marrow. Let go of any unnecessary tension. Rinse down through your vital organs. Feel your body as one radiant whole.
- Collect smiling energy at the navel into a warm, golden ball of energy. Use the pearl's warm vibration and light of awareness to open the points along the Microcosmic Orbit, so more qi can move through.

     Connect with the cosmic smile of your higher self several times throughout the day. Watch with loving acceptance as thoughts and feelings come and go, like clouds drifting in the vast, open sky. Open inner spaciousness. Make space for growing what you want to enhance in your life.

❀ Variations on the Inner Smile

The following variations can be practiced in addition to, or as variants of, the practice above.

● Wake-Up Practice

Before getting up in the morning, wake up your heart by connecting with it and smiling to it. Choosing to be happy will set the tone for your entire day.

     Immediately upon waking, breathe consciously. Put your hands on your heart. Smile to your heart and fill it with love, joy, and happiness. Radiate love to every gland, organ, and cell of your body.

● Mini Inner Smile

Smile down a waterfall of golden light, telling every cell, "I love you. Thank you for supporting my life."

     Melt down from the head to the toes with the relaxation response.

● Smile Down 1, 2, 3

I love this one. It is so easy and effective—as simple as 1, 2, 3!

1. Smile to your head and neck.
2. Smile down to your chest and arms.
3. Smile down to your lower abdomen and legs.

     Three into one: feel yourself as whole, relaxed, and grounded. Open, expand, include.

● Inner Smile with Sound or Music

Adding sounds or music can be a nice variation. Specific tones vibrate each organ. Tone or hum to vibrate smiling energy into your organs. Music is soothing for the organs and for the soul.

● Lotus Meditation

Your energy body is like a plant and your being is a complete ecosystem.

• Smile to your ovaries and sense them as the bulbs of your plant.
• Smile down your legs into the earth, sensing your roots.
• Smile up your spine, the stem of your plant.
• Smile into your heart and sense your heart's flower blossoming. Feel the fragrance rising to your head.

Your smiling energy is the sunshine beaming into your internal plant. Draw or paint your energy body as a plant and study the progress of your drawings.

Six Healing Sounds

The Six Healing Sounds release imbalanced weather conditions and emotional patterns that can be trapped in the organs. For example, excess heat can emerge as impatience or hastiness, while excess cold can manifest as fear. The practice doesn't simply relieve symptoms but gets to the root cause of the emotional imbalance on the mental and spiritual level. That is why we recommend continuing until you feel a shift.

After clearing dark, murky, dense emotion you want to immediately replace it with a higher-frequency energy—the "pure lights of the soul" or vivid colors as they appear in nature—to reprogram the system.

Benefits of the Six Healing Sounds

Releasing negative emotions benefits the body, mind, and spirit in a host of important ways.

RELIEVES STRESS ON THE ORGANS

With stress, the fascia (connective tissue) can cling to the organ so the organ feels trapped or like it is suffocating. It can become like a clingy plastic bag around bananas that makes them sweat and rot. While sweeping the organs with the eyes we can move the torso to internally massage and loosen the fascia.

LIBERATES SEXUAL ENERGY

Suppressed negative emotions lock our energy up in unhealthy ways. Releasing fear, anger, sadness, bitterness, and anxiety liberates bound energy and makes it available to our growing vitality. Women can experience more sexual pleasure and become more open to sensuality when negative emotions—especially fear and anger—are not creating contracting holding patterns in the body.

We tend to contract and tighten when we feel fear. In this way, fear freezes up the sexual waters and becomes a major obstacle to the expression of our sexuality. Be aware and feel your fear. Breathe deeply and expand around it.

It also takes a lot of energy to hold down suppressed anger. When this anger is released, like a pressure cooker, it liberates a lot of energy! The wood element, liver qi, is uprising and is responsible for erection. It is important to clear extreme anger before making important decisions, because clear decision-making abilities are also ruled by the element of wood. Let your yoni rise with passion rather than tightening the muscles with anger.

When the heart is bitter and feels separate, love is held back. The more love, the more orgasmic you feel! Releasing the delusion of separation, sexual energy generates love.

Anxiety brings us out of the present moment so we are not totally there to enjoy the pleasures of touch and sensation. Dampness dams up the water, and you might feel stuck or heavy or have yeast infections or fungal discharges. Let go of your worries so you can dance with the Sexual Qi!

Sadness is a sinking energy. The breasts and yoni can feel saggy, tired, and sad. Feelings of loss that persist will block you from recognizing all that you do have in this moment. Allow the tears to flow and the sun will come out after the rain.

The healing sounds can be used quickly in emergency situations to work with an individual emotion, so the entire sequence doesn't have to be used all at once. For example, taking a quick break from an argument to practice the healing sound of the liver can prevent the damaging effects of an emotion like anger from causing wounds in your relationship.

AIDS PSYCHIC DETOXIFICATION

The healing sounds help vent out trapped toxins and layers of suppressed emotion. Rather like a car, the body generates a lot of heat and needs a cooling system. The healing sounds serve this cooling function. (Western-ers tend to cool the body with ice water, but this forces the system to work hard bringing the water to body temperature. In China the national drink is hot water.)

Just as we clean our house every day of dust balls, the healing sounds can help clean our emotional body so that emotions do not build up into internal bombs that could explode with any trigger. This is preventive medicine!

Once you peel back the onion layers of more present emotions you can begin to clear emotions from childhood and past lives that still haven't been released or are in a dormant state. Emotional healing affects the past, present, and future. The healing sounds can be used to clear the negative emotions that accumulate from those around us, our partners, our parents, our ancestors before us, and even our children. Emotional detoxification of dysfunctional family patterns is important for the graceful unfolding of giving birth and raising children.

EMOTIONS AS MESSENGERS

What we call negative emotions are contracted in nature and positive emotions are expansive in nature. Both are important messengers for our soul and need to be honored. It takes a lot of energy to keep the lid on pent-up emotions. When we transform stuck emotions we liberate a lot of qi that can then be used for healing. Instead of suppressing negativity, we embrace our shadow and transform its energy into a more expanded form. For example, the liver energy can show up as anger or a tight fist; when this contracted energy is transformed, it can open into a caring, giving hand of kindness. Both arise from the same hand. Positive emotions also take energy, yet they uplift the spirit. Negative emotions tend to pull the spirit down when not spontaneously expressed.

Negative emotions are irrational and without a concept of time. Heal-ing happens in the moment and will heal past and prevent potential future stuck patterns from growing or crystallizing. If emotions have crystallized they can be triggered like a land mine.

The table that begins on the facing page shows both the positive vir-tues and the negative or acquired patterns of emotion associated with each organ.

EMOTIONAL SPECTRUM OF THE ORGANS—
VIRTUES AND ACQUIRED EMOTIONS

LUNG—VIRTUES

Physical: Cool, Dry, Strength, Prosperity
Emotional: Courage, Confidence
Soul, Spiritual: Discrimination, Integrity, Truth, Justice, Dignity, Responsibility, Righteousness

LUNG—ACQUIRED EMOTIONS

Physical: Tiredness, Weakness
Emotional: Sadness, Grief, Loss, Depression, Disappointment, Greed
Soul, Spiritual: Shame, Guilt, Disgrace, Self-righteousness

KIDNEY—VIRTUES

Physical: Cold, Wet
Emotional: Peace, Gentleness, Calmness
Soul, Spiritual: Self-understanding, Wisdom, Faith

KIDNEY—ACQUIRED EMOTIONS

Physical: Frozen, Isolation
Emotional: Fear, Loneliness
Soul, Spiritual: Paranoia, Existential fear

LIVER—VIRTUES

Physical: Warm, Moist, Steamy, Abundance of qi
Emotional: Generosity, Hope
Soul, Spiritual: Kindness, Decisiveness, Forgiveness

LIVER—ACQUIRED EMOTIONS

Physical: Frustration, Irritability
Emotional: Anger, Jealousy, Aggressiveness
Soul, Spiritual: Indecisiveness, Resentment, Overcontrol

HEART—VIRTUES

Physical: Hot, Dry, Warmth
Emotional: Joy, Happiness, Goodness
Soul, Spiritual: Love, Acceptance, Compassion, Beauty, Honor, Loyalty, Sincerity, Honesty, Appreciation, Gratitude, Humor, Respect, Reverence, Order, Harmony

HEART—ACQUIRED EMOTIONS

Physical: Overexcitement, Hastiness, Violence, Cruelty, Chaos
Emotional: Hatred, Bitterness, Impatience
Soul, Spiritual: Separation, Pride, Arrogance, Egotistic selfishness, Self-importance

SPLEEN — VIRTUES

Physical: Damp, Mild, Stability, Balance, Centeredness, Groundedness, Support
Emotional: Openness, Security, Empathy, Contentment
Soul, Spiritual: Trust, Fairness

SPLEEN — ACQUIRED EMOTIONS

Physical: Stress, Tension
Emotional: Worry, Anxiety, Scarcity, Self-doubt
Soul, Spiritual: Attachment, Addiction, Compulsion, Obsession, Over-thinking, Self-doubt, Neediness, Demanding, Consuming

TRIPLE WARMER — VIRTUES

Physical: Balanced heat, Survival
Emotional: Clear mind, Benevolent, Emotional balance
Soul, Spiritual: Integral, Wholeness, Stable consciousness

TRIPLE WARMER — ACQUIRED EMOTIONS

Physical: Overheated
Emotional: Busy mind, Distracted, Overwhelmed
Soul, Spiritual: Fragmented, Unstable consciousness

Eye Movement with the Six Healing Sounds

Sweeping your eyes back and forth as you scan inside your organs is a technique that was inspired by Eye Movement Desensitization and Reprocessing (EMDR) therapy. This technique helps you look deep inside to access your emotions, which may be hidden in the shadows. By sweeping our awareness with a subtle cradling movement we integrate and resolve our emotional experiences, which may be crying out for attention. When the baby cries, we cradle the baby. Normally we integrate our waking emotions when we dream at night. When we are in the dream state our eyes move rapidly back and forth in REM (or rapid eye movement) sleep. It is especially helpful to practice the Six Healing Sounds along with the sweeping eye movements before you go to bed so you can transform your emotions before you sleep. This way you will have less emotional processing to do in the dream state, which will allow you to sink into more profound levels of dreams and deep sleep.

Reprogram yourself by filling the organs with brilliant color and virtue energy. Through the Healing Sounds, we can empty the busy mind and relax the body, mind, and spirit.

Energetic Protection—
Your Radiance Is Your Best Protection

We are energetically protected by three Wei Qi fields that are filled with virtue energies (see fig. 2.1 on page 62). These layers of the auric field attract benevolent vibrations and filter energies to protect the three subtle bodies. If you have you ever felt thin-skinned, as if the emotions of others go right into you, you will understand the benefits of developing thicker, more radiant layers of your auric field.

Becoming aware of these levels gives us resources to sink into the hidden and mysterious causes of suffering and release them from there. You can strengthen these auric layers by practicing the Healing Sounds on all three levels.

Physical: The first energetic field is connected to the physical body and the lungs/corporeal soul, which help us incarnate and survive. This level is white like the metal element and acts like a second skin. It protects you with the virtues of truth and integrity. This auric field radiates about one to three inches from the body.

Start by touching and massaging your organs as you move side to side in a figure-eight movement that is in sync with the sideways sweeping of the eyes. The sound level for addressing this layer is obvious or out loud, vibrating the physical body.

Emotional/Energetic: The second energetic field is connected to the energy body and the kidneys. This level is blue like the water element and protects you with the virtues of self-understanding and wisdom. It radiates about twelve to eighteen inches from the body, acting as radar for our feelings.

Embrace the aura of the organ and sense how it grows bigger as you practice the sounds and fill your organs with pure colored light. Work on this layer with a sound level that is hidden or soft like a whisper. It works on the emotional and mental body and beliefs.

Soul Spiritual/Mysterious: The third energetic field is connected to the spirit body and the heart. This level is pink like the fire element and violet like the primordial light. It protects you with the virtues of love and compassion. This field can radiate about twenty-four inches to one hundred yards away from the body, according to the space you hold in your awareness. A performer is aware of the whole theater, and a mother is aware of her kids on the whole playground.

Work on this level with a sound that is silent or heard inside. This level works on spiritual and unconscious levels, addressing causal, karmic, and ancestral imprints.

✸ Preparation of Sacred Space

Prepare sacred space in which to work before you begin the Six Healing Sounds meditation.

- Connect with the earth, which is like a compost pit that neutralizes energy. Make a clockwise spiral with your hands to create a vortex into the earth for dark, murky energies to be transformed.*
- Call on the Divine to create a sacred space. Lift your hands up to the heavens and ask for the greatest healing in accordance with divine will. Connect with your higher guidance to help you release what you are ready to release.
- Connect with unconditional love and smiling energy to accept with compassion what arises in the practice.

✸ The Six Healing Sounds Meditation

Practice in the natural order of the creation cycle: fall, winter, spring, summer, Indian summer. Our breathing acts like a flywheel to get the healing process going, so we start with the lung sound. We complete the process with the triple warmer sound, which clears stress from head to toe and takes us into deep relaxation. This sound is often used to complete a practice session or at the end of the day before sleep.

● General Procedure for Each Element

- Hold the organ in your hands. Smile and breathe into it with loving acceptance. Sweep your inner eyes sideways, right and left inside your organ, looking for contracted, murky energy, which hides in the shadows.
- Lift your arms, stretch the organ, and open your eyes. Make the healing sound, releasing all the air, imbalanced conditions, and negative emotional energy like gray smoke into the earth.
- Slowly bring your arms down to the organ, breathing fresh energy into it.

---

*The right rule of thumb can be used to clarify the direction of how energy spirals. If you flip your right hand over so the thumb is facing down, the fingers are curling clockwise. With the right thumb facing upward, the fingers are curling counterclockwise.

Allow the organ to yawn and relax. Smile down and fill the organ with its corresponding bright color. Grow the positive virtues. Embrace the organ with colored light.

- With your hands on the organ or whichever level of the Wei Qi field you are working on, loosen up the fascia around the organ by moving the rib cage, while massaging and tapping the area to release toxins and stagnant energy.
- Go through all three levels of the Wei Qi field as described above for a deeper transformation of the organ energies. Then return to the physical organ, tapping and thanking it for all it does for you. If you like, you can make an affirmation.
- Rest and feel if there is more spaciousness in your organ.

● Lung Sound

- Smile into the lungs and scan for any cloudy gray energy, sadness, or depression.
- Lift your arms and turn your palms up, stretching the thumbs (the end of the Lung meridian). Exhale the lung sound, "ss-s-s-s-s-s," with your tongue behind your teeth (fig. 2.7).

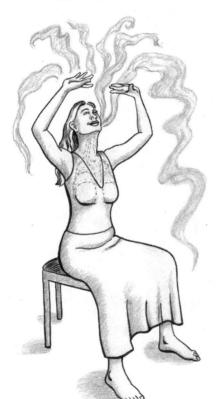

Fig. 2.7. Lung sound

- Breathe out excess cool dryness, smoky exhaust, and sadness. Turn your palms toward you and lower your arms to face the lungs, while keeping the lungs empty. Now, hungry for breath, breathe in fresh qi. Smile to your lungs. Breathe white light and courage into them. Stand up for what is right. *To my own self be true.*

● Kidney Sound

- Breathe into the kidneys while scanning for cold, contracted fear.
- Hold your hands below the knees and round your back to open the kidney area (fig. 2.8). Exhale the kidney sound, "choo-oo-oo-oo," blowing out excess cold wetness, murky colors, and fear. "Choo-oo-oo-oo" breaks the ice and gets the water flowing.
- Move your arms around to the back to face the kidneys. Breathe blue healing light into them.
- Smile and fill the kidneys with calmness and gentleness.

● Liver Sound

- Smile into the liver and scan for any contracted anger or pent-up steam.
- Interlace your fingers, turn your palms up, and stretch the liver on the right by leaning to the left (fig. 2.9). Look up and blow out the liver sound,

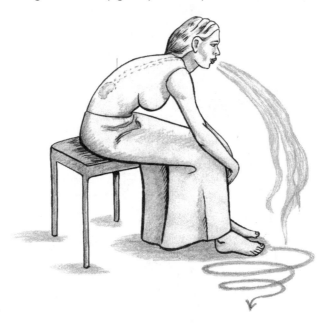

Fig. 2.8. Kidney sound

"sh-h-h-h-h-h," with back of your tongue near your palate, releasing excess steam and anger.

- Clear the space around you by lowering your hands with your palms facing out. Stretch the tendons in your hands.
- Breathe in green light and fill the liver with kindness.

● Heart Sound

- Smile into the heart and scan for overheated hastiness or separation.
- Clasp your hands and turn the palms up, stretching the heart on the left side (fig. 2.10). Make the heart sound with the mouth wide open, "ha-a-a-a-a-w," releasing excess heat, hatred, impatience, or separation.
- Lower your arms to your sides, stretching the pinkie fingers (the Heart meridian).
- Breathe rose, pink, or red light into the heart. Fill it with love, respect, and joy. Call the shen—the spirit—back home.

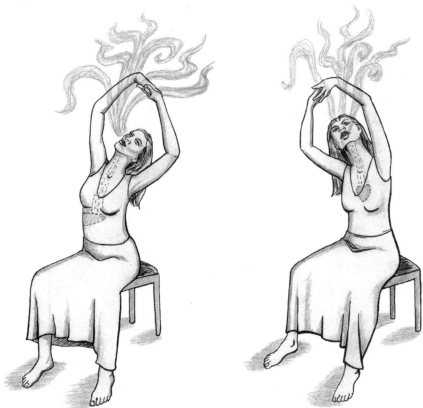

Fig. 2.9. Liver sound   Fig. 2.10. Heart sound

● Spleen Sound

- Smile into the spleen and scan for damp, foggy feelings of stress.
- Curl your fingers under the left rib cage (fig. 2.11). Make the spleen sound, a guttural vibration across the throat, "who-o-o-o-o-o," releasing congestion and worries. Toss out sick winds with a quick flick of the hands.
- Breathe in yellow light and fill the spleen with nurturing, balanced qi.

● Triple Warmer Sound

- Breathe up the three burners—belly, chest, and head—while lifting your arms above the head (fig. 2.12).
- Press down the length of the body three times: front, back, and middle.
- Exhale with the "he-e-e-e-e-e" sound. Smile wide like a Cheshire cat to feel a stretch behind your ears (the Triple Warmer meridian). Squeeze down mental, emotional, and physical tension, impurities, imbalances, and excess heat. Relax. Yawn out. Relax the chest, solar plexus, and abdomen.
- Flick excess mental, emotional, and physical tension out of fingers and toes. Bring excess heat down from the head to warm the lower burners and feet. (Ingredients for a good night's sleep include a cool head and warm feet: it is very difficult to fall asleep when the feet are cold and the head is too hot and busy.)
- Relax. Feel the energy and heat distribute in the body, the warmth brought down to the lower body and fresh coolness and calmness coming up into the head and chest.

❄ Variations on the Six Healing Sounds

The Six Healing Sounds practice can be modified to target particular traumas or to expand your healing experience.

● Healing Sexual Issues with the Healing Sounds

Practice with clear intention to transform triggers related to your sexuality. Do the Wands of Healing Light practice in chapter 3 to clear your womb.

Examples of fears related to sexuality could be fear of rejection, abandonment, performance, expression, penetration, intimacy, or surrender.

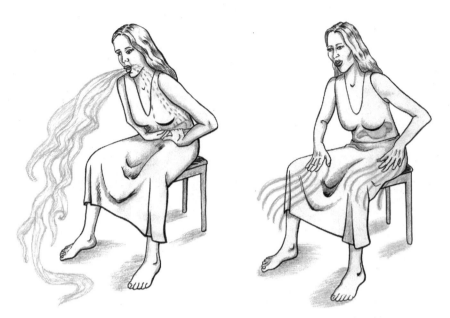

Fig. 2.11. Spleen (and stomach) sound and tossing out sick winds

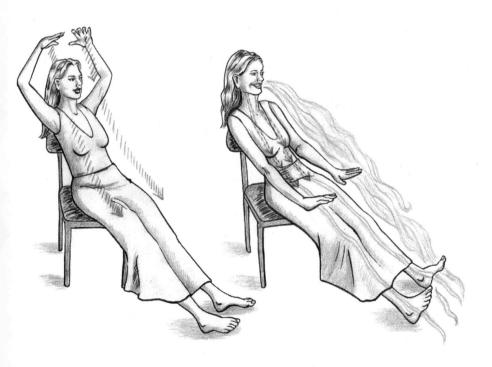

Fig. 2.12. Triple warmer sound

● Cosmic Healing Sounds

The planets are our cosmic organs, sources of feeling and of cosmic creative force.

> Lungs/Venus/white/integrity
> Kidneys/Mercury/blue/peacefulness
> Liver/Jupiter/green/kindness
> Heart/Mars/red/love
> Spleen/Saturn/yellow/stability

Practice this variation to evoke transformation from planetary frequencies.

- Call on the virtues of your higher self to transform and balance your inner life. Our egos do not have the power to transform their stuck patterns or negativity.
- Call on the spirit of the virtues to transform and heal.
- For each of the five major organs, connect with healing cosmic force from the galaxies, planets, and elements that correspond to that organ.
- Every sound has a shadow and light side, so the same sounds can be used to project the virtues, especially combined with the pure light colors. Beam the colored light of each organ through the palms/hands into the body. Bask in the virtue energy.
- Give your blessing of virtue. What you give, you receive. Amplify and multiply the virtue with the ripple effect.
- Receive the blessing of virtue. Absorb and embrace the vibration and aura of each organ.
- For the triple warmer, shower your front side with the light of purity, sealing the senses from harmful desires and temptations.
    Shower the back with a sense of balance—especially the kidneys, spine, and sacrum—to enhance the balance of yin and yang, heaven and earth.
    Shower the middle with clarity, clearing the Core Channel.
- Thank the air, water, wood, sun, earth, planets, and stars for greater purity, clarity, and balance.

● Affirmations with Sounds

As you beam virtue energies into your organs, affirm:
- "Courage fills me and goes with me every day" (lungs).
- "Gentleness fills me and carries with me all the way" (kidneys).
- "Kindness fills me and goes with me every day" (liver).

- "Love fills me and carries me all the way" (heart).
- "Trust fills me and goes with me every day" (spleen).
- "Balance fills me and carries me all the way" (triple warmer).

Offer each virtue out to all beings in the universe. Allow it to come back to you multiplied. Let it fill you and overflow into your auric field and into your daily life. Program the inner sounds to be self-sustaining and protect you from negativity.

● Navel Wind Gates

A lot of "undigested" life events and unresolved emotions sit like knots around the navel. When we clear these knots, the energy they release can radiate from the umbilicus (like the spokes of a wheel) into the organs. To open the passageway from the navel to the organs, we can use the healing sound associated with each individual wind gate and its corresponding organ.

The wind gates are located about one finger-width from the navel (fig. 2.13).

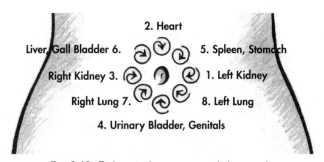

Fig. 2.13. Eight wind gates around the navel

- Using your sword fingers (the index and middle finger together), press into each wind gate.
- Press as deeply as you can relax into. With your intention, send the qi from the gate toward its associated organ, then exhale with the corresponding healing sound. Pause and melt, waiting for the release.
- Inhale, allowing the belly to pop open by itself.

For each wind gate, use the corresponding healing sound as listed below.
　Left of the navel—kidney—"choo-oo-oo-oo"
　Top of the navel—heart—"ha-a-a-a-w"

Right of the navel—kidney—"choo-oo-oo-oo"

Bottom of the navel—bladder and sexual organ—"choo-oo-oo-oo"

Top left of the navel—spleen and stomach—guttural "who-o-o-o-o-o"

Top right of the navel—liver and gallbladder—"sh-h-h-h-h-h"

Bottom right of the navel—ascending colon—"ss-s-s-s-s-s"

Bottom left of the navel—descending colon—"ss-s-s-s-s-s"

O Inner Empowerment

This variation on the wind gate exercise uses reverse or power breathing. It is energetic medicine for those who want to liberate themselves from victim consciousness. It is an empowering practice for people who have experienced sexual, physical, emotional, or mental abuse.

• Inhale and softly sink your fingers into the wind gate.

• Exhale and push your fingers out with your internal power by lifting the pelvic floor and bearing down with the upper diaphragm. This gesture empowers you to claim your inner space and healthy boundaries. The more you are able to push out with power, the more you are able to be soft and receptive.

OPENING CHANNELS

Flowing water never stagnates
and an active door never rusts.
When essence does not flow, qi stagnates.

CONFUCIUS

By clearing and harmonizing your emotions with the Inner Smile and Six Healing Sounds practices, you will make more energy available for opening the energy channels in your body. The Microcosmic Orbit meditation is the foundational Taoist practice for circulating and refining sexual energy in the body.

The Microcosmic Orbit meditation and its associated practices rely on one of the pillars of Taoist practice—the use of intention to move energy: "Where your mind goes qi flows." At first, creative intention may feel like you are imagining or visualizing the qi; over time this shifts into sensualizing or feeling the qi. With further practice, this experience shifts again into one of actualization, in which the qi becomes a vivid experience. This is another example of "fake it until you make it."

Microcosmic Orbit

Sexual energy is channeled, circulated, and refined in the Microcosmic Orbit (sometimes called the "multiorgasmic channel"), which runs in a circle up the spine to the brain and down the front of the body to the perineum, or up the front of the body to the brain and down the spine. Breathing in a circle refines your sexual energy and makes multiorgasmic bliss a possibility within your whole body. This is a powerful way to exchange and harmonize energy with your intimate partner during subtle-body lovemaking.

This Microcosmic Orbit practice balances cool yin and warm yang energy; circulating creative energy in this way cultivates the etheric body and the psychic centers, awakening the power of spiritual perception and creating a sense of wholeness. The Orbit pulls you together when you feel scattered. It seals the chakra openings with neutral qi so you do not feel so exposed. It helps contain your energy, making you feel safe in your body.

Prenatal Breathing

The Front and Back Channels of the Microcosmic Orbit are formed in the embryo as the first cells divide. Creative energy runs through the Orbit like a subtle breathing to facilitate the development of the fetus; for this reason, the circulation of energy in the Microcosmic Orbit is also called Prenatal Breathing. The Microcosmic Orbit links up the Governing Vessel in the back, which governs yang qi in the body, and the Conception Vessel in the front, which is a source of yin energy. The Conception Vessel ends in the tongue and the Governing Vessel ends in the palate, so putting the tongue on the roof of the mouth acts like a circuit breaker to link the flow together.

Water Cycle and Fire Cycle

There are two ways to circulate the qi in the Orbit: up the front and down the back, in a pattern known as the water cycle, or up the back and down the front, the fire cycle. The cycles vary through different phases of life. For example, in the womb the flow of the fire cycle activates our growth;

in childhood the flow of the water cycle helps develop our imagination; in adulthood the flow of the fire cycle develops our manifestation power; and in elders the flow of the water cycle enhances self-reflection and spiritual growth.

The water cycle has the effect of opening our psychic abilities as qi flows up to the third eye. It relaxes the nerves as you feel a waterfall of energy cascade down your spine. Placing your tongue in the Heavenly Pool on the soft palate will help shift you into this water cycle.

The fire cycle helps us awaken heightened awareness and grow our initiative in life. This flow can stir up stagnant emotions and purify them, just as debris is moved along by a current in the river. The fire cycle has the benefit of containing and protecting our energy field as we go out into the world. After energy healing sessions in which clients have become vulnerable and open, I always bundle them up with the fire cycle and collect their energy before they go out into the street. Placing your tongue in the fire position behind the front teeth will help shift you into the fire cycle.

If you are focusing on the Core Channel in the center of the body, align your tongue in the wood position—the center of your palate.

Benefits of the Microcosmic Orbit Practice

As you allow qi to move, it will work to bring you into balance. Often strange things happen! Consider these things as healing gifts and co-operate with them by holding space for the qi to do its magical work. A common experience is heat or shaking as the circulating energy breaks up resistance and blockages in the physical and subtle bodies. The heat is caused by friction as energy scrubs through the channels. When this energy is awakened it wants to heal and open the body. It has incredible wisdom and can do amazing work when you trust and let it happen.

The conscious circulation of energy is a safe way of cultivating Kundalini or primordial energy as it embraces both the ascension and expansion of consciousness and the incarnating and embodiment of the refined energy to grow and evolve all parts of ourselves. Once awakened, Kundalini—the power of evolution—is a profound catalyst for renewal on all physical, emotional, and spiritual levels.

Some of the benefits of opening the Orbit include the following:

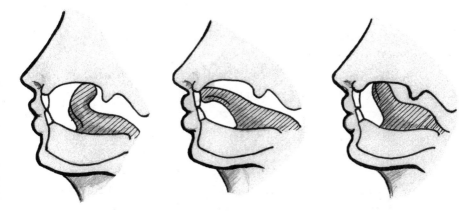

Fig. 2.14. Three tongue positions: water, fire, and wood

CIRCULATES THE LIGHT

Mantak Chia wrote that when people open the Microcosmic Orbit, profound shifts happen from within to awaken natural self-healing. The power of these shifts motivated Master Chia to bring these amazing teachings of Inner Alchemy to the West about thirty years ago. I personally experienced such a shift years ago, when my Microcosmic Orbit opened spontaneously.

> *Sitting in meditation, all at once a surge of warm energy rose up my spine to my crown and then fell like a waterfall down the front of my body. The energy took off, rising and falling in a circle with its own momentum, and caused my body to rock. I started to sweat even though the meditation hall was cool inside. The bell rang at the end of the sitting and I gathered qi in my navel into a ball of energy, a vibrant, golden pearl that sparkled like a diamond. What was this energy doing? Generating light, warmth, and life force!*

REFINES THE QI

Inner Alchemy is a way to transform something that is dense and dark into something that is penetrated with the light of consciousness, transparent and golden, filled with virtues and integrity. When raw sexual energy circulates through the Orbit, it moves through four pumps along the spine: the sacral, adrenal, dorsal, and cranial pumps, which pump the sexual waters upward. These energy pumps also refine the energy from a dense state in the lower centers to a more refined state as it moves through the upper centers.

GENERATES LIGHT

How does the Microcosmic Orbit generate light? If you put an electric wire between a positive and negative pole you can generate electricity. Our negative charged pole is in the perineum, called the Hui Yin or Meeting of Yin, and our positive charged pole is in the crown, called Bai Hui or Meeting of a Hundred Places. So when you circulate energy between these two poles you are a generator of free energy! The whirling action pulls in an abundance of energy from the heavens, earth, and human plane around us. Your center of gravity below your navel is like the magnetic core of the earth. As the moon orbits around the earth, so the orbit describes the phases of the moon. Imagine a ball of energy at the base of the spine as a new moon, which rises to your crown as the full moon, its most yang phase.

GENERATES LOVE

This circulation plays an essential role in cultivating sexual energy and is central in the practice of Tao Tantra. When a couple is conscious of exchanging energy during lovemaking, they can weave their Microcosmic Orbits together, joining at the heart, genitals, or third eye. Their light energy generates love so they can really "make" love, make joy, make courage, and grow limitless potential of creativity, wisdom, and bliss.

GENERATES LIFE FORCE

I have been practicing and teaching Taoist Inner Alchemy for more than thirty years, and I still close our practice sessions with circulating qi in the Microcosmic Orbit. The individuals or the group leave feeling calm, centered, and grounded. The practice embodies the realization that we are interconnected to all life, a microcosm of the whole universe. Through practice we generate light, love, and life force and expand our potential to heal ourselves and evolve the world.

INTEGRATES THE THREE DANTIANS

The Orbit weaves together and integrates the three dantians of the head, chest, and lower abdomen, which correspond to the zones of thinking, feeling, and willing, or intuition, feeling, and sensuality. It distributes qi to all the chakras and acupuncture meridians and nourishes the growth of our soul and spirit. It builds the energetic foundation for spiritual development.

LONGEVITY PRACTICE

The conscious circulation of qi in this way plays an important role in longevity. As we age, our energy tends to polarize, cold sinking and heat rising. Excess heat rising can lead to mental agitation and heart conditions, while excess coldness sinking can lead to weaker digestive fire and stiff joints, for example. The Warm Current meditation, another name for the Microcosmic Orbit, blends these hot and cold tendencies and makes us feel more balanced and youthful.

Energy Points and Pumps of the Microcosmic Orbit

Imagine the energy points and pumps as if they were jets, pumping the earth's sexual waters or jing—along with your own internal resources—up through the body, where they overflow at the crown and flow like a waterfall down the front.

If you pump water up a twenty-four-story building (the twenty-four vertebrae), it would explode at the top with the pressure of a geyser. Having multiple pumps along the route, however, ensures safe ways to regulate that internal pressure. The pumps help move the dense sexual energy upward against gravity and through the vertebrae.

These pumps are also refinery stations that purify the crude raw energy into the more delicate essences of the higher centers. Then, by bringing the energy down the front, the refined essence is integrated into the whole body. If you do not refine the energy sufficiently, you can end up with excess raw energy in the intricate instrument of the brain, where it can lead to migraines or Kundalini crises.

The fourteen points of the Microcosmic Orbit are described below. Note that they are listed in the order of the fire cycle; the order would be reversed for water cycle practice.

NAVEL

Location: At the navel center

Characteristics: The umbilicus is the place where you access your Original Qi and the center where you can digest your life. It is an alchemical kitchen. The navel point is the starting and ending point of Microcosmic meditation. Energy can be collected and stored here without ill effects. The organs in the belly are hollow and are designed to store nutrition

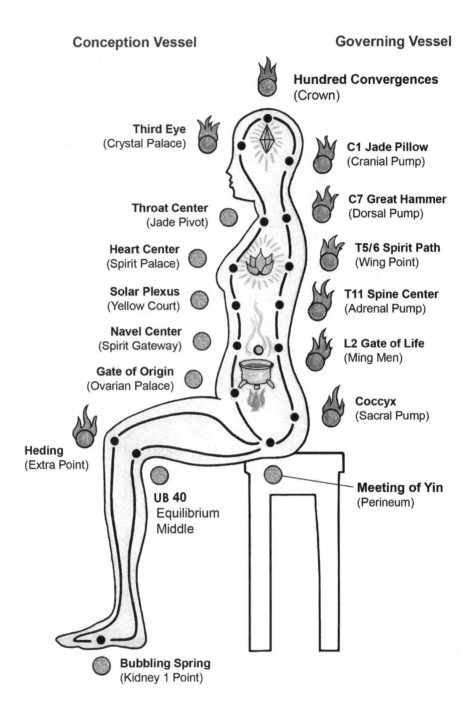

Conception Vessel

Governing Vessel

Hundred Convergences
(Crown)

Third Eye
(Crystal Palace)

C1 Jade Pillow
(Cranial Pump)

C7 Great Hammer
(Dorsal Pump)

Throat Center
(Jade Pivot)

T5/6 Spirit Path
(Wing Point)

Heart Center
(Spirit Palace)

Solar Plexus
(Yellow Court)

T11 Spine Center
(Adrenal Pump)

Navel Center
(Spirit Gateway)

L2 Gate of Life
(Ming Men)

Gate of Origin
(Ovarian Palace)

Coccyx
(Sacral Pump)

Heding
(Extra Point)

UB 40
Equilibrium
Middle

Meeting of Yin
(Perineum)

Bubbling Spring
(Kidney 1 Point)

Fig. 2.15. Microcosmic Orbit, energy points, and pumps

and qi, like a gas tank. You don't want to store energy in the brain or heart because you would "cook" them.

When open, the navel point balances and centers you. There is a sense of abundance from the universe through this energetic umbilicus. When it is closed, there is sloppy, picky, distracted behavior.

OVARIAN PALACE—THE SEXUAL CENTER

Location: Guan Yuan/Ren 4, four finger-widths below the navel. Create a triangle with your hands, thumbs touching at the navel. Where your index fingers touch is your uterus and under your pinkie fingers are your ovaries. (In men, the Sperm Palace is located at the point Middle Pole/Ren 3, one thumb-width up from pubic bone.)

Characteristics: The Ovarian Palace is a meeting of the Kidney, Liver, and Spleen channels. The womb is your powerhouse: it contains a lot of initiative and the will to manifest your creative impulses.

When the sexual center is open there is a sense of being connected to creative, passionate energy. When it is closed, it is hard to enjoy life. There is a sense of self-destructiveness, negativity, and listlessness. It is possible to become allergic to your own energy, which can amplify negativity.

PERINEUM—THE GATE OF LIFE AND DEATH

Location: At the perineum, between the vagina and the anus

Characteristics: The perineum center connects the soul and the ground and has a close relationship with earth energy. Note that energy can escape from this point when the lower gate is not energetically sealed.

When this point is open, there is feeling of being grounded, stable, and peaceful. You feel like you belong on Earth and that you are supported. When it is closed, there is a feeling of being insecure, fickle, and lonely. You may feel as if you don't belong here, and you may fear change.

SACRAL PUMP—THE DOOR TO IMMORTALITY

Location: This pump is activated by squeezing your yoni and anus. The coccyx (tailbone) tucks under slightly and opens the sacral hiatus opening, a little trap door into the spine.

Characteristics: *Sacrum* means "sacred bone." It is the door that connects us with the sacred earth, the center from which you can propel earth force up through your body. The sacrum is the rudder of your boat, helping to steer the energy where you want it to go. The Taoist principle of movement is essentially as follows: life force is rooted in the feet, propelled by the sacrum, and expressed by the hands.

The sacrum is a good place to store solar energy, which will warm the Sexual Palace from behind. (See the Inner Sun practice on page 118.)

When the sacrum point is open, you enjoy life! It provides momentum for life and helps use the past as a resource. Just as an animal's tail provides balance, so does this center. When it is open there is a potential to draw Kundalini energy up to the higher centers for continuation of consciousness through all states (waking, dreaming, and deep sleep). This portal makes it possible for Shakti power to rise and merge with Shiva, the consciousness pole at your crown to illuminate the body-mind.

When this point is closed, the past is a prison and unconscious fears and hopelessness may arise.

KIDNEY POINT/MINGMEN—DOOR OF LIFE

Location: This point is directly behind the navel at the back of the waist.

Characteristics: Mingmen is the moving qi between the kidneys that provides balances for the rest of the body. It is often used as a venting point if someone has a panic attack or energy deviations like extreme emotion, shaking, or too much energy in the head. Hold this point to give stabilizing support.

When the Door of Life is open, there is connection to Source Qi. Your instincts are intact and you are able to inherit the gifts from your ancestors. The point has a sense of openness, generosity, abundance, and gentleness. When it is closed, there is a feeling of imbalance and a particular fear of being taken advantage of. Old fears may return.

ADRENAL PUMP

Location: This pump is directly behind the solar plexus at T11, on the spine.

Characteristics: The adrenal glands are the body's alarm system, triggering hormones that help us respond to crisis. However, the adrenals are easily abused, especially by coffee and tobacco, which artificially trigger the alarm system and exhaust adrenal energy. Then the energy is not there when you need it.

The adrenal pump is the place where the upper and lower body link; it is a place to project the power of the legs up through the arms.

When the adrenal pump is open, there is a feeling of personal power. You feel energetic and confident, able to sense your individuality and uniqueness. This pump activates the heart. When it is closed, there is a feeling of being hyper, listless, or fatigued.

WING POINT/SHENDAO—SPIRIT PATH

Location: T5/6, the back door of the heart chakra, between the shoulder blades

Characteristics: This is where the wings of your heart extend, so it governs how you are flying into your spiritual path and highest destiny. We often don't focus too much on this point because it can overheat the heart.

When the Wing point is open, it serves as a portal for receiving inspiration and love. You can embrace life and be socially connected. This area can help you feel free—like a heart with wings. When it is closed, emotions can get stuck here. Often it closes when there is heartbreak and you want to prevent further wounding.

DORSAL PUMP—GREAT HAMMER

Location: C7, the big bone or dorsal prominence at the base of the neck, directly behind the throat

Characteristics: This point is sometimes called the "hugging point"; from here energy moves into the arms and hands. It is the hub of the tendons and the yang arm meridians.

When the dorsal pump is open, communication is expressive, like a caricature of someone who speaks with dynamic arm gestures. This point enables us to embrace each other with our humanity. You can embrace life and share openly about yourself. When it is closed, there is denial, a feeling of not fitting in, and the likelihood of being entrenched in your patterns. Stubbornness can show up here in someone who does not embrace change (e.g., "redneck").

CRANIAL PUMP/MOUTH-OF-GOD POINT—JADE PILLOW

Location: C1, occiput, base of the skull

Characteristics: This point is opened up by lightly tucking your chin in or pressing GV 26 (the end of the Governing Vessel) under the nose above the lip. Pressing the tongue on the roof of the mouth also helps open this pump, which conducts energy and cerebrospinal fluid up to the brain.

When the cranial pump is open, inspiration can be received from the spiritual world. The back of the brain controls involuntary functions like breathing and heart rhythms, so when it is open you can be spontaneous and respond to your intuition. You can channel your rational mind. When it is closed, there is a sense of burden and suffocation.

CROWN/PINEAL POINT—HUNDRED MEETINGS

Location: Crown of the head

Characteristics: As the seat of Original Spirit, this point is a main receptor that serves as an inner compass. It is the wisdom and direction point, allowing you to know where your spiritual home is (like a homing pigeon) and to have direction from lifetime to lifetime. In higher practice, the spirit can leave through this center at will.

When the crown point is open, there is a connection to your higher guidance. It helps you see auras and "the light." When it is closed, there are a lot of delusions, illusions, headaches, erratic mood swings, and victimized feelings.

THIRD EYE/MASTER GLAND—CRYSTAL PALACE

Location: On the centerline of the forehead, between the eyebrows

Characteristics: This pituitary point is known as the Crystal Palace that reflects light from the cosmos into the body. Imagine light reflecting off a prism inside your head, refracting rainbow light into the body. This control tower networks the pineal, pituitary, hypothalamus, and thalamus glands—the master glands that activate sexual and growth hormones and govern water metabolism.

When the third eye is open, there is a sense of purpose. Through your wisdom eye your intuition becomes clear and you know what is good for you from moment to moment. When it is closed, there is a sense of indecisiveness: the mind wanders and is directionless.

THROAT CENTER

Location: In the dip at the base of the throat, between the collarbones

Characteristics: The throat is a center for communication and dreams. When this point is open, there is flow of expression and a greater lucidity in dreams. We are able to communicate through our creative voice. When it is closed, there is a feeling of being choked up and an unwillingness to change.

HEART CENTER

Location: In women, two finger-widths above the lower tip of the sternum

Characteristics: The heart is the seat of joy, respect, and surrender and is the home of the spirit. It is where you point when you point to yourself.

When the heart is open, there are feelings of honor, love, and respect. You are connected to your truth and who you are. When it is closed, there is a feeling of being under attack, sorry for yourself, unloved, and incapable of love.

SOLAR PLEXUS

Location: Halfway between the sternum and navel

Characteristics: There is a complex of nerves, lymph, blood vessels, and energy channels here. It is your moving center. If you made a cross of the arms reaching upward and the legs reaching downward, they would cross at the solar plexus.

When this point is open, there is a feeling of personal power, self-control, freedom, and courage. There is an awareness of the space around you and your personal boundaries. There is a sense of feeling open and trusting. When it is closed, there is a sense of anxiety, worry, and self-doubt.

✸ Circulating Qi in the Microcosmic Orbit

Focus the qi at each point and let it vibrate or spiral there. *Chakra* means "wheel of light," so it is natural for the points to spin like vortexes of light. Be aware of what direction they want to spin. At any time during the practice you may feel warm energy rise up the spine to the head or up the front to your heart. This energy can be used for self-healing and divine purpose.

- Relax your whole body with the Inner Smile practice. When you are relaxed, qi moves with natural ease.
- Bring your awareness to your navel. Breathe into the navel to gather the essence of the breath.
- Exhale down to the Sexual Palace and continue to breathe there. Let the energy gather, vibrate, and awaken this energy center.
- Exhale down to the perineum. Let the earth energy gather in your root. Feel the perineum lift subtly on the inhalation and stay buoyant on the exhalation, like a trampoline of the spirit.
- Use your PC pump (pubococcygeal muscle, between the pubic bone and the coccyx) to uplift the sexual energy. First squeeze the yoni and perineum, then squeeze the anus and the back part of the anus—a point called Long Strong, below the tip of the tailbone. When you inhale, squeeze up the urogenital muscles, which tucks the tailbone. Relax and smile on the exhalation. This tailbone action is like drinking nectar with a straw from the pools of yin.
- Rub your sacrum to build warmth as warmth naturally rises. Smile and welcome the Shakti energy to move.
- Inhale up the spine to the each successive point, breathing in and out of each point until you reach the crown.
- Breathe in and out of the crown to gather heavenly energy. Breathe through the third eye to gather smiling energy. Touch your tongue to the roof of your mouth. Exhale down to the throat and clear this center with your breath. Exhale down to the heart and breathe loving energy in and out of the heart. Exhale down to the solar plexus and softly open this center as you breathe. Gather more qi power as you breathe into the navel.
- Then sip with tiny inhalations through your nose, like sipping up a straw, all the way up the spine and cascade down the front with a long exhalation. Subtly roll your eyes to guide the qi around, looking in and up the spine as you inhale, looking down the front as you exhale. Another way to keep the qi pumping is to allow qi to rock your pumps in a wave forward and back, like the currents of water moving seaweed.

In the beginning, your sexual energy may feel dense and thick like molasses. As you circulate it, it melts into refined, golden, liquid honey. Saliva will flow abundantly as you circulate sexual energy, so consciously swallow it down to the navel before you collect the qi.

● Freeing the Qi

Qi can potentially flow as fast as the speed of light; that's why this practice is often called the "circulation of light." However, our breath and thoughts can slow down the qi flow. It is good to free up the connection between qi and the breath so that the qi can flow as fast as it wants to. To disassociate qi circulation from your breathing, imagine that you are riding a bike. The pedaling of your legs is like your breathing, and the fast spinning wheel is the qi flow. Move the qi many times around the Orbit as you inhale and many times around as you exhale.

Your qi may entrain with the speed of your blood by tuning in to the heart's pulsation behind the navel. The heartbeat of the navel becomes the rhythm behind the qi flow and the entire Orbit. It will help focus your mind behind the navel so you observe the Orbit from there. Then let it take off at its own pace. You can accelerate and pull in the influx of energy from the three sources as if you were reeling in a big fish from the universe.

● The Water Cycle

Reversing the Orbit helps cleanse the channel—like scrubbing in both directions when you clean a bottle with a bottle brush. The water cycle has a relaxing effect on the nervous system. Recall a time when you were tenderly stroked down your back.

Not Feeling the Qi?

If you are not feeling the qi, be assured that "something" is holding you up and grounding you at the same time. Sometimes if your body and channels are nice and open, there is less resistance and the flow can be more subtle.

If your kidneys are weak and hungry for qi, your body will feed them, rather than sending qi moving up the spine. Build up more qi in your core, be patient, and welcome the Shakti energy to move and dance around your Orbit.

❀ Variations on the Microcosmic Orbit Practice

After you have become familiar with circulating qi in the Microcosmic Orbit, you can try the following variations.

● Spinning Dragon Pearl

This ancient method for circulating qi in the Orbit comes from the Wudang Mountains. Michael Winn's version—with a spinning dragon to propel the life force—brings an extra spin to this practice!

- Expand your pearl to the size of a tennis ball. Get it spinning in a mini Microcosmic Orbit, up the back and down the front.
- Call on the sexual essence of the earth to rise up like pink steam into your pearl and form into a dragon. Observe the dragon somersaulting inside the qi ball as though chasing and eating its own tail. This ancient Ouroboros symbol represents the eternal cycle of renewal and enlightenment, where consciousness and energy merge into a dynamic whole. Figure 2.16 shows the sexual waters of Ouroboros rising and the fire of love descending in a continuum.
- Spin the dragon in the qi ball at each of the energy centers along the orbit to break up blockages.
- Spin the qi ball slightly outside of your body so it pulls in external qi and mixes it into the internal qi.
- Spin two pearls, a blue yin dragon coming up from the earth and a red yang dragon coming down from the heavens. As one rises the other descends; the male and female dragons chase after each other and their sexual mating dance generates orgasmic energy! Be aware of both the rising and falling simultaneously until your whole Orbit is a continuous river of golden, pink, liquid light.

Cosmic Ouroboros

Life force, a cosmic serpent,
Spirals through cellular space,
uniting us beyond skin.

Love, a life-saver
ready for passionate souls
rising through the storm.

Light, an endless torus,
A halo glowing with stars,
opening the portal of mystery.

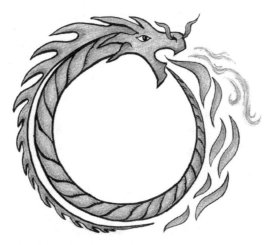

Fig. 2.16. Ouroboros: dragon eating its own tail

● Macrocosmic Orbit

The Macrocosmic Orbit includes the arm and legs routes, which are streams that feed into the big river of the Microcosmic Orbit. It is very grounding to connect the flows from the earth and the heavens through the arms and the legs.

- Induce the flow by breathing down to the palms and soles of the feet.
- Breathe up from the big toes and middle fingers, streaming into the spine, up to the crown, and down the Front Channel. This will make a figure eight that crosses at the perineum. (See fig 2.15 on page 100.)
- Flow with the meridians: down the insides of the arm and up the outsides, down the backs of the legs and up the insides of legs. If you run the water cycle, it does not cross at the perineum but simply washes up the front of the body and down the back (palms facing back). Practice the Spinal Pelvic Rock exercise from chapter 6 while running the qi in the Macrocosmic Orbit.

Absorbing the Energy Generated by Your Circulation Practice

After any practice session it is good to absorb the high-quality energy you have generated. The art of storing is essential as women tend to be big givers and big spenders! Tell the qi to stay for a while and build up the reserves in your core. "It takes money to make money," so you need qi to attract and transform qi. When you have a lot of loose cash you tend to spend it, but when you have it in a savings account, it grows.

✼ Centering

When you feel centered you can meet life with acceptance and respond spontaneously.

- As you circulate qi in your channels, simultaneously sense your center, your home base. The pearl in your center is continually being nourished by the seven directions; heaven, earth, the four cardinal directions, and the center.
- Slow down the qi flow and start filling a pool at the bottom of a waterfall in your navel center.
- Breathe in peace and blue light, drawing them into your kidneys; breathe out strength and golden light, sending them into your core. You can also breathe out trust, health, or an affirmation that means something to you.
- Simply fill your abdomen with breath and life force and then blow down internally into your core, concentrating the qi there. While doing other things, be aware of conscious breathing to stay centered.

✼ Collecting Energy

Remember the law of physics called the "right rule of thumb": force moves in the direction of the thumb and spirals in the direction of the curled fingers. With your right hand at your navel, point your thumb outward. Energy expands out from the center counterclockwise, up the left side of the navel and down the right side of the navel, like opening a jar. In this direction, earth (vagina, feminine) expands from your core to the vast heavens.

With your right hand at your navel, now point your thumb inward. The forces of the vast heavens (penis, masculine) contract to the center of the earth in a clockwise direction—up the right side of the navel and down the left side, like closing a jar.

- Place your hands over your navel. Spiral the energy from the root of the navel, in your core, to a hand's-width-diameter circle around the navel at the level of the skin (fig. 2.17).
- Spiral the energy back into the center of the body; gather it with the action of a funnel, vortex, or tornado. Condense it into a qi ball or pearl. Good energetic grammar is putting a period at the end of the sentence!

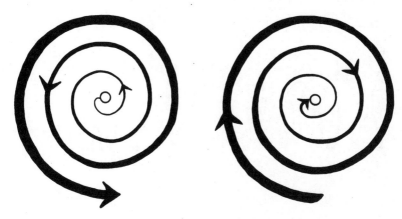

Fig. 2.17. Collecting energy: spiraling outward and condensing inward

● Quick Collection

Collect the energy by first spiraling outward from your navel in a counterclockwise direction. Spiral nine times. Fuse heaven, earth, and your Original Qi together.

Then gather qi like a lasso, spiraling in clockwise, condensing qi into your navel nine times. Condense the energy into a beautiful golden pearl (see fig. 2.18 on page 112). Nine is the number of completion; counting in sets of threes naturally spirals, like dancing a waltz!

● Longer Collection

You can acknowledge the specific charge of your gender by spiraling more in that direction. Women begin by spiraling counterclockwise thirty-six times (solar number) and then spiraling clockwise twenty-four times (lunar number).

● Golden Pearl

Swallow the sweet nectar in your mouth to nourish the pearl. The pearl is a condensation of your awareness and energy. Circulate the pearl in the Microcosmic Orbit. The nectar refines and distributes evenly. The nectar thins into a river of warm light. Let the qi circulate freely in and around the body.

Return the pearl back to your center, where it floats in the essence within your cauldron. Imagine your mini-self within your pearl, smiling with contentment and the blissful harmony of yin and yang.

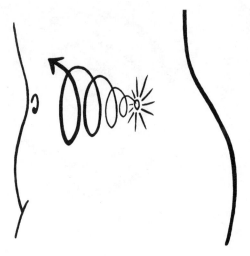

Fig. 2.18. Collecting energy into a pearl

● Rest

Give your loving attention to the pearl in your center. Come to total peace. Affirm whatever quality you would like to cultivate and empower it with your breath and smiling energy—for instance, affirm "I am centered and strong." Notice the centered, calm state of your mind and body so you can tap into it anytime during the day.

Enjoy deep yin relaxation in a sitting posture or lie flat and allow the earth to support your body. You can also lie on your side and spoon yourself.

❋ Closing Your Microcosmic Orbit Meditation

At the end of a circulation session, you will want to spread the qi you've collected into your whole body.

● Brush Down

Rub your hands together. Place your palms over your eyes, breathing in the warmth. Replenish the senses. "Wash" your face with the energy in your hands, brushing them over your ears and down your neck. Your sexual energy is your best cosmetic! Brush down the chest, bringing excess energy down from the head to the navel to safely store it there. Wash the body with the refined, divine energy gathered during meditation.

● Qi Shower

For a more energizing closing, slap or tap your whole body to vibrate the qi into your bones and organs. You can also use bamboo or wire hitters. (See Tapping Practice in chapter 8.)

● Stroking the Meridians

Stroke down the insides of your arms (the yin meridians) and up the outsides (yang meridians). Then stroke down the outsides and backs of your legs (yang meridians) and up the insides of your legs (yin meridians). Distribute the qi and charged blood evenly into the body. Rub the "ground wires" in the soles of your feet.

● Triple Warmer Sound

Articulating the triple warmer sound brings down excess heat to promote restful sleep. This variation of the healing sound acts as a divine blessing.

* Sweep down the front, middle, and back of the body while making the healing sound, "he-e-e-e-e," in a soft, whispering voice.
* Inhale and bring your arms up, palms down to shoulder height and then palms up to above your head. Imagine you are embracing the ocean, forests, mountains, and sky.

   Lower your arms and bring down the qualities of the Divine Feminine through you as you make the descending sound "she-e-e-e-e."
* Repeat the inhalation step, then bring down the qualities of the Divine Masculine as you exhale and make the descending sound "He-e-e-e-e."
* Repeat the inhalation step, then bring down the qualities of divine love and union as you exhale and make the descending sound "we-e-e-e-e."
* Bow. Give thanks to yourself, your loved ones, your community, and the vast universe for supporting your life.

   Bring the creative energy into your day!

> *"A lotus for Thee, a Goddess to be."*
> *We all honor the Goddess in our own way.*
> *We are all fingers of the Great Goddess's hands!*

TAO TANTRIC YOGA

Embodying the Shamanic Power of Animals

Tao Tantric Yoga exercises provide another way of boosting and circulating your sexual energy. The postures below will help you embody the power of animals and the greater cosmos.

The animal nature within us is sexual, innocent, and pure in expression. When we move like animals, raw instinct fills us with sexual power and sensuality. Our awareness embraces the movements with dangerous beauty: we awaken our ability to ravish and be ravished. We come alive by returning to nature and moving beyond habitual contractions.

Recall a time when your beloved was coming toward you. Feel the excitement in your heartbeat and the rush of blood as you run to him or her! It is spontaneous and alive!

✳ Butterfly

Sit on the floor with the soles of your feet together, knees out to the side. You might need to sit on something. As you bend your head toward your feet, press your knees down to open the hips. In this posture, practice the Crane and Turtle Neck to open the throat chakra. This wave makes the spine fluid, the superhighway for your energy.

✳ Crane Neck

Begin with the Butterfly posture. Bend forward with a flat back, reaching your chin out to open your throat chakra. Exhale down the front of the body. Drop your head, chin in. Inhale up the spine, rolling up with a round back. Press your knees down to open your hips. Lengthen your neck at the top. Circulate qi in the fire cycle—up the back and down the front.

This practice can also be done in a standing position.

✳ Turtle Neck

Begin with the Butterfly posture. Exhale and curl down, melting your solar plexus. Stick out your chin to come up, like a turtle emerging out of its shell, as you inhale (fig. 2.19). Press your knees down to open your hips. Roll down with a round back and rise up with a flat back. Circulate the qi in the

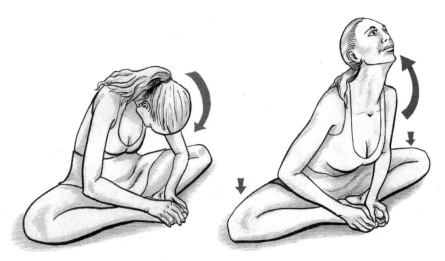

Fig. 2.19. Turtle Neck in Butterfly position

water cycle—up the front and down the back. Stretch the Conception Vessel (Front Channel) by stretching your tongue into the Heavenly Pool (back palate) as if you were licking up an ice cream cone or a lingam!

This movement reminds us how a baby is born. As if you were coming out of the womb, tuck in your chin, then brush along the inner sacrum and lift your back crown to emerge. Breathe in a circle and make a small circle with your nose like you are nuzzling up to your lover. Gather qi in your saliva and gulp it down. Swallow down the flavors. Brush down your chest.

❋ Dragon Awakens

Clasp your hands behind your head. Pull your sexual energy up the Front Channel, lifting your sternum and forehead. Exhale, dropping your sternum and head. Repeat this cycle two more times. After the third time, open your elbows and press the back of your head into your hands. Hold your breath for three counts, then flare your arms open and make a surprising sound, "HA!" The dragon flares its hood!

❋ Wild Cat

Get on your hands and knees with your legs hip-width apart. Arch your back to the ceiling as you inhale, tucking in both your chin and sacrum (fig. 2.20).

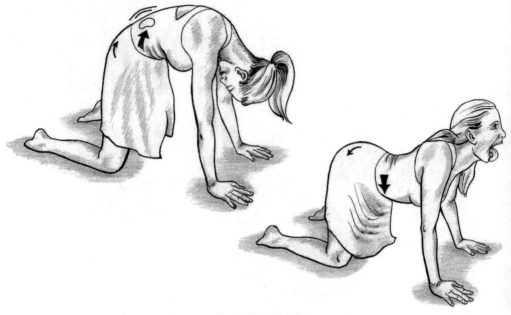

Fig. 2.20. Wild Cat

Pull up your navel. Squeeze your yoni and pull sexual energy up your spine. Hum sound vibrations up the spine as you arch up—"Hummmm."

Your exhalation expands the groin; use this expansion to widen your hips. On the out breath, feel your hips widen as the belly drops (reverse breathing). As your belly drops, open your mouth, stick out your tongue, and say "Maaah!" Let your wild cat out!

● Cat Licks Milk

Repeat the Wild Cat stretch above, but move the spine in a circle as you arch and say "Hummmm," lifting the urogenital muscles. Sweep across the ground sideways as you lick "milk" with your tongue—"Maaah!" Feel every rippling muscle in your body. In between each round of the exercise, breathe into the groin.

✸ Crouching Tigress

Kneeling with your knees wide and your elbows and hands on the ground/ mat/bed, you can move your spine in many ways: Crane Neck, Turtle Neck, skipping rope, circles, and sweeping sideways like a snake. You can brush your breasts on the ground and massage them as you move. This is great practice for massaging your lover with your breasts!

�֎ Dolphin

Lie on your belly with your toes curled under your feet. Let your hands form a triangle under your forehead. Inhale up the front of the body to lift the elbows. Exhale and bear down to lift your buttocks.

● Dolphin Comes Up for Air

Place your hands under your shoulders. Lift the upper body higher, keeping elbows on the floor. Exhale and bear down to lift the dolphin's tail fin.

● Dolphin Rides Bigger Waves

Now push all the way into a cobra by straightening your arms as much as you can. Seesaw between lifting your buttocks and lifting your upper body.

Massage up and down your belly with this movement.

✖ Cobra Opens Its Throat

Lie on your belly with your toes curled under your feet. Place your hands under your shoulders and lift your upper body, keeping your elbows on the floor. Rise up effortlessly with juicy sexual energy rising up the stem, and open your heart like a flower. Smile! Elongate your stretchy digestive tract, inhaling. Squeeze your yoni to draw up sexual energy. Look up.

Lower as you open your throat with the heart sound, "ha-a-a-a-a-w."

● Love Cobra Growls

Begin as above. Curl your toes under and start the inhalation with your toes. Grip your buttocks. Flare the cobra hood at the back of your neck by tucking in the chin and opening the cranial pump.

Stick out your tongue as you growl, "ha-a-a-a-a-w." Stretch your eyes up toward your crown. Expand your sexual power into all the tendons. Suspend the out breath for three counts, creating empty force, which sucks the sexual energy up the spine.

Inhale and expand the belly with qi; lower slowly as you exhale.

❀ Rocking Child

Push back into Child Pose, kneeling with your forehead on the floor and your arms extended. Wiggle your hips and wag your tail to loosely rock the spine and head sideways.

❀ Turtle Breathing

This exercise squeezes groin and lymph areas, stimulating the lymphatic system. In this posture, the kidneys are wide and open to receive qi. It is very comforting in times of shock, panic, or fear, as if returning you to the safety of the womb.

In Child Pose, with your arms on the floor behind your buttocks, palms up, keep your arms relaxed and let your shoulders drop forward. With a rounded back, widen the lower rib cage; breathe into the kidneys and upper back, simulating a turtle's shell. Exhale mental tension from the forehead into the ground. Sweep the breath like a wave from the pelvic basin up the back.

Embodying the Cosmos

In addition to embodying animal energies, we can also resonate with other forces of nature and the cosmos.

❀ Inner Sun and Moon Channels

Our Inner Sun Channel flows through the heart on the left side (fig. 2.21); our Inner Moon Channel flows on the right side. Practice Alternate Channel Breathing to balance inner masculine and feminine energies. (For more details about this practice, see the Triple Purification exercise in chapter 6.)

- Inhale, squeezing your Jade Fountain, and make fists. Pull sexual energy up the Left and Right Thrusting Channels.
- Exhale as you pull your head to the left side with your left hand over your head. Close your left nostril with the middle finger. Press the LI 20 point, "Welcome Fragrance," in the nasolabial groove. This is the end point of the Large Intestine meridian. Press your thumb and index finger to stimulate the starting point of the Large Intestine meridian, which runs along the shoulder to the outside of the nostril. Drop your shoulder.
- Repeat on the right side.

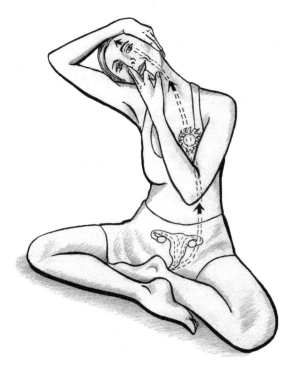

Fig. 2.21. Opening the Inner Sun Channel

❈ Pine Tree

Clasp your hands behind your head, chin tucked in. Inhale, squeezing your anus, and pull sexual energy up to the head. Hold the breath in the spine. Press the back of your head into your hands. Feel yourself standing like a pine tree, firmly in the wind.

Release your head down and rock it from side to side.

❈ Volcano Rises from the Sea

Imagine the heart of the earth rising to heaven to feel the warm sun on her hills. She then sinks down into the valley of her womb. This is a whole-body movement using massage to connect the qi of the earth and the sexual center up through the heart and crown, opening the front of the body. The rising bliss of the wave then washes down and penetrates the sides and back of the body.

• Lie on your back with your legs in Butterfly position, soles together and knees out to the side (fig. 2.22). Inhale and stroke or scratch up the inner thighs (Liver meridian).

- Squeeze your yoni while stretching your legs out on the floor. Send a fountain of energy up to the heart, lifting your chest as you do in the Fish Pose in yoga.
- Let your head tilt back so your crown touches the earth. At the same time, massage up over your breasts.
- As you exhale, stroke down the sides of the ribs, pressing your lumbar spine down to the floor.
- Draw your feet up again as you stroke down the sides of your legs. Tilt your pelvis up and look down by pressing your feet into the floor.
- Lie flat and feel the pulses in your body as the qi spreads evenly through it.

YOUR BODY IS YOUR TEMPLE

Your body is a sacred temple, worthy of great care and love. It is a receptor and transmitter of qi and consciousness as well as a vehicle for movement, sensation, and communication. The feminine is the body to be played!

It is important to nurture yourself with a good diet, self-massage, and acupressure.

Dietary Support

When we feel content internally we are less hungry for the kinds of external stimulation that can be harmful to our body-minds. When we are truly nourished, we don't need to stuff down our sexual energy with unhealthy foods.

Balancing the cleansing and tonifying aspects of food is quite an art and requires a willingness to experiment and observe which foods energize you. As you explore the power of deep nourishment, the following points may help:

- A healthy, balanced diet prevents excess toxins, fats, and estrogens from building up.
- Meat and dairy products often have steroids, which can throw off your natural hormones.
- Foods that tend to dampen sexual energy are excessively cooling and sweet and often contain refined flour, dairy, and/or soy milk ingredients.

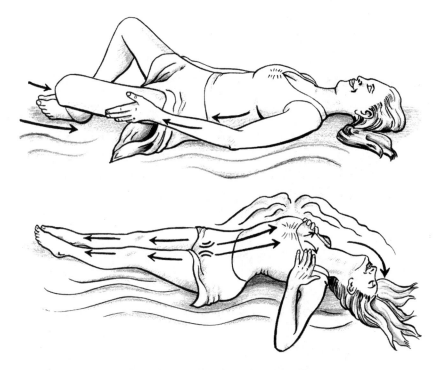

Fig. 2.22. Volcano Rises from the Sea

⚔ Ginger counteracts internal dampness and can feel warming during menstruation.

⚔ Fresh greens help mobilize the liver, which moves sexual energy.

Benefits of a Beauty Facial

Sexual Energy Is Your Best Cosmetic!

Beauty comes from within, and your face reflects your health. There is a Qigong expression, "young face, white hair," which describes the youthful glow you can emit even after your hair has turned white.

If the uterus is loose, your facial skin will sag. To prevent the "sag and spread syndrome," rejuvenating energy needs to be uplifted. The face-lifting exercises that follow can be done after you put on your moisturizer and clean your hands.

Your cells are eavesdropping on what you say inside, so try this affirmation and see what happens: "I feel younger and more beautiful every day!"

✤ Your Beauty Facial Routine

Before each practice, pull sexual energy up to your face and rub warm qi into your hands. This beauty facial tones the face with a natural face lift.

● Cosmic Egg Drop

Inhale as you lift your arms. Clap your hands above your head and crack the cosmic egg! Stroke the golden liquid light down your face to the navel. Clap and stroke over your ears, neck, and shoulders. Clap and stroke the qi conditioner down the back of your head and neck.

● Facial Stretch

Use your thumbs to pull up the skin under your eye sockets, lifting the corners of your eyes. Pucker your lips, like you're whistling: feel how the other sphincter (ring) muscles in your eyes and perineum also squeeze together. Tauten your facial muscles and slowly release them on the exhalation.

● Facial Toning

Hook the corners of your mouth with your index fingers. Provide resistance as you widen and narrow your mouth. Notice how the anal sphincter/qi muscles also squeeze and release.

● Cheek Squeeze

Hook your index fingers into the inside center of your cheeks. Squeeze your cheeks around your fingers and slowly release. Notice how your pelvic floor squeezes and relaxes.

● Tongue Press

Press fingers under your chin to give resistance. Pull up your perineum. Tone the tendon connection between your sexual organ and your tongue by stretching the tongue out, then curling it back to press and release on the top of your mouth. Press and release the tip of your tongue first on the water point in the back palate, then on the wood point in middle palate. Continue with the fire point behind your upper teeth. See tongue positions in fig. 2.14 on page 97.

Qi Self-Massage

Light touch massage, as with a silk cloth, stimulates the yang, protective qi at the surface of your body. Deeper massage stimulates the internal, yin qi and the physical body. Tender touch tells the body that it is loved and cared for. Touch nourishes the earth element. Touch stimulates the anti-aging hormones and promotes good circulation and a youthful glow.

Don't just wait for someone else to touch you; your own qi is your best body-worker! Listen to the qi and allow yourself to be guided into giving what your body needs through touch. Through regular self-touch, you will get to know your body and your body's signals.

✺ Your Qi Self-Massage Routine

This is a good routine to follow just before your jade egg practice.

- With or without fragrant massage oil, rub your hands until they are warm.
- Smile down with love to the area being massaged.
- Pull up the sexual energy by squeezing the Jade Fountain with each inhalation, drawing qi to each area.
- Massage qi into the sexual organs and surrounding area to increase qi circulation. Follow the steps below.

Stoke the stove. Place your fingertips about three finger-widths below the navel. Press into the Sea of Qi point to send in heat as you make the fire sound, "ha-a-a-a-a-w." This helps relieve abdominal aches and cramps due to excess coldness.

Warm the stove. Place your right hand over your sexual organs and circle your left hand around the stove and cauldron, just below the navel. Stir the fire below the cauldron, spiraling counterclockwise. Stir the pot of elixir above the cauldron in a clockwise direction, increasing sexual vitality. Breathe deeply and feel the warm qi spread into your body.

Massage the Ovarian Palace between the ovaries. Make a downward triangle with your thumbs at the navel. Your index fingers point to the Ovarian Palace and your pinkies rest on the ovaries. Place your left hand over the Ovarian Palace, and place your right hand on top of the left hand. Massage counterclockwise (bottom to the left) and then clockwise (bottom to the right).

Massage the ovaries in circular motions with your palms. Massage outward nine times to open the center. Massage inward nine times to draw in warm qi.

Lightly tap the ovaries to release stagnation and stimulate them. Wake up their energy!

Cleanse the uterus. Sweep your palms down in front of the uterus, palm over palm. Clear any stagnant blood to prevent it from settling and causing endometriosis. Thank your body for cleansing impurities, excesses, and imbalanced qi.

Massage the labia. Locate about six spots on either side of the vaginal lips between the perineum and the clitoris, and massage them with little circles. This releases stagnation and improves circulation. Roll the vaginal lips (labia) along the clitoris.

Massage the perineum. The perineum, located between the anus and vagina, is the known as the "trampoline of the spirit." Massage it by spiraling with the fingertips. Then massage around the anal sphincter muscles (also called "qi muscles"), which pump qi up into the body.

Massage the Rushing Gates, the creases on either side of the groin, to open the pelvis and stimulate the yin meridians of the kidney, liver, and spleen. This massage increases circulation in the large lymph nodes.

Massage the inner thighs. Stroke the yin flows up along the inner thighs, between the muscles.

Massage the knees. Rub your inner, upper knees in circles until they are warm.

Massage the sacrum. Rub your sacrum with your knuckles to stimulate the flow of energy up the spine and to soothe lower back pain. This is also great for relieving menstrual cramps.

Massage the kidneys. Massage your kidneys warm with a circular massage. This relieves lower backache. When the kidneys are warm, the body will be more relaxed for the jade egg practice.

Self-Acupressure

The acupressure points described below are particularly beneficial for healthy menstrual flow and blood circulation. Specific points can also help you alleviate pain, become more fertile, and calm your mind.

Warning—contraindicated points for pregnancy: Do not press these points if you are pregnant: LI 4, UB 62, CV 4, SP 6. If you are pregnant, find a qualified acupuncturist to assist you through your pregnancy.

✹ Acupressure Practice

In order to stimulate acupressure points, follow these simple guidelines:

- Apply pressure with your fingertips or your thumb for about one to two minutes. If you feel pain or discomfort, decrease your pressure. These points will be sensitive, but intense pain may be a sign of stagnation in the meridian or the associated organ.
- To disperse stagnant qi, use a counterclockwise spiraling motion. To tonify or strengthen weak qi, spiral clockwise.
- Make sure your nails are clean and well trimmed and do not jam your fingernails into your skin.

● Balancing Sequence

Refer to the point descriptions that follow, then follow this sequence for grounding, balancing, and healing.

- Rub your hands until they are warm and vibrant with qi.
- Open the "tiger's mouth" by pressing He Gu.
- Massage from the back of your Qi Belt (kidneys) to the front dantian. This will include the following points: Door of Life, Kidney Shu Point, Bladder's Vitals, Sea of Qi, Gate of Origin, and Curved Bone.
- Massage down the yin channels along the inside of your legs to the soles of your feet. This will include the following points: Rushing Gate, Yin Wrapping, Sea of Blood, Sea of Nourishment, Three Yin Crossing, and Shining Sea.
- Smooth out the channels with a Qigong movement called "Descending Yang, Ascending Yin":
    Stroke down the back and sides of your leg to the Calm Sleep point.

Pick up Earth Qi around your toes and stroke up the inside of the legs. Stroke around the Qi Belt (waist) and rub qi into your kidneys.

The Acupressure Points

HE GU • *JOINING VALLEY* • LI 4 (LARGE INTESTINE 4)

Location: At the end of crease between the index finger and the thumb (fig. 2.23)

Functions:

⚔ Regulates the defensive qi and adjusts sweating

⚔ Alleviates pain like abdominal pain, headaches

Method: Press with your thumb and shake, making the metal sound, "ss-s-s-s-s-s."

MINGMEN • *DOOR OF LIFE* • GV 4 (GOVERNING VESSEL 4)

Location: Directly behind the navel on the spine (fig. 2.24)

Functions:

⚔ Governs the moving qi between the two kidneys

⚔ Acts as a venting point for energy that is overheated

Method: Knock on the Door of Life by tapping with loose fingers.

SHENSU • *KIDNEY SHU* • UB 23 (URINARY BLADDER 23)

Location: At the waist, above the hip bone, two finger-widths from the spine (fig. 2.24)

Functions:

⚔ Shu (back) point for the kidneys

⚔ Addresses abnormal vaginal discharges, irregular periods, cold uterus, lower back pain in women

Method: Rub from the spine outward to warm these points.

BAOHUANG • *BLADDER'S VITALS* • UB 53 (URINARY BLADDER 53)

Location: In the dimples of the upper sacrum, behind the ovaries; sometimes called the "sex points" (fig. 2.24)

Functions:

⚔ Benefits the bladder and relieves stiffness and pain in the lower back

Method: Rub these points with your knuckles.

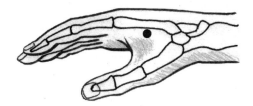

Fig. 2.23. Joining Valley, LI 4

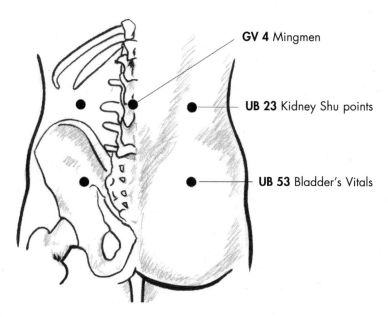

GV **4** Mingmen

UB **23** Kidney Shu points

UB **53** Bladder's Vitals

Fig. 2.24. Mingmen, Kidney Shu points, Bladder's Vitals

QIHAI • *SEA OF QI* • CV 6 (CONCEPTION VESSEL 6)

Location: Two finger-widths below the navel (see fig. 2.25 on page 129)

Functions:

- Fosters Original Qi and tonifies qi
- Tonifies the kidneys and fortifies yang
- Regulates qi and harmonizes blood
- Prevents coldness and alleviates cramps

Method: Stoke your "stove" by pressing your fingers into this point and making the fire sound, "ha-a-a-a-a-w."

GUANYUAN • *GATE OF ORIGIN* •
CV 4 (CONCEPTION VESSEL 4)

Location: Four finger-widths below the navel (fig. 2.25)

Functions:

- ⚔ Fortifies the Original Qi and benefits essence
- ⚔ Tonifies and nourishes the kidneys
- ⚔ Warms and fortifies the spleen
- ⚔ Benefits the uterus and assists conception

Method: Exhale and push your belly out against your fingers (reverse breathing) as you make the fire sound, "ha-a-a-a-a-w."

QU GU • *CURVED BONE* • CV 2 (CONCEPTION VESSEL 2)

Location: Just above the pubic bone (fig. 2.25)

Functions:

- ⚔ Sometimes called the "B spot" as it encourages deep breathing from the groin
- ⚔ Warms and invigorates the kidneys
- ⚔ Relieves dryness and pain in the genitals
- ⚔ Relieves difficulties with urination, including dribbling or hesitant urination

Method: Exhale, pressing with your fingers in and slightly up above the pubic bone. Inhale, pushing your fingers out with your belly.

CHONGMEN • *RUSHING GATE* • SP 12 (SPLEEN 12)

Location: In the fold beside the pubic bone, feel the pulse of the femoral artery (fig. 2.25).

Functions:

- ⚔ Sometimes called "hip wind gate": allows sick winds from the abdomen to flow down the legs and out the feet
- ⚔ Invigorates blood, regulates qi, and alleviates pain
- ⚔ Drains dampness, clears heat, and regulates urination

Method: Tap in the crease with loose fingers.

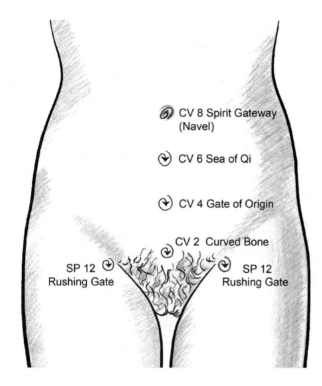

CV 8 Spirit Gateway
(Navel)

CV 6 Sea of Qi

CV 4 Gate of Origin

CV 2 Curved Bone

SP 12
Rushing Gate

SP 12
Rushing Gate

Fig. 2.25. Sea of Qi, Gate of Origin, Curved Bone (B spot), and Rushing Gates

YINBAO • *YIN WRAPPING* • LV 9 (LIVER 9)

Location: Three finger-widths above the kneecap, in between the muscles of the inner thigh, about a quarter of the way from the knee to the groin (see fig. 2.27 on page 131)

Functions:

- Regulates irregular menstruation and disorders of menstruation
- Alleviates lumbosacral pain extending to the lower abdomen

Method: Sit cross-legged and lean into these sensitive points with your elbows and make the liver sound, "sh-h-h-h-h-h."

XUEHAI • *SEA OF BLOOD* • SP 10 (SPLEEN 10)

Location: In the tender depression beside the inside padding of the knee, four finger-widths up from the kneecap. When sitting with your hands on your knees, the point is where your thumbs naturally rest (see fig. 2.27).

Functions:

⚔ Invigorates the blood, dispels blood stagnation, cools blood

⚔ Harmonizes menstruation

Method: Massage this point with your thumbs in a circular motion.

ZUSANLI • *SEA OF NOURISHMENT* • ST 36 (STOMACH 36)

Location: Four finger-widths below the kneecap on the outer edge of the tibia (fig. 2.26)

Functions:

⚔ This point is also called "Leg Three Miles": massaging it is known to give you the strength and endurance to walk three extra miles!

⚔ Fortifies the spleen and resolves dampness

⚔ Tonifies qi and nourishes blood and yin

⚔ Alleviates pain

Method: Tap this point with fists and loose wrists to help yourself ground.

SANYINJIAO • *THREE YIN CROSSING* • SP 6 (SPLEEN 6)

Location: Four finger-widths above the inside ankle bone (fig. 2.27)

Functions:

⚔ Resolves dampness

⚔ Harmonizes the liver and tonifies the kidneys

⚔ Regulates menstruation and benefits the genitals

⚔ Helps prevent stagnation, which can lead to masses like tumors, fibroids, and cysts

Method: Massage this point with your thumbs toward the shin bone. Exhale while pressing and inhale while releasing in a pulsing action.

ZHAOHAI • *SHINING SEA* • KD 6 (KIDNEY 6)

Location: One thumb-width below the inner ankle, in the groove (fig. 2.27)

Functions:

⚔ Benefits the throat

⚔ Nourishes the kidneys and clears deficiency heat

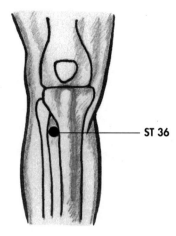

Fig. 2.26. Sea of Nourishment (Leg Three Miles)

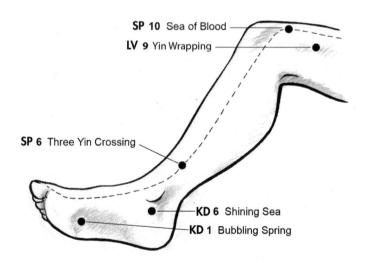

Fig. 2.27. Yin Wrapping, Sea of Blood, Three Yin Crossing,
Shining Sea, and Bubbling Spring

⚔ Calms the spirit

⚔ Regulates the lower abdomen

Method: "Saw" both sides of the ankles with the outside edges of your hands.

SHENMAI • *CALM SLEEP* • UB 62 (URINARY BLADDER 62)

Location: In a depression between the outside ankle bone and the heel

Functions:

⚔ Calms the spirit, promotes good sleep

⚔ Activates the water element and alleviates pain

Method: "Saw" both sides of the ankles with the outside edges of your hands.

YONGQUAN • *BUBBLING SPRING* • KD 1 (KIDNEY 1)

Location: In the dip below the ball of the foot, where the earth energy bubbles up into the body (see fig. 2.27)

Functions:

⚔ Descends excess energy from the head

⚔ Calms the spirit

⚔ Grounding

Method: Massage and warm this point before sleep.

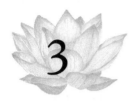

3

Heart and Healing

*The lifelong art of loving
carves gems with our hearts.
Out of our raw essence
The beauty reveals itself.*

Sexual energy cultivation fuels the fire of love. How can we grow and radiate love? By opening our hearts and healing the emotional scars that prevent us from fully embracing ourselves and others. The more love, the more orgasmic our experiences become. Feeling orgasmic also increases our cardiovascular strength.

THE HEART

Palace of the Spirit

Inside your heart is a sacred treasure.

Where do you point to when you point to yourself? Most of us will point to our hearts, not our heads. The seat of consciousness sits in the heart, which the ancients called the "Palace of the Spirit." The heart connects us with the violet light of the primordial wisdom of the universe. This light educates our soul and spirit about the great mysteries of life and death.

The heart communicates with our other organs, embodies our wisdom, and radiates love and compassion. When our heart spirit is happy, we spontaneously smile. Our real nature is happiness. Happiness is central to everyone's sense of well-being. Let your heart breathe freely and set yourself free. To be loved, to love, and to be free are essential gestures for feeling happy.

The Sovereign Heart

An Organ of Perception and Communication

The heart is the sovereign that rules the whole body and communicates with every cell. When you communicate with your heart, you communicate with your whole body. When the emperor is not happy, the whole kingdom is not happy. When the emperor is feeling good, you feel good. The heart is the conductor of your internal orchestra and is central to creating a harmonious state of being.

The heart is an organ of perception, which perceives the feelings arising in the other organs. Although the heart is considered a pump, blood that bypasses the heart during heart surgery in fact moves faster than blood that goes through the heart. So the heart actually regulates the blood, allowing it to perceive the feelings in the blood.

Negative emotions, like impatience and hatred, contract the heart and the rest of the body as well. When we feel angry our face turns red and our hands clench into fists. There is a lot of energy, but there is resistance and closure in the heart. This contraction can be harmful for the heart and creates damaging cholesterol. On the other hand, appropriate anger is the first line of defense, which protects our heart.

Love and Compassion

The heart is like the sun, which brings out the beauty of nature. Have you noticed that more people are smiling on a sunny day? The heart thrives on love. Married people tend to live longer lives. Divorce or the death of a loved one can become a medical emergency. Creating a loving atmosphere in the family and community plays an important role in our health.

Love brings out the best in us. When we smile with love and appreciation to someone, that person feels good and will work better. When you smile to your organs, they will work so much better in supporting your life. When we smile to our heart and shine love to our other organs, it brings out the virtues and balances any excess negativity that may be held there.

The heart is the center of compassion; its compassionate embrace holds space and presence for our emotions to move and transform. Through spiritual practice, the fire of passion is transformed into the warmth of compassion and the light of wisdom. We grow compassion by integrating the virtues of all the vital organs. The compassion becomes balanced and has integrity, strength, gentleness, fairness, respect, and kindness.

Laughter and the Heart

Laughing plays a big role in creating a happy heart. It vibrates joy and lightness throughout the body and uplifts the spirit. Laughing is one of the most contagious conditions!

- Laughter is very good for us. It can lower blood pressure and reduce stress hormones. It gives a boost to the immune system—increasing T cells to fight infections, gamma-interferon proteins to fight disease, and the antibodies called B cells that destroy disease. Laughter is so powerful that it releases stagnant suppressed emotions, which can cause cancer.
- Laughing releases endorphins, natural painkillers. Have you ever laughed a bit when you stubbed your toe? Laughing in times of trouble makes a shift in consciousness and puts our life in a bigger perspective. We see the hidden blessings in our challenges. You develop the control to shift your emotions into a mood of acceptance.
- We need to have faith that we can heal ourselves. Genuine laughter shows our faith in the Divine and our ability to let go and be positive.

❀ Laughing Qigong

Qigong is a way to express loving connection with nature and our bodies through energetic movement. It empowers you to manifest compassion in your actions. Laughing Qigong does not require stimulation from the outside; just simply laugh!

Laughing Baby. Lie on your back. Wiggle your arms and legs in the air and laugh like a baby! This practice is great for releasing tension in your womb and increasing blood circulation and lymph drainage. Let your inner child freely laugh!

Happy Boobies. Hold your breasts, then shake and laugh! When you laugh wholeheartedly all your cells are vibrating like an orgasm! Imagine your boobies are bouncing upward, "Up, up, up, I feel good, good, good!"

Heart's Call to Love

Love Is the Great Healer. Healing starts with self-love. The healing journey takes us to the heart of truth. When we feel the love behind it all, great resolution happens.

Listen to Your Heart. Listening and following our heart's messages is very important to our spiritual path. When you get a *"Yes to life!"* notice how your creative energy rises to meet and serve your heart's calling.

Calm the Blood, Calm the Ego

The heart is the seat of consciousness, compassion, and unconditional love. The practices below are designed to balance fire and water by calming the heart with water and warming the kidneys with fire. This prevents the heart from being "cooked" by false fire or overstimulated by adrenaline, external stimulants, and stress. Make the blood peaceful.

The seat of the ego is in the physical heart. When we feel separate from the world, the ego—which works through the muscles—creates a subtle contraction in the heart. When the ego aligns with the higher good, there is less personal tension. The ego relaxes.

✸ Heart's Flower

Sense a flower with twelve petals in your heart chakra (fig. 3.1). Each petal has a virtue energy: love, goodness, beauty, truth, respect, devotion, compassion, happiness, joy, honor, gratitude, or harmony. Has the growth of any of these petals been stunted by some form of negative contraction? Smile deeply inside and unfold each petal, creating an even, balanced flower with a center of pure golden light.

✸ Great Heart Breathing

This Qigong practice connects your personal heart with the heart of the universe. When we connect with the vast universal heart—the love that binds all beings—our heart expands.

- Hold a lotus in your hands. In prayer position, touch your pinkies and thumbs together and open your fingers like an open flower. Smile inwardly to your inner heart as you inhale.

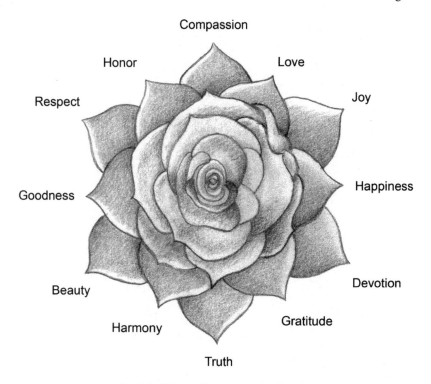

Fig. 3.1. Heart's flower, petals of virtue

- Exhale and make the heart sound, "ha-a-a-a-a-w." Open your arms out to the side, radiating love and compassion. Expand the love into your body and legs, pressing your feet into the ground and growing tall. Open your eyes and palms. Imagine you have a thousand arms, like Avalokitesvara, the Bodhisattva who embodies the compassion of all Buddhas.
- In each hand is an eye that sees what is needed in the world, so you can serve with wisdom (see fig. 3.2 on page 138). Receive the information back into your heart, soften the front of your body, look into your lotus, and sense your inner heart. This gesture is very important for taking to heart what is really happening around you and offering your energy wisely.

Heart to Sex

Dear Sex, I invite you to rise,
To nourish all of me,
To open my flower,
And give me energy to multiply
So my light shines on all beings.

Dear Heart, I invite you to shower me
With your love, encourage my flow,
Turn on the tap of my creative juices,
To grant me the permission
To express my passion for life.

We are married in the embrace
Of consciousness and life force.
Together we make the world go round.
Let us join in the core and
Unite our divine qualities into One.

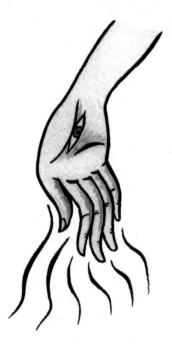

Fig. 3.2. Eye in the
heart of the hand

✻ Heart and Yoni Breathing

It is possible to have sex without love, yet the more we love, the more orgasmic we become. This simple yet profound practice heals the delusory split between love and sex by allowing your heart to speak its longing to your sexual organs and your sexual organs to share your deepest secrets of sensual desire.

When the fire of the heart and the water of the sexual organs join forces, we have the alchemical power of transformation.

- Smile down to your Jade Fountain. Place your right hand over your heart and your left hand over your yoni (womb). Bring loving qi down to warm up your sexual waters.
- You can also put your right hand on your yoni to send passion up to the heart to grow compassion.
- Breathe up and down between these two centers and allow them to communicate with each other.

When we feel appreciation, compassion, and kindness, our hearts open. When our hearts open, our yoni opens. Try to do this practice every morning when you wake up. Smile and breathe. Connect love in your heart with the creative life force in your Jade Fountain. This will set the tone of loving acceptance for the day.

THREE FIRES OF TRANSFORMATION

Keep your fires burning!

There is no transformation without fire—the spark of the Divine, love of life, flaming enthusiasm, and passion to be alive! Taoists consider the three fires to be essential for transforming and transporting jing, qi, and shen throughout the body. These fires assist in evaporating water and transforming bodily fluids, and they are also vital for circulating the energy that sustains the human soul.

Do you feel that you are burning your candle at both ends? Do you need to warm your feet on your lover? Women can be very devotional, often giving their fire away without knowing how to replenish it. The Three Fires practices described below will help you nourish your inner fire and support your many transformations.

❄ Three Fires Meditation

The three fires meditative practice is used for sexual energy cultivation and spiritual liberation. It builds fire for the alchemy of fire and water inside. It ignites the will for transformation.

● Dantian Fire

The dantian fire is located in the lower abdomen above the perineum. This fire heats the internal organs of the lower burner, evaporates water, and transforms bodily fluids. It transforms jing into qi—essence into energy.

- Visualize this fire under your cauldron at the navel center cooking your sexual essence. A dynamic visualization of this fire is an orange volcano under the blue ocean generating steam from below. This fire is the yang within the yin.

● Heart Fire

The heart fire is also called the Imperial Fire, Emperor's Fire, or Sovereign Fire and is located in the center of the chest. It heats internal organs in the upper burner and energizes thought and emotion. The heart fire transforms qi into shen—energy into spirit.

- Visualize your heart fire as a green dot of light in the red glowing sun. This is the compassionate essence of the heart—the yin within the yang.

● Mingmen Fire

The Mingmen fire is located at the Door of Life between the kidneys. It is also called the Ministerial Fire or kidney/adrenal fire and is the yang fire within the yin water element. It heats the internal organs of the middle and lower burners and is the root of the body's Yuan Qi (Prenatal Qi).

- Visualize the Mingmen fire as a violet flame—a pilot light that keeps us alive. Violet is the color of the primordial Yuan Qi. This fire creates a balance between the yin dark blue kidney and yang bright blue kidney. See the discussion of yin and yang kidneys in the section "Building Your Core Reserves" in chapter 8.

  The Mingmen fire is a major motivating force of the body. When deficient, this fire may lead to gray hair, wrinkled and prematurely aging skin, and decreased sex drive and frigidity. When in excess, sexual drive and sexual obsession are increased. Stress in many forms can lead to adrenal burnout. When your adrenals are tired and over- or underproducing your hormones, you will start to look and feel as overworked as your adrenals are.

❦ Stephanie's Journey of Inner Fire

I had been working on clearing the belief "I am not good enough" from my subconscious. One morning I awoke and I could feel the remnants of the painful emotions that resulted from this belief hiding inside my body. I smiled with love down into the places it was hiding in my left pelvis and ovary. I knew that this energy was calling to be loved and transformed. I prepared to enter a shamanic journey right there in my bed and called in the assistance of the directions and my power animal.

The wolf came to me in the journey and took me deep into a cave. The ground began to shake. "Don't worry," she said, "we are safe here." It was as if there were an earthquake happening all around us. The ground cracked and shifted as orange and red molten lava seeped up through the cracks. The lava, I was told, would not hurt me. I allowed it to rise up into my body, up my feet and legs. It filled my pelvis, my ovaries, and my whole body.

The "I am not good enough" energy was burned up in the lava and all that was left was a steam that rose out of the ashes. I immediately felt the steam enter the Microcosmic Orbit and circulate around and around my body, transforming what used to be a heavy and dense energy into high-frequency light. This light was focused into my heart, where I had also been holding the belief, and it began to fill the space in which it once lived. What happened then was the light began to transform the belief and harden it into a diamond, reflecting all the colors of the rainbow.

The heart-shaped diamond was drawn out of my body through a point above my heart on my chest called "Spirit Burial Grounds," which has the qualities of letting go of the past and boosting self-esteem. I felt the light energy in this diamond on my chest connect down my left arm into my out-stretched hand. From here on I felt the compassionate capacity to reach out to receive others' love. I also became a mirror for others struggling with the same issue, reflecting back to them the pure, innocent, and radiant joy of true love that we really are.

STEPHANIE LAFAZANOS

❋ Burning Up Delusions

Use your creative intention to burn up imbalances within the fires.

Point with both hands into each center and practice bellows breathing to fan your fire. Imagine that you are stoking your inner fire.

- Burn up self-destructive desires in the dantian fire.
- Burn up selfishness and ignorance in the heart fire.
- Burn up burdens of our past and unresolved ancestral imprints in the Mingmen fire.

✴ Balancing Three Fires Practice

In this practice, you use the water cycle (up the front and down the back) to breathe alchemy among the three fires. The water cycle calms the heart fire and warms the kidney fire. As you circulate qi among the three fires you generate what is called "True Breath" or "Holy Fire." When True Breath weakens, one develops unease, and when it gathers, one feels tranquility.

- Practice the Spinal Pelvic Rock as described in chapter 6: Lying down with your knees up, inhale the warmth of the earth through your hands and feet. Arch your back as you inhale, drawing warm steam from your dantian up to your heart.
- Exhale, pressing your lower back down to the floor; bring the heart fire down to the Mingmen. Continue to exhale down to the lower dantian. As you exhale, spread the warmth from your core out to the periphery of your hands and feet. Continue to breathe in this triangle, generating a warm pink and golden glow.
- Smile down from your crown with a transcendent violet light. The "Celestial Fire" in your upper dantian transforms shen into Wuji—spirit into primordial universe, boundless infinite.

For another alchemical experience of fire within water, practice this exercise in the bathtub with your jade egg. Pull the string attached to your jade egg as you exhale and press your midback down. This can also be done without movement in a meditative posture.

✴ Black Pearl Process

Have you ever felt a deep loneliness that you believe can never be satisfied? Do you always "need" to be in a relationship? Try this Black Pearl practice to transform your lonely and needy energies.

- Create a black pearl in the cauldron behind your navel. Imbue it with the qualities of black obsidian to absorb the shadow from your organs. Move the black pearl from organ to organ and use the healing sound to release excess negativity from the lungs, kidneys, liver, heart, and spleen into the pearl.
- Bring the black pearl to Mingmen, Gate of Destiny—portal into Wuji, supreme creativity, unmanifest spaciousness. Allow it to receive all it

needs from the vast realm of infinite possibilities. The pearl absorbs all the virtues and light that will make it balanced and whole. Watch how the color changes into gold. Gold is the preciousness within that never tarnishes. Circulate the golden pearl around the Microcosmic Orbit to distribute this high-quality energy through the body-mind.

How have your beliefs about yourself shifted? Transform the loneliness into longing and spiritual awakening. Give your gifts from infinite sources of loving abundance.

TRANSFORMING THE PAST AND THE FUTURE
Ancestral Healing

Your ancestors are in your DNA right now! Their energy can be unwound to reset your evolution.

Ancestral healing works to free you of the energetic cords that tie you to old patterns. Cords are like weeds that are rooted in the generational pain body and tend to be passed down like family feuds. They feed on negativity—like unhealthy attachment or resentment. They filter and limit our thoughts, feelings, and perceptions. Cords are sticky and glued into the body-mind with sexual essence. They dissolve when the people on both ends of the cord let go and return to love and compassion.

Bonds based in unconditional love are free. The possibility of transformation allows you to free yourself from conditioning and repeatedly attracting the familiar energies of your parents or generational pain body. Free yourself to attract a lover who will support your evolution. When you liberate these ancestral knots, there is a potential for you to liberate blockages in the whole generational line—including all future generations.

❋ Ancestral Healing Practice

This healing process is best to do with both parents, one at a time. If your grandparents or another family member raised you, the same practice applies. Once the connection with one parent is liberated, the second process will reveal deep interconnections. You can process this yourself but having someone holding space for you is a great support.

● Invocation

- Call in the presence of your guides and the guides of your parent. Call on divine guidance for the best possible resolution between you and your ancestors. Imagine that your parent is sitting in front of you.
- Wrap yourself and your parent in three Wei Qi fields. (See Drawing from Three Sources exercise in chapter 2.)
- Create a clockwise spiral vortex into the earth for recycling blocked energy.
- Forgiveness is the energy for growing beyond the hurt. Circulate energy in the orbit between you and your parent: a wheel of forgiveness, compassion, and unconditional love moving up your Core Channel and down his or her Core Channel. Imagine a river of rainbow light that clears debris and stagnant qi. Set your intention to nourish the highest in your ancestral line and resolve negative patterns.

● Connect to the Stages of Life

For each stage of life listed below, connect with yourself at the time and with your parent(s).

- **Before conception.** Intuit why you chose this being to be your parent. Feel the connection between your parents. Thank your parents for conceiving you.
- **In utero.** Get a sense of your father's or mother's emotions during pregnancy. Get in touch with your mother's emotions through her breath, heartbeat, and the contractions and expansions of her belly. You would feel your father's emotions also through the mother's responses.
- **Early childhood.** Circulate light energy to clear dark and hurtful memories. Give thanks to your parent for raising you. If you experienced abuse and you are ready to release this energy, make any primal sounds from within or healing sounds to clear suppressed hurt, anger, shame, fear, or frustration. A child picks up on the shame or guilt of the abuser, so it's important to clear that. Even if there was no actual physical or emotional abuse, children are sensitive enough to pick up hurtful thoughts and intentions.
- **Teenage years.** This is a time when the rise of sexual energy and the power of change and self-assertion naturally create feelings of rebellion. Say what you always wanted to say but held back.

You can also use the healing sounds to clear emotional imprints. If you felt loving support, for instance, you can express the heart sound. If you felt separation, the heart sound can also express your lack of connection. How did your parent support you as you came through puberty and during your first romances and sexual encounters? Breathe and move through it. Give thanks to your parent for seeing you through this challenging time of your life.

- **Adulthood.** Feel your independence and your first steps onto your own life path. How did your parents deal with your transition into this stage of your life? How did they respond to your life choices, education, career, boyfriends, marriage, children, and/or divorce?

If your parents have passed over, your love can continue to grow. If they are on their deathbed, what can you say to resolve any regrets and come to peace with them?

● Resolution Prayer

> *"I'm sorry, please forgive me.*
> *Thank you, I love you."*

This Ho'oponopono prayer came from Hawaiian shamans. Use it to say any of the following: *"I'm sorry"* (meaning, "I take responsibility for the role that I play in the pattern that has been created"). *"Please forgive me"* (for my judgments and/or any harm that has been afflicted upon us—past or present.). *"Thank you"* (for being a mirror, for being here to help us heal, for the opportunity to share my gratitude for the gift that is presented). *"I love you"* (I feel the love flowing).

- Say this prayer to your parent and imagine your parent is saying it back to you. Your witness or support person, if you have one, can say this back to you on behalf of your parent.
- Sense your Core Channel and that of your parent as pillars of light, aligning each of you with your highest destiny.
- Bow with reverence to your ancestors and to the power of healing. Place your hands and your head on the earth and let go.
- Your support partner can wash down your back in the gesture of letting your past wash behind you. If doing this by yourself, you can make the triple warmer sound, "he-e-e-e-e, " to clear from the heavens down through the body.

- Come to peace with your past.
- Do Spinal Cord Breathing to build courage for the next process with your other parent.

● Releasing Cords and Reprogramming

The energetic cords that may be attached to old patterns can be released through the portals of the Lung 1 points under the collarbone. The right lung has to do with your father and male ancestors. The left lung has to do with your mother and female ancestors.

This exercise is best practiced in a lying-down position.

- Have your partner pull the energetic cords from your Lung 1 points. It feels like pulling out weeds or roots. Every cord has a mysterious story. Draw the cords out from the pain body with the lung sound, "ss-s-s-s-s." To loosen the soil and the roots, your partner can tone another healing sound for the lungs—"shaaang"—over your belly and chest.
- Pull the cords again with divine assistance. Sweep down the left or right Lung meridian, down the inside of the arm, out the thumb, and into the earth. Let go of the heaviness of the past like releasing a waterfall. Then repeat on the other side.
- Form a white qi ball above your chest with the strengths and gifts of the ancestors. Breathe it in by gently pressing it into your chest.
- Thank your guides, guardians, and angels. Request that your work today may serve all beings.

HEALING FROM SEXUAL TRAUMA

If we look into the collective consciousness of our feminine history, we will touch upon many forms of sexual trauma. When a woman has been entered too soon, this shock requires trust to open to pleasure again. If we consider the lives of our mothers, grandmothers, and female ancestors, how much of these painful imprints are we carrying? I believe that we have the consciousness and compassion at this time to shift these archaic dynamics of victim and perpetrator. Secret doors are opening for our collective wounds to be exposed and healed.

We all want to feel safe and guard against attacks and invasion, whether real or perceived. When the masks or walls we built in order to cope crack, the emotions emerge. It is necessary to *feel it to heal it.* Tracing back to the root of suffering, we peel back the physical, emotional, mental, and spiritual layers. Returning to love, understanding, and compassion, resolution is possible.

Remember that it is important, once you start this unraveling process, to guide yourself through into finding the love. Avoid stopping halfway, because unprocessed emotions may cause you to linger in a half-cooked state and become retraumatized. Victim consciousness can eventually come out as aggression, hence turning the wheel of suffering again. You will know when you have come to full resolution when your body no longer cringes while thinking about the traumatic event or the person involved. This resolution process can be done for the sake of all beings to break the wheel of suffering.

The muscles of the body hold memory and trauma, which is called "armoring." That is why it is important to include in this process healing self-massage or bodywork. Loving touch will de-armor any blockages that were created to protect against hurt, transforming victim consciousness into co-created love and trust.

With compassion, patience, and gentleness, our emotional body matures and we start to understand the whole picture from a higher perspective. This healing journey is best done with a witness holding space for you to unravel any knots of fear, shame, and guilt that may be tied up in your sexual organs and body. If you would like to embark on this journey by yourself, you can call on your guides, guardians, and angels to be present and assist you to resolve what you are ready to resolve at this time.

✷ Sexual Healing Practice

Remember to go through all the steps of the practice, so that you come to full resolution.

● Dissociation and Grounding

When abuse or trauma happens, we tend to go out of body so as not to feel the hurt. We then continue to dissociate during sexual connection; what was once a way of coping becomes an impediment to receiving loving penetration from a lover.

The way back into the body is being totally present, breathing and smiling deeply into frozen, contracted areas to melt them into an expansive form. Hold your healing hands over any contracted areas and be patient until the energy shifts. You can ask the area, "What is here now?" Continue to ask, layer upon layer, until you are complete. Ask for divine assistance to help you release what you are ready to release and transform at this time.

Iron Shirt Qigong practices like Embracing the Tree (see chapter 8) are particularly beneficial for establishing solid roots and the confidence that you are not a pushover. Breathe in all the support you need to come to peace with your past and be open to love in the present.

● Unveiling the Mask

In social situations, we often put up masks to cover up our pain or to defend and justify our position. When you have the courage to take off this mask, release it to the light. Imagine an angel bringing a mirror for you to see your authentic self. You will be amazed at how beautiful you truly are! In the vulnerable moments when we reveal our authentic emotions, we invite true intimacy. In this way we can reclaim our innocence, love, and respect!

● Transfiguring the Goddess

It is incredibly healing to be heard and seen for who you really are. Find a friend who will allow you to look into her eyes, see through all the pain, all the masks, into the spark and depths of her beautiful soul. Transfigure her into her unique Goddess self. In this way, we give each other the resources to move beyond traumatic patterning into the free expression of who we really are.

● Resolution through Compassion

- Listen inside for a trauma that wants to come up to be healed. Imagine the person or people involved standing in front of you. For auric protection, wrap yourself and that person in bubbles of golden light or in the three Wei Qi fields. Connect your higher self and their higher self with a rainbow of compassionate light between you.
- Return to that moment in time when the trauma happened. Reconnect with repressed emotions such as anger, fear, and desperation. Make spontaneous sounds to clear the energy.
- Step into their field for a moment and feel their emotions behind the superficial layers; sense their deep fear. How are they suffering? Then

step out of their field again, brushing off your hands. This will invoke understanding and compassion in you.

- Imagine that person in their childhood and the emotional state in and around them. Through this reflection, you will understand the roots of their problems, creating a compassionate opening inside of you. Give that person all the love and compassion they need, which could have changed their life—and still could change it. Imagine you are embracing that child and watch how their expression shifts. Understand the pain in both of you. Be grateful for the spiritual meaning of this event and how it strengthened some quality in you.

● Releasing the Cords

Astral cords are rooted and hooked into the vital organs; they need to be loosened to be released. The toughest cords with people are the ones built on negativity; it takes a sincere resolution to transform them. There are astral beings or entities who "eat" sexual energy that is bonded with negativity. These entities want to be fed with negative emotions, addictions, and thought forms in order to survive.

Have you ever had an argument, then broken into tears and come to some truthful realization that returned you to love? Our hearts are broken so they can expand in love.

The cycle for emotional resolution begins with the liver and moves in a backward direction around the creation cycle from liver to kidneys to lungs to spleen to heart, as we want to get to the bottom of it; under the grief there is love. We grieve due to the depth of our love and the loss or damage of love. Everyone deep down is love, a divine being on a spiritual level. We need to go back to experience that person's divinity to come to peaceful resolution.

Go through the whole creation cycle in reverse, beginning with the liver:

> Transform the anger in the liver into kindness.
> Break the frozen ice of fear in the kidneys and transform it
>   into wisdom and understanding.
> Let go of sadness and tears in the lungs and transform it into
>   the courage to love.
> Release attachment and worry in the spleen and take
>   responsibility for this karmic connection.

> Heal separation and hatred in the heart and transform it into love and compassion.

- Make a golden ball above your body to contain negative energies with love. Scan your body and observe where the cord is attached. Cords are attached to tension throughout the body. Pull the cord, pulling out all that does not belong to your evolution from the past, present, and future time.

- Clear negative emotions around this person or event from your vital organs with all six of the healing sounds. Use the healing sounds to breathe the cords out as murky smoke, into the golden ball. Make the sounds for the sake of all your relations and all women who have experienced sexual abuse. Especially, clear any shame or guilt you may have picked up from the association with this being. Guilt is the energy of feeling that you did something wrong. Shame sits deeper in the heart as the feeling that you are wrong or bad.

- After clearing excess negativity from one organ, hold it and fill it with the associated virtue and pure color.

- Place your hands over your heart and smile deeply into your heart. Forgiveness here is the energy to grow beyond the hurt, the ability to let go so you can move on.

- Make the heart sound softly—"ha-a-a-a-w"—as you forgive yourself, accept the situation, and forgive the abuser. Be grateful for all the hidden blessings and lessons learned.

- Pull the last cords out into the golden ball. Ask for a divine being to help you cut the cord. Cut the cord with a strong heart sound—"ha-a-a-a-w"—and a cutting arm gesture. The golden ball ascends and merges with divine light, which bursts into fireworks. Compassionate energy showers down as crystal droplets of rainbow light. Breathe it in as healing mist. Fill all the areas of your body where dark emotions were once hidden with compassionate light.

- Reprogram with a high-frequency virtue of worthiness—worthy of being respected, honored, and loved. Fortify your Core Channel, which runs through your sexual organs, heart, and crown, with the white golden light of integrity.

- Pull down the heavens with the triple warmer sound ("he-e-e-e-e"). Circulate qi in the Microcosmic Orbit and collect the energy. Come to peace. Bow and give thanks to your guides for assisting in this liberation and transformation.

HEALING THE WOMB

Before practicing with the jade egg and circulating sexual energy, it is best to practice emotional clearing. Sexual energy amplifies our emotions, so if old anger is trapped in the sexual organs, you can get passionately angry if you don't first transform that anger into kindness.

After one jade egg workshop, a woman called me and said that she was so angry, swearing and throwing things! Then she said, "I have never felt so good!" Now I make sure to do some clearing work to prepare for the jade egg practice.

Going into the dark side of sexuality can be like opening Pandora's box, so you need to be well grounded and have positive resources like memories of loving connection that you can use to center yourself. Substantial experience of emotional transformation using the Inner Smile and Six Healing Sounds practices is necessary preparation before embarking on this level of healing.

Many women have deeply rooted trauma from sexual repression and relationship disharmony—culturally, ancestrally, and individually. When we heal these wounds we can alleviate generations of suffering and open the way to more harmony in this world.

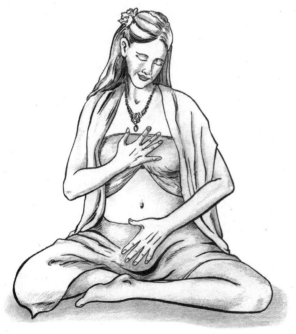

Fig. 3.1. Embodying Self Love

During an abusive situation a woman may have dissociated or gone "out of body." To access these painful memories, one needs to get into a trancelike state in a trusting and safe atmosphere. By understanding the deeper meaning in the whole picture, the suffering in the pain body unravels. Ask the Divine to liberate whatever is ready to be liberated to avoid retraumatization. Always find the love, compassion, and gratitude for this lesson behind the whole scenario.

One in three women on the planet will be raped or beaten in her lifetime. That is about one billion women.*

❇ Womb Healing Practice

Free yourself from the negative downward spiral of trapped emotions like fear, rage, violence, hatred, worry, shame, guilt, and depression.

● Invocation

Create sacred space as described in the Energy Massage for Your Lover practice in chapter 9. Say, "I dedicate this practice to liberating all women and men from the chains of painful memories held in their body-mind. May this practice bring the best possible healing, for the sake of all beings."

This invocation will create a safe and sacred space for the trauma to be revealed and resolved.

● Womb Cleansing

- Make a clockwise vortex for toxic qi to be transformed in the earth.
- Smile down with the sense of forgiveness, compassion, and gratitude for the lessons learned and inner growth.
- Emit qi with what is called a "double beam" by placing your right hand over your left hand, facing your womb. Brush down and clear out cloudy, murky energy with a descending "Yoouuu" sound.
- Rinse with refreshing blue water qi.
- Rub your hands to generate fresh warm energy. Fill the womb with the golden light of compassion.
- Notice if your womb feels more transparent and spacious.

---

*See www.onebillionrising.org.

● Wands of Healing Light

This profound practice was developed with Shashi Solluna in our Sacred Femininity training for women. It can be practiced to clear ancestral imprints of past lovers or to clean the nest emotionally and energetically for a new being to grow there if you want to become pregnant. This practice is also helpful for healing from sexual abuse or abortion, transforming feelings of loneliness, hurt, or sexual frustration, and clearing any negativity you might have absorbed from sexual encounters.

Emotions may arise during PMS to be cleared through menstruation. Yet deep residues can still remain, requiring conscious intention to be released. Women find it supportive to practice this together and then celebrate their liberation through dance and song.

Sense what emotion is most prominent in the moment. You can start the emotional resolution from there and then move through the creation cycle, or you can start with the lungs or the kidneys. Use the individual healing sounds and associated colors to clear the negative emotions into the earth—for example, blue wands and the "choo-oo-oo-oo" sound to clear fear from the water element.

- Sit on a chair or kneel with your knees out wide. Make a clockwise vortex for toxic qi to be transformed in the earth. Connect with your higher guidance to assist in clearing what you are ready to clear.
- Lift your hands to heart height with your fingers connecting to the heavens. Ask the Divine to extend the aura of your fingers into wands of pure colored light. At the same time, radiate from your Core Channel the virtue energy and pure color light into the aura of your fingers. Comb with the wands of light up through your vagina, uterus, and ovaries.
- Lift your hands to the height of your Sexual Palace. Turn the palms facing down as if holding a colored qi ball, holding your breath and pulling up your perineum. Sweep down through the sexual organs as you make the healing sound. Continue repeating the sound until you feel an energy shift. If memories arise, let them go with the sound. Trust in the process and do not get caught up in the stories. Spiral down and touch the earth to let go.
- Rub your hands to build neutral energy. Gather the pure colored light and natural elements from the earth. Hold your womb area and absorb the positive emotion. You can recall a time when you felt this virtue.
- Repeat these steps for each element, until you have completed the creation cycle. Finish with the triple warmer sound.

• Hold your hands over your yoni and fill with golden light and compassion. Notice if you feel more transparent, sparkling clean, and free. Circulate energy in the Microcosmic Orbit and collect the energy to seal the aura.

Metal element: Clear sadness from missed opportunities, loss of old relationships, loss of love, loss of youthful desire, depressed passion, disappointment, shame or guilt, victim or martyr consciousness.

Fill with courage to step into the unknown.

Water element: Clear sexual fears and trauma, fear of sexual expression, feelings of power and surrender, rejection, abandonment, loneliness, frigidity.

Fill with flow and gentleness. Come to peace with your sexuality. Have faith in the continuation of your spirit.

Wood element: Clear sexual frustration, anger, jealousy, aggression, explosiveness, as well as overcontrolling and overprotecting behaviors.

Fill with passion and kindness, following your bliss.

Fire element: Clear separation, loveless sex, violence, generational hatred, impatience with your sex life.

Fill with love and compassion.

Earth element: Clear sexual hang-ups, worry about smell or performance, attachments, mothering, smothering, neediness, possessiveness, self-doubt. Transform "I am not good enough" to "I am worthy of touch."

Fill with openness, safety, trust.

Triple Warmer: Clear out with the wands of crystal light any negative energy that does not belong to you: conditioning from media, family, peers; karmic imprints from past lovers; negative emotions from past sexual experiences. Also clear any desires or broken dreams that do not support your higher destiny.

Fill with balance and clarity.

● Alchemical Womb Transformation

Fire from the heart descends to warm any excess coldness in the womb and clear excess dampness.

Bring down the love of the heart to transform fear in the sexual organs.

• Stroke down from the heart with the "ha-a-a-a-w" sound. Bring down a red, fiery pearl from the heart into the blue, watery uterus.

• Allow the inner fire to evaporate excess coldness and dampness in the womb. Allow steam to wash in and around the uterus, vagina, and clitoris.

• Come to balance and rest.

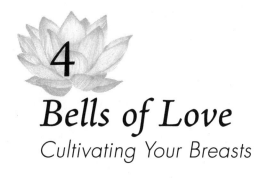

4

Bells of Love
Cultivating Your Breasts

The ancient Taoists called the breasts "Bells of Love."
Breasts are gateways to the heart center and female orgasm.
Feel your breasts from within. Ring your bells!

After you have become comfortable transforming emotions and circulating energy in the Microcosmic Orbit, you can actively cultivate sexual energy. This chapter will lead you through many exercises for enlivening, healing, and energizing your breasts. Breast massage opens the heart and nourishes self-love, preparing the way for cultivation of the yoni, which we will cover in the next chapter.

The breasts are essential for cultivating female sexual energy. They are intimately connected to the endocrine glands that produce hormones, which is sexual energy in modern science. Taking good care of our breasts and preventing stagnation is vital for our emotional, energetic, and physical health and well-being.

The breasts are symbols of sexuality. When we take pleasure in our own breasts and body we feel sexy. We give loving energy to our lover through our breasts. They are the nurturers in our body and embody motherhood. When we accept the size and shape of our breasts we have a positive self-image.

The divine Sophia was often pictured as a woman with infinitely large breasts, from which all of humankind suckled wisdom. Embody the qualities of a goddess of compassion to raise the frequency of Mother Earth. Give thanks to your breasts for all they give to you, your possible children, and lovers.

Free Up Your Breasts

Tight bras can restrict circulation in the breast area and compress the tissues and have been linked with breast cancer. Metal also disturbs the qi flow, so I suggest removing the underwire in bras. Just make a small hole on the side and pull the wire out. Feel the freedom of your breath and qi flow when you take off your bra to massage your breasts.

BREAST MASSAGE BASICS
A Practice of Self-Love

The breasts are the gateway to female orgasm. When they are opened with love, the heart opens and the yoni—the Jade Fountain—becomes receptive. Explore the dynamic dance of Healing Love single and dual cultivation practices with openness and playfulness. Your love life will be greatly enhanced!

Benefits of Breast Massage

Regular breast massage has the following beneficial effects:

Replenishes the heart. Breast massage develops more softness in the chest area to help open the heart. Women tend to be givers and are devoted to serving others. When we massage our breasts we give back loving attention and replenish our heart, right between the breasts.

Supports our "melting pots." Sexual energy amplifies our emotional state, so it is very important to transform any excessive negative emotions into virtues. The breasts are like melting pots for the virtue energies of the vital organs. Breast massage with attention to our emotions brings out the healing qualities of the organs' energy.

Cleanses and stimulates. Breast massage is a pleasurable way to improve qi circulation and break up stagnation, which can form into cancer. It liberates suppressed emotions, which can accumulate into various forms of dis-ease. Massage makes the body feel loved, which releases growth and antiaging hormones. Breast massage stimulates many erogenous zones and acupressure points around the breasts including points on the Kidney, Spleen, Stomach, Liver, and Pericardium meridians.

Regular practice also helps early detection of anything unusual in the breast tissues. Please share these practices with other women!

Transforms blood into qi. The more we pull our sexual energy up to the breasts, the less blood and qi we lose through menstruation. When a woman lactates, her energy is drawn to the breasts to nurture a child. We can similarly draw energy upward to nurture our inner child.

> *The Feminine Treasures work is pertinent to my hormone-related issues with my health. I really need this; so many women do as we age. All the underwire bras and breasts that are not free! My mom's breast cancer was right where the underwire would be in the bra. The lymph can't drain properly. Having such a strong family genetics with breast cancer makes me really want to love my breasts. All women need to. This is so important, the self-love and touch, so basic really to life."*
>
> MARTA HERNANDEZ,
> CERTIFIED QIGONG INSTRUCTOR

When and How to Practice Breast Massage

Over the years, I have found the following guidelines to be helpful for getting started with a regular breast massage practice.

Morning and Evening Tune-ups

Breast massage is a great practice first thing in the morning—before, during, or after a shower or bath. Say "good morning" to your breasts and you'll have an uplifting start to your day! In the evening, when you remove your bra, your breasts are happy to be released and free to move. This is an excellent time to practice massage again, to release stagnation and stress that have accumulated over the day.

Besides these twice-a-day "quickies," we recommend nurturing yourself with a longer healing or enlivening massage session at least once a week. It is also a good idea to do this practice whenever something arises that asks for attention. For example:

- When you feel emotional, practice a longer breast massage with healing sounds to release emotions.
- When you are feeling pretty balanced and you want to boost your natural self-confidence, practice the breast massage that grows courage and positive emotions around the creation cycle.

⚐ Breast massage is an excellent Metta (loving-kindness) meditation for growing compassion that can be integrated into your spiritual practice.

Massage Oil

Use massage oil with aromatic essential oils—like clary sage, geranium, fennel, and ylang ylang—for promoting hormonal balance. Practicing breast massage in the bath with essential oils is absolutely delicious. Enjoy a massage with coconut, jojoba, or almond oil before or after you bathe. If you need more warming qualities, sesame oil is excellent in cold climates.

Silk Cloth

Silk conducts the smooth flow of qi. When you massage your breasts through a silky scarf or piece of lingerie, you will find that your movements develop a sensual quality.

> *This powerful and playful practice has stayed with me over the years and I have passed it on to many other women in healing circles and communities all over the world. Thank you! I think of you every time I practice and pass it on.*
>
> Biz

Preparing Yourself for Breast Massage

Whenever you practice breast massage, keep in mind the following:

Maintain grounded posture. Sit on the edge of your cushion, cross-legged, if this is comfortable for you. Or sit in a chair with your feet firmly planted on the ground. Let your heel or a rolled-up towel create gentle pressure on your clitoris. You can also make yourself comfortable by lying in your bed, on moss, or against a tree. You can also stand in a wide horse stance that helps you ground and connect with the earth.

Warm hands. Pull up sexual energy by flexing the PC muscles. Squeeze the energy into your hands and rub them warm. Use fragrant massage oil if you like.

Deepen awareness. Feel your breasts with your hands. Then shift your awareness to feel the energy of your hands from the inside of your breasts. This awareness can help you feel connected if your breasts have become desensitized. With this heightened awareness, breasts become more sensitive to touch.

Love your breasts. Love and accept your breasts as they are. Breathe through the tiny holes in your nipples. Breathe into your heart center. Blossom a deep red rose. Spread its fragrance of beauty and goodness through the breasts. Smile down and feel the breasts glowing with warmth.

Clear the chest. This is an effective way to release any heavy emotions that sit on your chest. Place your hands on your chest and blow out "who-o-o-o-o" three times into the earth. Rub your hands warm and massage your breasts in both directions (see the Dispersing and Gathering Qi practice below).

Come to peace. Coming to peace with yourself is the best way to master sexual energy. Yin stillness, emptiness, and receptivity are the womb that gives birth to yang substance and activity.

✸ Dispersing and Gathering Qi

When you massage the breasts in both directions,
the breasts become firmer and fuller!

Drawing energy from earth and heaven allows for balanced circulation in the breasts. Spiraling your hands outward will disperse heavy, stagnant energy, making the breasts firmer, while spiraling inward gathers energy, making them fuller.

● Drawing from the Earth

Earth energy builds the blood and substance of the body and sustains it. The earth is a watery planet, with about 72 percent of its surface covered by water. The human body is also about 50 to 70 percent water. The essence of the water is very cleansing and dispersing.

- Draw energy up from the earth to nourish love, joy, and compassion in your heart center. Visualize/sensualize/actualize a geyser rising up from the earth through the Bubbling Springs points (KD 1) on the soles of the feet and up your legs.
- Stroke qi up from the Jade Fountain (vagina and uterus) to your heart center, over your breasts, and down the outsides of the breasts, in flowing circles.

This direction of qi circulation around the breasts will disperse stagnant and excess qi and cleanse the breasts. It can help prevent cancer. If you practice frequently in this direction, your breasts may become smaller and/ or firmer. This direction is self-nurturing because it is like a fountain drawing up from the nourishing earth.

● Drawing from the Heavens

Heavenly energy recharges the body as if you were plugging yourself into the universe. As a baby, you had a soft fontanel to receive heavenly energy through your crown, activating brain growth. The fontanel generally closes by the age of two. Cranial sutures, though, can remain flexible into adulthood, usually hardening when the bones stop growing.

• Draw heavenly energy from above by opening your crown to the light of the stars, sun, moon, and planets.
• Draw that qi down through the master glands, down the center of the chest, around the bottoms of the breasts, and up the outsides.

This inward spiraling of qi around the breasts will gather energy. Stroking down the middle of the chest funnels Heaven Qi into the crown, stimulating growth hormones in the master glands. This enhances your ability to grow your breasts fuller and helps build a sense of confidence in your body.

�֎ Up and Down the Mountain

This practice balances both directions of spiraling. Imagine your breasts are two mountain peaks. Start your journey with your fingers on the heart center in the valley between the mountains. Connect with your longing for a heightened state of aliveness. Start massaging up through the valley and down around the sides and base of the mountain in wide circles. Start climbing in a spiral around the mountain in smaller and smaller spirals until you come to the peaks. Use your middle finger to spin in ecstasy at the peak of the mountain with a sensitive touch.

Then reverse direction and spiral bigger and bigger circles down the mountain with a wider touch down through the valley and up the sides again. End with your hands touching your heart and smiling to the beautiful landscape of your body.

We all long to be on top of the world and bring the heavenly bliss back to our heart!

❄ Deer Breast Massage

This breast massage practice was originally called the "Deer Exercise" because the deer is the shamanic animal for the gentle kidneys. This practice balances the left and right sides of the body. It links up the sexual organs with the heart. It opens the Left and Right Thrusting Channels.

Place your left hand over your Ovarian Palace as your right hand massages your right breast in circles. Squeeze your Jade Fountain as you inhale and draw the qi up to the inside of your right breast. As you exhale stroke down the outside of the right breast. Breathe deeply and relax. Compare the two sides and feel the warm tingling sensation in your right breast. The wide-open right nostril is a sign that your Right Thrusting Channel opened more. Change hands and place your right hand above your pubic bone and massage your left breast in the same manner. Remember to smile as you massage your breasts!

❄ Three Hearts, Two Breasts, One Love

In this exercise, we draw heaven and earth energies into loving, compassionate heart shapes within our bodies.

● Earth's Heart

Rub your hands warm. Stroke the qi from your Jade Fountain up to your heart. Circle in a heart shape over your breasts and return back to a point at the Sexual Palace. Inhale with the "choo-oo-oo-oo" sound (like sucking water up a straw) and exhale down.

● Heaven's Dewdrop

Start with your hands in a prayer position above the crown. Stroke down the centerline of your body, drawing from the heavens a shower of beautiful, loving light to awaken the heart. Circle your breasts and stroke with the backs of your fingers in a dewdrop shape—up the outside of the breasts to a point above your crown. Exhale with the "ha-a-a-a-w" sound as you stroke down, and inhale as you stroke up.

● Embracing Heart

Stroke your hands over the top of your breasts from your heart center. Embrace all the good things in life with your arms in front of you. Bring your hands together pointing forward, completing a horizontal heart shape. Then pull the good qi toward your heart.

✸ Breast Breathing

Take a full breath from the earth to the breasts. Feel your breasts becoming firmer and more resilient.

Take a big breath from the heavens. Fill your breasts with abundant cosmic energy. Hold your breath and condense the qi. Expand your breasts elastically on the exhalation. Feel them become fuller and more beautiful.

✸ Cloud Hands Breast Massage

Move your hands as in the Taiji movement called Cloud Hands, first around one breast, then around the other. The left hand makes a circle toward the right, then the right hand makes a circle toward the left. Cloud Hands protects the torso with a shield of moving qi, and this flowing massage is great for clearing the lymph and moving qi within.

- First the right hand strokes over the top of the left breast and down the outside.
- Then the left hand strokes the top of the left breast and down the middle line.
- Repeat around the right breast, reversing the hands.

✸ Breast Massage Quickies

The following short massage practices are great for tuning up in the morning and relaxing in the evening. They feel great anytime during the day when you want a quick pick-me-up. These exercises focus on breathing and sound to nourish your breasts and direct the flow of qi.

Happy Boobies. Hold your breasts and shake them lightly up and down. Giggle or laugh and fill them with happiness! This is a great immune booster!

Transforming Sadness. Medical Qigong uses the lung sound ("ss-s-s-s-s-s") during breast massage to relieve grief and sadness that might have settled in the breasts. Cradle your breasts or chest, rocking left and right while chanting another powerful healing lung sound, "shaaaang." Then fill your breasts with white light, courage, and inner strength.

Sing to Your Inner Child. Cradle your breasts, rocking side to side, like you are cradling your inner child. Chant "maaaang": "ma" for mother and "ang" for heart opening. Let the area resonate with loving-kindness. Sing the tone F, the archetypal tone for the heart chakra. Nurture your inner child with a heart song.

Smiling from Nipple to Nipple. Sweep lightly with your fingers a big smile from nipple to nipple, dipping all the way down across your clitoris. Chant "shoeng," the vowel pronounced like the vowel in *burst*. The image is of bursting blossoms. Go down and up the scale: F, E, D, C, D, E, F. It sounds like a Gregorian chant, though I am quite sure the nuns did not do this!

Breast Stretch. Pull your nipples as you inhale. Keep the stretch as you exhale while your sternum sinks a bit. Breathe three times and relax. This brings qi and blood to the breasts.

Quick Circles. This is one of the best stress relievers! Take a massage break and rub your breasts in circles, six, twelve, or thirty-six times each way. By the time you hit thirty-six you will most likely be smiling!

Brush Down. Stroke down from the heart center to the Ovarian Palace. Channel love down to transform lust. Bring the impulse of compassion into your desires. Chant the heart sound, "ha-a-a-a-a-w," as you stroke down.

IN-DEPTH
BREAST MASSAGE PRACTICES

The following exercises provide step-by-step instructions for the cultivation of deep and powerful sexual energy. It is a good idea to begin with the nipple/gland massage before massaging the body of the breasts, because the nipples are triggers for pleasure through their connection with the clitoris and the endocrine glands.

✳ Love Bud Massage

Nipples are "love buds." Touch them lightly.
They awaken the glands, opening like buds in the light.

● Nipples and Endocrine Glands

Both the nipples and the clitoris contain reflex zones of your glands. By acknowledging and stimulating the whole endocrine system you create a natural balance of your hormones (fig. 4.1).

- Smile down to your nipples and the tip of your clitoris. Gently kiss with your lips and notice your vagina squeezing around your clitoris simultaneously—as above, so below. All ring or sphincter muscles serve as orifices to the world. They like to move together. For example, if you wink your right eye, you will feel the right side of your anus squeeze! If you make a "hummmm" sound, your vagina will hum too! Kiss above and below!
- Place your warm hands over your breasts. Breathe deeply and relax. Pull up sexual energy by squeezing the PC pump (the muscles running from the pubic bone to the coccyx) and drawing qi up to the nipples.
- Gently massage up the medial side of the nipples and down the outside in a circular motion. Massage gently to avoid overstimulating the very sensitive nipples. Pull up sexual energy to the glands as you continue to massage around the nipples.
- While pulling up to the following glands, feel them as buds, drinking in the sexual waters, becoming full and juicy. You can empower and enhance each gland's inner qualities and physical function.

● Pineal Gland

Under your crown is the pineal gland, related to the thousand-petals lotus and the Hundred Meetings point (Bai Hui). This gland illuminates your inner compass and time clock. It connects you to your higher guidance. Use this gland as an antenna to pick up the clear violet light of the stars. Affirm your direction in life.

As you pull energy up to your pineal gland, massage the tips of your nipples with the heart of your hands—the center of your palms—in light circles. Affirm, "I am aligned with my highest guidance."

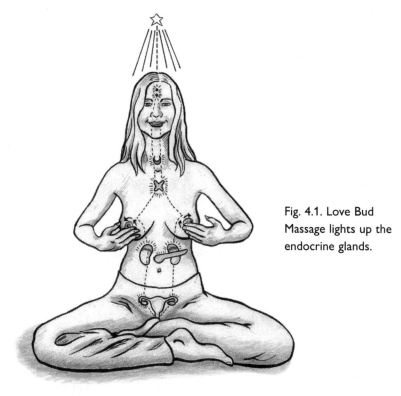

Fig. 4.1. Love Bud Massage lights up the endocrine glands.

● Pituitary Gland

The pituitary gland is behind the third eye. It empowers your inner vision and psychic ability. Intuit what is appropriate for you in the moment. Affirm, "I can intuit what is good for me from moment to moment." Open your wisdom eye. Activate your master gland. Enliven bliss to nourish your higher destiny.

When you bring your awareness to the pituitary gland, pluck your nipples with your fingertips—like you are playing a beautiful instrument. Pull all of your fingertips together and away from the nipples, releasing stagnant energy and allowing your breasts to breathe more freely. Notice a similar movement in your vagina. This movement also expands the auric field of your breasts. With this awareness you can turn on your high beams or low beams!

● Thyroid and Parathyroid Glands

The thyroid and parathyroid glands are located in the throat and are related to the throat chakra. Empower your creative expression and your dreams. Activate your metabolism and prevent thyroid imbalance, weight gain, and sluggish energy.

Massage the nipples gently in circles with your middle fingers. Affirm, "I express myself clearly and creatively. I live my dreams."

● Thymus Gland

The thymus gland, located behind the breastbone, is considered the upper heart and the center of the immune system. It produces T (thymus) cells. Blossom a golden flower to awaken your healing power.

As you pull energy up to your thymus gland, roll your nipples between the thumb and fingers like turning a doorknob. Open the doors to inner mysteries and remind yourself, "My immune system is strong and vital. My body can heal itself."

● Pancreas

The pancreas, which is located at the solar plexus, often gets tight due to stress, worry, and overcontrolling.

As you pull energy up to your pancreas, activate your digestive juices and personal power. Circle the base of the nipples with the fingertips and say, "I am open and trusting that the universe supports my life."

● Adrenal Glands

The adrenals are in the lower back above your kidneys. Unwinding the adrenals will quicken your yang, kick-start energy, and replenish your fight-or-flight responses. It will also allow your vagina to relax and surrender to the natural flow of energy.

As you pull energy up to your adrenal glands, circle the base of the nipples with your fingertips and say, "I can easily relax. I am ready for action. I access the strength of inner peace."

● Ovaries

Feel your ovaries vibrate with pink light. Feel them responding to your touch and make the conscious connection to stirring the abundance of sexual energy stored in your ovaries.

Circle around your nipples and sense energy circling around your ovaries. Affirm, "I have an abundance of creative energy and enjoy my life!"

● Uterus

Gently squeeze your nipples as you exhale "mmm" and feel the uterus contract. Release the nipples as you inhale and feel your uterus expand with qi. When a baby suckles on a mother's breast, the uterus responds.

● Heavenly Shower

- Raise your hands above your head and bring them down your midline (see Shower of Yang in chapter 7). Shower the violet light of the primordial energy from the heavens down into your glands.
- Reverse the direction of the spiral: massage up the outside of the nipples and down the inside in a circular motion, but keep your fingers a little bit off the skin. This ethereal massage will help you feel and move the qi.
- Draw heavenly energy down to each individual gland to grow its potent potential. This shower through the center of the brain stimulates the anti-aging human growth hormones. Open your crown and invite sparkling violet starlight to shower down and charge up each gland, down to the clitoris. Light up each gland like a star and sense your unique constellation of stars!

● Rest

- Cross your arms and rest with your hands over your nipples.
- Give thanks to all the glands working together for your health and well-being.
- Allow them to come into a natural hormonal balance.

※ Breast Massage with the Six Healing Sounds

This variation of the Six Healing Sounds uses the control cycle to dissolve excess negativity. If negativity is suppressed it can get stuck in the breasts and can lead to cancer. Instead, the breasts can become cauldrons for fusing and transforming energies.

- For each element, put one hand on your Jade Fountain and your other hand on the associated organ. Breathe murky colors out through your skin as you shake and tap your organ to loosen up any stuck energy.
- Move that energy into your breasts to be fused with the other energies and transformed.
- Massage your breasts up the middle and down the outside to disperse energy while exhaling with the healing sound.
- Open your eyes. Breathe in the associated virtue as pure colored mist.
    Fire element: Breathe impatience out of the breasts with the heart sound, "ha-a-a-a-a-w." Breathe in the brilliant rose red of love.

Metal element: Breathe out sadness with the lung sound, "ss-s-s-s-s-s." Breathe in the brilliant white light of courage.

Wood element: Breathe out any frustration with the liver sound, "sh-h-h-h-h-h." Breathe in the vivid green light of kindness.

Earth element: Breathe out any worry with the spleen sound, "who-o-o-o-o-o." Breathe in the radiant yellow light of openness.

Water element: Breathe out any fear with the kidney sound, "choo-oo-oo-oo." Breathe in the calm blue light of peace.

● Shower from the Heavens

- Reverse the direction of your massage, stroking down the inside like a shower of light from the heavens.
- Pull down yang energy to strengthen the hormones. Smile and draw down the heavenly energy with an ethereal massage, barely touching the skin. Sensualize the virtues as colored steam, mist, or fragrance—like a pink fragrant mist infusing the cells of your breasts.
- Massage your breasts down the middle and up the outside to gather the virtue energy. Close your eyes.

● Mix the Virtues into Compassion

- Feel the breasts glow with pure golden light. Breathe and build confidence to bring compassion into your life. Become a goddess of compassion with all her attributes.

● Rest and Absorb

- Cross your arms over your heart in a protective and containing gesture. Lay your warm hands over your breasts. Radiate love, peace, and acceptance to yourself. Absorb the virtues deeply into your soul.

Ancient Arousal

The Queen of Egypt awakens
with arms crossed
her staffs drop open
cupped hands feel her warm, full breasts
nipples poke out of her mummy bandage.
Rising like an earthquake,
the Phoenix emerges.

❄ Purging Channels Breast Massage
Getting It Off Your Chest

This variation of the Inner Smile meditation uses the control cycle to toss out excess psychic toxins from the breasts down through the channels and out the fingers and toes. Then we hold points on the breasts to feel supported.

In preparation for this practice, create a sacred space by connecting to your higher guidance to help you release what you are ready to release.

- Create a clockwise energy vortex directed into the earth to transform and neutralize energy.
- Connect with a cosmic source of unconditional love.
- Beginning with the fire element, follow the control cycle as you complete the Inner Smile practice to purge negative emotions. You can refer to the table of the negative and positive emotions on pages 83–84.

● Heart/Small Intestine

- Smile down and place your hand on your heart. Sweep your eyes sideways through the chambers of your heart, getting in touch with any impatience, hatred, arrogance, separation, or selfishness.
- Massage your breasts in big round circles—up the middle and down the outside (the dispersing direction)—as you make the heart sound, "ha-a-a-a-a-w," to clear these emotions from your chest. Repeat this three times.
- Cross your hands and bring your thumbs into your armpits, touching the Heart 1 points. Stroke down the Heart meridian along the insides of your arms, down to the pinkie fingers. At the same time, let the heart sound chase the sick winds down. Brush the pinkie fingers, then blow and flick the toxic energy down to the earth.
- Stroke up the Small Intestine meridian from the pinkie fingers up the outsides of the arms to the Small Intestine 11 point on the shoulder blades. Hug yourself. Smile and fill your heart with a warm rose or red color, as well as with all the virtues of the heart—love, joy, and respect.

● Lungs/Large Intestine

- Smile down and place your hand on your lungs. Sweep your eyes sideways through the right and left lungs, getting in touch with any sadness, tiredness, or depression.
- Hold your breasts and move them in round circles—up the middle and

down the outside—as you make the lung sound ("ss-s-s-s-s-s") to clear these emotions from your chest. Repeat this three times.

- Cross your hands over your heart center and bring your thumbs into the armpits. Stroke along the Lung meridian down the insides of the arms to the thumbs as you make the lung sound. Blow and flick the stuck energy down to the earth.

- Stroke your pointer fingers along the Large Intestine meridian—up the outsides of the arms to the first point on the Lung meridian, which is located in the groove under your collarbone. Find this point on both sides. Smile and fill your lungs with a pure sparkling white light and all the virtues of the lungs—courage, strength, and integrity.

● Liver/Gallbladder

- Smile down and place your hand on your liver. Sweep your eyes sideways through the liver, getting in touch with any anger, frustration, or irritability.

- Massage around the nipples vigorously, making about six little circles—like flower petals. Make the liver sound ("sh-h-h-h-h-h") to clear the emotions from your chest. Repeat this three times.

- Massage up the insides of your breasts, squeezing your yoni to send a jet of energy upward. Then let the energy flow down around the outsides of the breasts, then down the Gall Bladder meridian—along the rib cage and the sides of the legs to the fourth toe. Blow and flick the stuck energy down to the earth.

- Stroke up the Liver meridian, from the lateral side of the big toes up the inner legs through the ovaries and belly to the chest. Cup your breasts and allow yourself to be supported by the uplifting energy of the wood element. Smile and fill your liver and breasts with a bright emerald green light and all the virtues of the liver—kindness, generosity, and abundance.

● Spleen/Stomach

- Smile down and place your hand on your spleen and stomach. Sweep your inner eyes sideways through the spleen and stomach, getting in touch with any worry, anxiety, or attachment.

- Loosen and shake off the grip of these emotions. As you shake and vibrate your breasts, make the spleen sound ("who-o-o-o-o-o") to clear these emotions from your chest. Repeat this three times.

- Massage up the insides of the breasts, squeezing your yoni at the same time to send a jet of energy upward. Let the energy flow down the outsides of the breasts, then along the Stomach meridian—down the rib cage and the front of the legs to the second toes. Blow and flick the stuck energy down to the earth.

- Stroke up the Spleen meridian from the inner side of the big toes up the insides of the legs, through the groin crease and belly, to the chest. Cup your breasts and allow yourself to be uplifted by the unconditional support of the earth element. Smile and fill your spleen and breasts with a bright yellow light and all the virtues of the spleen—openness, trust, and stability.

● Kidney/Bladder

- Smile down and place your hand on your kidneys. Sweep your inner eyes sideways through the kidneys, getting in touch with any fear or loneliness.
- With a silky gentle touch, circle around the base of the breasts and up the Kidney meridian along the sternum. Make the kidney sound ("choo-oo-oo-oo") to clear these emotions from your chest. Repeat this three times.
- Stroke upward through the insides of the breasts to the forehead, then stroke down the Urinary Bladder meridians on the back of the head, the back, and the legs to the pinkie toes. Blow and flick the stuck energy down to the earth.
- Stroke up the Kidney meridians from the arch of the foot up the insides of the legs to the breasts. Cup your breasts and allow yourself to be supported by the floating, calm water element, like floating water lilies. Smile and fill your kidneys and breasts with a deep blue light and all the virtues of the kidneys—peace, calm, and gentleness.

● Pericardium/Triple Warmer

Smile down and place your hand over your pericardium—the protective sac around the heart. Sweep your inner eyes sideways through the heart area, getting in touch with any pessimistic feelings.

- Massage the base of your breasts in large, wide circles—up the middle and down the outside, in the earth or dispersing direction. At the same time, make the pericardium sound, "he-e-e-e-e," to clear excess heat from your chest. Repeat this three times.
- Cross your hands over your heart center and bring your thumbs into the armpits. As you make the pericardium sound, stroke down the Pericardium

meridian—along your inner arms to the middle finger. Blow and flick the stuck energy down to the earth.

- Stroke up the Triple Warmer meridians, from your ring fingers and outer arms to the Heavenly Bone point, TW 15, on the back of the shoulder. Smile and fill your pericardium with a clear light and all the qualities of the pericardium and triple warmer—balance and clarity.

✵ Five Element Breast Massage

Feminine Meditation for Cultivating Compassion

Sexual energy amplifies our emotional state, so it is very important to transform any excessive "negative" emotions into virtues. Instead, the breasts can be cultivated as melting pots for the virtue energies of the organs.

In this massage, we pull sexual energy up to the vital organs and fill the breasts with virtue energy. The order is the creation cycle—the cycle of the seasons—to enhance the growth of virtues and to generate all the five elements. The basic practice for all of the elements and organs is as follows:

- Pull sexual energy up to the organ, then massage the high-frequency energy/virtue/pure color/light of the organ into the breast. Use the massage techniques recommended for the individual elements.
- Massage around the breasts, circling up the inside and down the outside, like a fountain rising from the earth and the Ovarian Palace.

● Fire Element

Expand the heart's love into the breasts with warm outward movements. Smile down with sparkling eyes. Pulse the tongue. Fill the breasts with a rose red or pink glow.

● Earth Element

Swirl saliva and gulp down golden nectar to the spleen to nourish empathy and trust. Breathe up from the earth and pull up the left side of the anus to pump up to the spleen. Pull sexual energy up to the spleen and then up to the breasts. Cup the breasts and shake them. Shimmy the flesh in your breasts to release stress and sticky stagnation. Release anxiety. Vibrate the spleen's openness and nurturing qualities into the breasts. Trust that the universe will support you. Feel yellow light expand in the breasts.

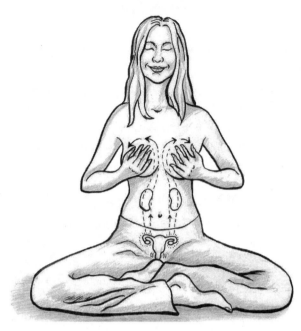

Fig. 4.2. Drawing the water energy of the kidneys into the breasts

● Metal Element

Pull up to the lungs. Breathe the lungs' strength, courage, and confidence into the breasts by cupping the breasts and moving them in big circles, breathing up and down. Feel your skin breathing. Surrender to the intelligence of the qi. Fill the breasts with a white glow.

● Water Element

Pull up the back of the perineum/anus to pump qi up to the kidneys. Stroke the gentleness of the kidneys around the base of the breasts, into the lymph nodes around the armpits, into the rib cage and the Kidney meridian along the sternum (fig. 4.2). Be gentle with yourself. Fill the breasts with a calm blue light. Relax and slow down.

● Wood Element

Pull up the right side of the perineum/anus to pump up to the liver. Generate the kindness of the liver with rolling, kneading circles—as if you have six petals around each nipple. Fill the breasts with vibrant green light. Check for any lumps or anything unusual in your breasts. Disperse stagnation. Fill the breasts with a green glow.

● Fusing Virtue Energy in the Breasts' Cauldrons

• Reverse the direction, stroking down the inside, like a shower of light from the heavens. Smile inside and draw down golden light with an ethereal massage, barely touching the skin.

- Mix the virtues into the golden glow of compassion. Feel like a goddess of compassion, like Kuan Yin. Imagine being the divine sophia with all of humanity suckling wisdom from your breasts.

- Rest your hands over your breasts and absorb the compassion deeply into your soul. Radiate love, peace, and acceptance to yourself.

🔥 Breast Massage Testimonial

Miracles are happening inside of me! I was familiar with some of the other energy work but had never really worked with my breasts before. My first reaction to the intentional focus on them was to ignite a deep yearning for love. I was filled with such sadness and loss for I had never loved my breasts or really felt them for many years. This was reflective of how I felt about myself. I had never really felt my worth or truly loved myself. I cried and cried as I infused myself with self-love.

I recently understood why I had never felt the fullness and beauty of my breasts. When I was going through puberty, I had been teased about my "high beams," meaning the reaction my nipples would have to stimulus such as my clothing or a cute boy. I felt embarrassed and learned to "turn them off." I was so successful, I turned off all feeling. I could never understand why women enjoyed the sexual stimulation of their breasts! To me, they were just there.

Now, not only do I honor and love my breasts as I learn to better honor and love myself, I have feeling in them! I further understand their subtle yet deep connection to the clitoris and the circulation of the Sexual Qi for higher and more loving connection. I am cultivating a deep love and appreciation for myself as I learn to honor my sexual energy, instead of running from abuse of it. My heart is filled with deep gratitude.

FEMININE TREASURES STUDENT

BREAST MASSAGE
AS ENERGY MEDICINE

Breast Massage is powerful medicine that can help prevent cancer and other unwanted conditions. If you have cancer, breast massage can be a nourishing addition to your other treatments.

Cancer Prevention

In the practice of Chinese medicine, breast cancer is understood as an excess condition in which stagnant qi and suppressed emotion become trapped in the breasts, forming into a body or mass. The three main internal causes for breast cancer stem out of imbalances in the earth, wood, and metal elements.

- When the earth element (stomach and spleen) is imbalanced, there is an accumulation of dampness, which is fertile ground for growths—like mushrooms growing on a damp forest floor. The corresponding emotion that arises from an imbalanced earth element is worry.
- The wood element (liver and gallbladder) moves our emotions. When we are not allowing our emotions to be moved, they tend to rise to the breasts and get trapped.
- When there is excess sadness or depression in the lungs (metal element), the breasts become tired and deficient and have less resistance to sick cells forming there.

Through breast massage in the dispersing direction, we prevent accumulation of dampness, loosen stuck emotions, and wake up the immune system, thus preventing it from sleeping on the job.

Cancer: Treating the Whole Person

Rather than just treating cancer, the whole person needs healing on physical, emotional, and spiritual levels.

- If you have cancer and are concerned about it growing, it is recommended to massage the breasts energetically—off the body—in the outward dispersing direction.
- Smile down to your thymus gland to boost your immune system to dissolve the sick cells. Affirm your body's ability to heal itself. Talk to your cells, reminding them to come back to normal function.
- Practice the Six Healing Sounds to transform the emotional root cause.
- To clear excess stagnation, practice the Qi Shaking exercise that appears in chapter 7. You can also practice the Laughing Baby, where you lie down and shake your arms and legs up in the air and laugh to drain the lymph (see chapter 3).
- Meditate, connect with, and call on your higher power, whatever that means to you.

The Power of Sound

Since stagnation of the liver can rise up and settle in the breasts, Medical Qigong uses the liver sound ("sh-h-h-h-h-h") during breast massage. The breasts resonate with loving-kindness if you cradle them while singing the healing sound "shaaaang." Sing this chant to your inner child in the F tone, the archetypal tone for the heart chakra.

Musical tones make healthy cells radiant, while unstable cancer cells can explode with sound frequencies. Fabien Maman's research shows that the consciousness in the human voice can powerfully dissolve a cancer cell in about nine minutes, while musical instruments can do the same in fourteen to twenty-one minutes.*

❀ Self-Healing Practice for Breast Cancer

To open the doors for excess trapped emotion, put your hands on your breasts and open the palms outward—as if opening a door—while chanting "shaaaang," a powerful healing sound for the lungs.

Open your eyes when you are clearing the energy, and close them as you bring your palms back to the breasts. As your palms return to your breasts, breathe in white light and the courage to heal.

● Self-Healing with Jade Egg Practice

In conditions of excess, blockage, and stagnation, like endometriosis, fibroids, and cysts, women should follow the complete protocol of Inner Smile, Three Fires Transformation, Opening Channels, and Healing the Womb before practicing with a jade egg.

The jade egg practices in chapter 6 will bring awareness to open this area, which could have been closed in some way. In the jade egg practice we use intention to also cleanse the area of blocked energy. The energy is circulated so if the river is dammed up and too full in an area we get the river to flow again! If a woman has cancer in the sexual organs I would recommend energetic massage, not even touching the skin.

---

*See *The Tao of Sound* by Fabien Maman for more information.

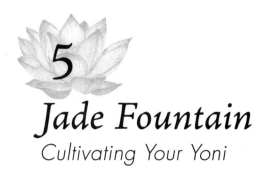

5

Jade Fountain
Cultivating Your Yoni

The yoni is naturally beautiful
like a conch shell or an unfolding bud.
Through the yoni we can drink
the fertile nectar from Mother Earth.

The yoni is an interconnected web, a source of pleasure and creative power. It is our wellspring of sexual energy. By subtly articulating the Jade Fountain we can move our creative juices through the channels and throughout the body. Being aware of yoni reflexology, we can make conscious connections between the clitoris and hormonal activation, as well as between the yoni canal and the organs. Having a loving relationship with your yoni is vital for your physical and emotional health. This chapter includes a full range of ways to breathe with your yoni and circulate sexual energy.

The yoni is also the entrance to your Core Channel. Along the Core Channel are the sexual organs of the chakras. If you imagine the chakras as flowers, their stem is the spine, their flowers extend to the front, and the stamen and pistil (sexual organs) sit in the Core Channel. By raising the sexual energy, we water these flowers and make them blossom!

✳ Exploring Your Inner Landscape

● A Journey to the Jade Fountain

The ancient Taoists regarded the feminine genitalia with respect and admired her natural beauty. They studied her landscape as an art and science. Indeed, the entrance to the yoni temple is a beautiful, natural creation similar to those found in rock crevices, hollows in trees, conch shells, and opening flowers.

The following descriptive journey into the yoni is inspired by the eloquent, poetic, erotic Chinese language. The terms in italics are direct translations from Chinese; the other imagery is my own. Descriptive terms are followed by the Latin or English equivalents in parentheses.

- Let's go on a journey to the headwaters of the *Jade Fountain* (vagina). Imagine you are the size of a pearl, walking through the *fragrant grasses* (pubic hair). Our legs tingle with delight in the swish of the long grasses. Our toes sink into the soft *moss* (pubis). We rest on the *hill of long grasses and rushes* (mound of Venus) and sigh, "Ahhh." Approaching the *Jade Gate* (labia majora), we hear a trickle of water along the smooth pink rocks. Beads of sweat form on our brow as we pass this sacred threshold. The *red pearls* (labia minora) stand like guardians of the temple and invite us in.
- We are greeted by the *lute strings of the water goddesses* (the little piece of flesh in the cleft where the labia minora meet near the clitoral crown). Looking up, we see the arch into the *dark garden* (clitoral hood) and sense the majesty of the *God Field*. The *magic jewel* (clitoral bulb) is glowing and seems to change color! This is truly a magical garden! The wind is fluttering the blanket of lichen draped over the branches (hymen) as we dance through the entrance. Perhaps the veil was broken by another traveler?
- We climb onto the *golden jade terrace* (legs of the clitoris) and sit on the *seat of pleasure* (clitoral glans). We stroke along the two smooth railings as we climb up the stairway to bliss (erectile tissue of the clitoris). It takes us higher to new plains of joy. On the *sun terrace* (vulvovaginal glands), on the sides of the tunnel walls, we drink a thick fragrant nectar (protein-rich secretions) that nourishes our journey.
- Entering the *secluded valley* (vestibule), we discover a *heavenly courtyard* with fountains flowing from the rocky walls (mucus-secreting glands). The *Jade Fountain* is magnificent, with deep folds along the tunnel where we bathe naked under the waterfalls (the tunnel traveled by menstrual fluids, ova, sperm cells, and the birthing baby). It is lit up by jewels, leading us deeper.
- Finally we arrive at the *goddess spot* (urethral sponge), and we meet the goddess of love pouring her *love juices* (orgasmic fluids from the Skene's glands) for us. Looking up, we see dripping luscious vines. We run our

fingers along the spongy surface on the tunnel's roof, which comes toward us. It feels like the ridges of a sandy shore shaped by sensual waves in an internal sea.

- We feel with our fingers a round portal. In the center there is a tiny opening, which has appeared to be closed since giving birth (external os, the opening of the cervix). Looking through the tiny peephole, we see into the red chamber, into the mystery we are graced to revisit. We slide along the pear-shaped curves of the *jewel enclosure* (uterus). We find the jade vines (fallopian tubes) and are guided to the *source of feminine yin qi* (ovaries). With gratitude we embrace the pulse of life within these two hidden gems.

- We retrace our steps carrying the gift of life and land on the *meeting of yin* (perineum). We feel as if we always belonged here. We rest at the crossroads of the infinity symbol (pelvic floor muscles), the ground of infinite possibilities. We can go anywhere from here.

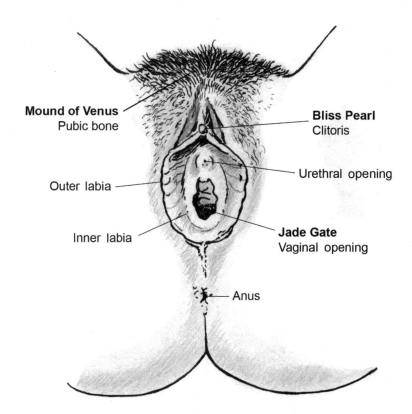

Fig. 5.1. Jade Gate, entrance to the sacred temple

THE WOMB

Palace of Creative Power

The uterus is like an upside-down pear, which sits behind the bladder and in front of the rectum. If the uterus hangs on the bladder, women experience difficulties with urination like incontinence. When the uterus is toned, the face is toned.

The qi and blood of the twelve primary channels pass into the uterus via the Thrusting Channels and the Conception Vessel. Each of the organs and channels can affect the quality and regulation of menstruation, as follows.*

- ✄ The liver provides and moves the blood.
- ✄ The heart's blood and yang nourish the uterus.
- ✄ The spleen keeps the uterus in place.
- ✄ The kidneys supply jing to the uterus.
- ✄ The Conception Vessel supplies qi to the uterus.
- ✄ The Thrusting Channels supply blood to the uterus.
- ✄ The womb is the temple of conception and the entrance of the human soul into earthly life.

❄ Baking the Sexual Palace

Place your left hand over the Sexual Palace (uterus/womb). Place your right hand over the sacrum. Rub in circles. Feel the warmth breathing between your hands. Smile to your place of creative power.

Place your right hand over your ovaries and the left hand over any part of your body that needs some healing energy; pulse the energy to that spot. Breathe and smile into the area.

SEXUAL REFLEXOLOGY

The sexual organs are like a microcosm of the whole body: in the part, there is the whole—just as a single leaf has the same shape as the whole tree. The natural healing art of reflexology is based on the principle that there are reflexes in the feet, hands, ears, and yoni that correspond to

*See *Chinese Medical Qigong Therapy*, volume 1, by Jerry Alan Johnson.

every part, gland, and organ of the body. Application of pressure on these reflexes is meant to relieve tension, improve circulation, and help promote the natural function of the related areas of the body.

The three rings of muscles inside the vagina reflect the three dantians—lower, middle, and upper. The clitoris reflects and activates the glands. Squeezing the vagina develops the strength and agility of the genitals. Yoni Breathing and jade egg practices stimulate the organs and glands by activating and massaging the reflex zones.

How genius is the design of the supreme Creatrix! The reflexology zones in the male and female sexual organs match up to each other during deep penetration (fig. 5.2). In the center of the head of the penis is the heart zone; the lungs are like wings on the sides of the heart. This heart zone meets the female heart zone near the cervix. Lovemaking is a deep inner massage of these zones.

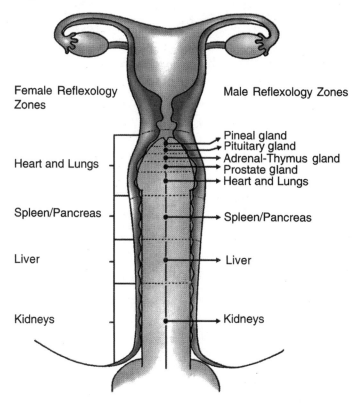

Fig. 5.2. Interaction of female and male reflexology zones
(Illustration courtesy of *Sexual Reflexology* by Mantak Chia and William U. Wei)

Making Love, Making Music

Following our heartbeat brings us
into the heat of the swelling clitoris.
Drumbeats of excitement accelerate,
with a crash of a cymbal, the strings kick in,
Playing the emotional push-pull of tango.
Building into a crescendo, the violin soars,
Whirling celestial sounds in higher octaves.
Celebrate the glory of our divine lovemaking!

THREE GATES OF THE YONI

Becoming Multiorgasmic

Becoming aware of the three gates of the yoni will help you activate the jets within the three tiers of your Jade Fountain. These jets can be stimulated in any order and in any combination. The natures of these fountains are expressions of whole-body bliss: the clitoral jet has a lubricating function; the G-spot jet is an orgasmic, pleasurable gushing from internal sources; the cervical jet is the blissful consecration of nourishment offered before entering the sacred womb.

First Gate: Clitoris

Location: The clitoris is the nodule located between the inner folds of the vulva (labia minora), at the top. The glans of the clitoris is similar to the head of a man's penis yet more sensitive. The tip of the clitoris or "bliss pearl" is like the tip of an iceberg: long legs or roots of the clitoris reach into the entrance of the vaginal canal (fig. 5.3). During sexual arousal, the vestibular bulbs fill with blood, causing the tissue to become erect. This puts pressure on the clitoral legs, which spread and appear to fly like quivering dragonfly wings inside! The blood inside the bulb's erectile tissue is released to the circulatory system by the spasms of orgasm. If orgasm does not occur, the blood exits the bulbs over several hours. Massage will help to move this blood.

Self-healing: Begin with a soft, spiraling massage off the body in the Wei Qi field. Gently massage the area of the outer and inner labia without touching the clitoris first as it can be ultra-sensitive. Then you can gradu-

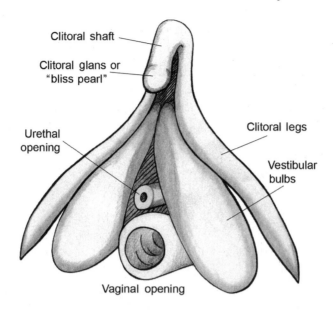

Fig. 5.3. Flying clit: bliss pearl, clitoral legs, and vestibular bulbs

ally spiral down onto the physical body like a butterfly softly landing. Be aware of which spiraling direction feels good.

Clitoral Orgasm

When most women think of orgasm they refer to this short-lived physical bliss. The aroused qi builds up in the swollen mound of Venus into a potent volcano. When she erupts there is a quick rush of intense pleasure! The clitoris is on the outside of the body, so it can be stimulated by a finger, penis, or dildo. This external part of the body is as much for the woman's pleasure as it is for the man to play with. Often, a woman will know how to best stimulate herself to climax.

A clitoral orgasm helps a woman connect with herself as a physical being capable of amazing pleasure. It is an exciting gate that awakens the sex hormones triggered by the master glands. This prepares the body for deeper journeys and higher bliss. Unfortunately, it is common to stop here due to the misconception that this is the only peak experience. Some women feel like they still are not satisfied and intuitively know there is something more.

The condition for a clitoral orgasm is to get down into your body and senses. A practice that can help induce this orgasm is to smile down to your Sexual Palace with a readiness for whole-body arousal. This is like your warm-up to dance with your partner or with yourself. Another essential way to wake up the clitoris is to practice nipple massage; these two areas of the body are linked through reflexology with each other. You can massage the nipples and the clitoris at the same time to wake up their connection.

Nectar of the first gate: The nectar secreted from the first gate or clitoris is a clear fluid that invites further entry into the sacred chamber.

Second Gate: G-Spot (Goddess Spot)

Location: You can find the G-spot by curling your middle finger into your vagina and stroking toward yourself on the upper wall—as if saying "come." If your partner is doing this, he can also make the curling finger movement. You will feel that the texture of the G-spot is similar to the ridged feeling of the roof of your mouth.

Self-healing: The G-spot can be numb or painful if it has not been awakened. This can be a sign of stagnant qi, accumulation of contracted emotion, and/or crystallized sediment from old blood. You or your partner can gently massage this area to clear blockages. It may take five or more times until you experience sensation or pleasure. Make sure you have a lot of lubrication.

G-Spot Orgasm

Simultaneous stimulation of the clitoris and the G-spot area, which is in the area of the urethra, will help induce a G-spot orgasm. A G-spot orgasm stimulates the liver zone. You will tend to grip and move a lot as the qi moves through the liver and into the tendons throughout the body.

The liver qi moves our emotions and ignites passion, so this kind of stimulation can be a passionate push-pull tango dance. There is an intense and urgent sensation like you have to pee. (Best not to go pee then, however, as you or your partner would need to start the arousal all over again! Keep reading for more about female ejaculation.)

The condition for a G-spot orgasm is intense movement and friction. A woman may want to move her body into different postures that will invite stimulation. There may be a lot of resistance that she has to move through because this gate is like opening a dam of emotions. On this part of the journey, a woman may feel like she is sweating and bushwhacking through a dense forest, before reaching the beautiful vista. With the female ejaculation there is an intense cleansing of the soul that clears the way for a spiritual orgasm.

❈ Goddess Awakening

You can help induce this intensely blissful state with a jade egg practice that is similar to rebirthing. For basic instructions on inserting and working with the jade egg, see chapter 6.

Suck up the jade egg and then pull the string in a push-pull action near the G-spot. Breathe quickly, filling up with qi on the inhalation and letting go with the exhalation. Exhaling with your mouth open will release sound and emotion. Allow your breath to speed up into a crescendo. There will be a natural, peaceful bliss afterward.

Another practice is to dance like a wild passionate animal. The effort needed to climb the mountain is contained in the instincts of the animal—it bypasses all rational thought. This wild-animal energy is needed for your eventual spiritual goal of merging with the light. So let down your hair, be wild, and be aware!

Nectar of the second gate: female ejaculation. The nectar from the G-spot is ejaculated from the Skene's glands, sometimes called the female prostate glands (see fig. 5.4 on page 186). The G-spot will swell like a bulbous sponge and may spray like a shower head, as there are many ducts within the Skene's glands. This sweet fluid has a lot of glucose in it and can have traces of urea depending on how much urine was in the bladder before ejaculation. I like to call it "sweet water."

Even though it feels like you are going to pee, this fluid is not urine. The Taoists consider it to be water essence that is released from the kidneys through the bladder and the Skene's glands. If you pee before you make love or self-pleasure, then you can be confident that this pressure is not from a full bladder, and you won't have to stop to run to the washroom.

The kidneys need to feel safe to allow ejaculation. If the kidneys are too afraid, then the fluid is frozen with fear. Feeling safe melts the ice and allows the internal waters to flow. With the contractions of the uterus during orgasm, the bladder will also contract, causing the ejaculation to

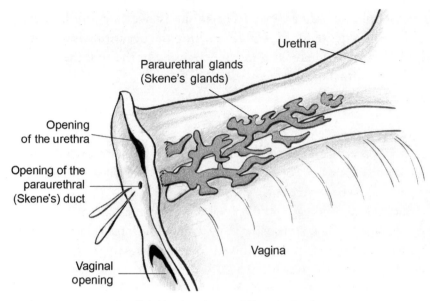

Fig. 5.4. Urethra duct and Skene's glands

flow in waves. With these orgasmic contractions there is a bearing down or pushing out sensation as if you are giving birth to your own orgasm.

Third Gate: Cervix

Location: The cervix is the entrance into the uterus, located at the very top of the yoni canal. It feels like a hard doughnut or a ring with a small opening. This opening has its own wisdom and knows when to open for conception and menstruation and ovulation.

The cervix is the reflexology area of the heart, and with loving deep penetration the heart opens. It is also the opening to the Core or Central Channel, and through this telescope we can experience the heavens. If thrusting is too aggressive and not done with love, however, the cervix shuts down and with it the heart.

✳ Feeling the Life Pulses

You can feel the life pulses of the cervix, the heart, and the master glands all at the same time.

Place one hand on your belly and one hand on your heart. Feel the pulsing of the three dantians together. Allow these areas to resonate like octaves in the same sound column. When these three centers are consciously linked up, it will induce what the Taoists call self-intercourse. (See the Divine Union Meditation on page 349.)

Cervical Orgasm

Ahhh! We made it to the top of the mountain! The vista is vast and open, and we feel at one with all of life. The bliss of being on top of the world! The heart bursts open with tears of release and joy and feels as vast as the universe. All boundaries may dissolve between yourself and your partner, and you can soar freely together in ecstasy. A fountain of bliss bubbles up through your body and encompasses both of your auras in an embrace of sublime unity. The echo of this experience is a feeling of wholeness—a full and satisfied glow that may last for days. The condition for a cervical orgasm is surrender to your natural longing to unite with the Divine. No expectation, trusting in the Divine, pure openness, allowing yourself to be taken—all of these help in letting go. As you can't fall out of the universe, you will become one with it.

Practices to induce cervical orgasm involve making space for the Divine to happen through you: prepare for grace with meditation, dance, and creativity. The practice of Unwinding allows the qi to move you spontaneously (see page 320). This requires you to surrender to the spirit and allow yourself to be taken on a journey.

Nectar of the third gate: During a cervical orgasm, the nectar called the "liquid pearl" emerges. This cervical fluid is white and thick and is nourishing for the sperm. It can also be a sign of readiness for spiritual rebirth. The liquid pearl is the cherry on top!

❀ Self-Love Awakening

We are practicing with awakened and warmed-up sexual energy, like melting a frozen iceberg of potent sexual waters and allowing it to flow. You can induce lightly aroused energy with the joy and love of your inner smile. Shine on your flower and it will rise and open to the light!

Hold one hand over your yoni and the other hand over your heart or breast. Wait for Shakti, life-force energy, to awaken, and simply allow the energy to move—no force, no push. She will quicken and rise to dance! Smile and welcome her to fill your body with delight!

Whenever you practice, it is good to remember the following:

⚔ Fantasies can bring you away from the present moment and your energy tends to be projected onto those whom you are fantasizing about. Where your mind goes, qi flows.

⚔ Do not expect or have the goal of an orgasm each time you practice!

⚔ Listen and make space for the natural wisdom of your energy.

Multiorgasmic Journey

Clitoral Orgasm: personal, physical, excited, quick rush
> Prepare to go on a journey with your water bottle!

G-Spot Orgasm: interpersonal, soulful, cleansing, energetic, emotional, engaged, tango, passionate
> Climbing the mountain, sweaty and intense!

Cervical Orgasm: transpersonal, spiritual, ecstatic, oneness, expansive, blissful
> You are on top of the world!

YONI EXERCISES

Exercising the muscles of the pelvic floor, yoni, and Sexual Palace will build your sexual energy and your overall vitality. A strong physical foundation gives you the means to reach greater heights of ecstasy!

✸ Pelvic Floor Articulation

Articulation of the pelvic muscles tones the pelvic floor, upon which all the organs rest. A strong pelvic floor supports all the organs from the base.

● Five Magic Points

The pelvic floor looks like a diamond between the pubic bone and coccyx and the two sitz bones. An infinity symbol wraps around the anus and vagina, crossing at the perineum (fig. 5.5).

Squeeze gently in pairs: the clitoral ligament and the anus toward each other, and then the two sitz bones toward each other. Then squeeze up

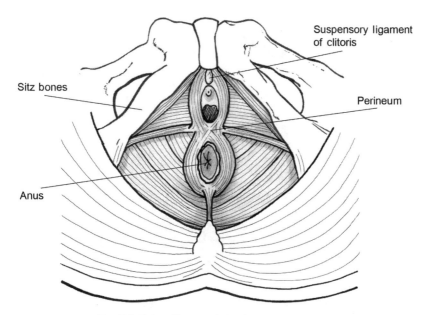

Fig. 5.5. Pelvic floor and the five magic points

the middle—the vagina and perineum—to pull up the whole diamond in one piece. Move your pelvic floor like a trampoline, which I like to call the trampoline of the spirit!

● Pelvic Floor Toner

This practice tones your pelvic diaphragm and helps lift the uterus so it does not hang on the bladder.

Press your fingertips above the pubic bone as you inhale. Suck in your lower belly by humming "hummmm." Exhale strongly with the "ma" sound while pushing your fingers out with your lower belly and the power of your pelvic diaphragm. The perineum stays buoyant.

● Relax Your Butt

If someone is a "tight-ass," their mouth will also be chronically tight. When we clench our buttocks we want to protect something or project something, but it is good to be able to relax our glutes and not remain continuously "uptight."

Allow your butt to relax to receive the Earth Qi and yet have elastic tone to uphold the organs.

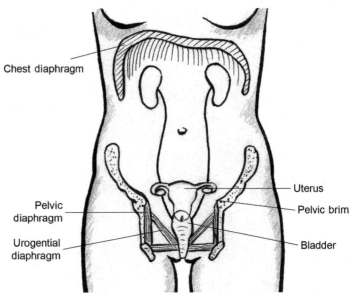

Fig. 5.6. Female pelvic diaphragm and urogenital diaphragm

● Wink Ups

If you wink with your right eye, notice how the right side of your anus contracts.

• Wink with the left eye to pull up the left side of the PC muscle, then the right eye to pull up the right side of the PC muscle. Feel the connection up to the brain.

   Winking will never be the same again! It is actually pretty sexy to wink!

● Peeing Practice

This practice can be done when you pee to test the strength of your pelvic floor and to exercise your urogenital diaphragm (fig. 5.6). Toward the end of urination pull up to stop the flow as you inhale. To accelerate the flow of urination, exhale and bear down into the dantian. If you can't stop the flow of urination, then you really need to practice with the jade egg to build the strength of the pelvic floor and lift the bladder off the uterus. This can prevent and heal incontinence.

● Uterus Lift

With gravity gradually bearing down on their bodies, many women get the "sag and spread" syndrome. Without the uplifting force of qi, the organs

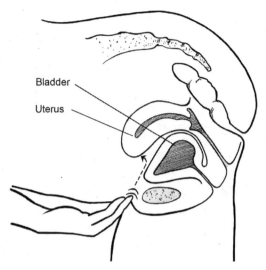

Fig. 5.7. Lifting the uterus off the bladder

can prolapse and start to drop and hang. To counterbalance this tendency you need the uplift or levity of the life force, like a tree growing up against gravity.

The purpose of the uterus lift is to lift the weight of the uterus off the bladder so the bladder can function properly.

- In a standing position, cross one foot in front of the other. Inhale as you lift your arms up to lengthen the spine.
- Bend forward at the hips, lowering your arms as you exhale. Hook all four fingers of one hand above the pubic bone (fig. 5.7).
- Inhale, bending your knees slightly. Then exhale, pressing your feet into the ground and straightening your legs as you pull your uterus up off the bladder, saying "lift." Trust that your uterus will respond to the encouragement of your mind.
- Repeat the above steps several times, then uncross your legs so your feet are hip-width apart. Hold on to the kidney and bladder points around the back ankles. Wag your tail/sacrum from side to side. This releases the spine, tones the Urinary Bladder channels, and releases tension in the pelvic floor.
- Push your feet down against the floor as you roll up slowly, inhaling. Roll your shoulders down your back.
- Repeat on the other side. After finishing both sides and returning to a

standing position, enjoy the rising sensation like mist rising up, clearing your head.

✳ Yoni Toning

*Become as articulate with your yoni
as you are with your mouth!*

Singing reduces the stress hormones cortisol and cortisone, relaxes the nervous system, and boosts the immune system. These practices integrate our sexual and throat chakras to empower our creative voice. They also tone our muscles as we tone or sound to accompany our movements.

Our orifices connect us with the world. The sphincter muscles around the orifices like to move together; "as above, so below." Make the sound "mmmmm," like you are kissing. Notice what happens to your yoni.

● Seed Syllables

Keep your right hand on your lap with the palm up to ground the rising tones, while the left hand moves up the chakras. Sing up the scale, using the note names in parentheses as your guide:

- Place your left hand in the right palm in front of the root chakra and sing "lam" (do).
- Place your left hand on your yoni and sing "vam" (re).
- Place your left hand on your navel and sing "ram" (mi).
- Place your left hand on your heart and sing "yam" (fa).
- Place your left hand on your throat and sing "ham" (sol).
- Place your left hand on your third eye and sing "om" (la).
- Sing "so hum" (ti do)—liberation! Touch your crown with "so" and reach up with "hum." Take your hat off to the Divine!

Clear down with rainbow light, sweeping your left hand down in front of your chakras. Hum "mmmm" down the scale. Switch hands and repeat.

✳ Strengthening the Ring Muscles

The following exercises focus particularly on the three rings of muscles inside the vagina. By engaging these muscles, you learn to ride your sexual energy like a horse. You can give direction by pulling the reins with muscle control. When you are in tune with your horse power, it will respond to just your mind. As they say in Zen, "The horse (the body-mind) responds to the shadow of the whip."

● Suck Nectar with a Kiss

Draw energy up through your yoni like sucking nectar up a straw. Do not oversqueeze like a "sourpuss" or a "tight-ass!" Smile inside and squeeze your yoni like a kiss.

● Reverse Breathing

This breathing increases the suction of qi into the body. Women can use this exercise to tone the sexual organs, especially after childbirth. It will help uplift the uterus so it does not hang on the bladder. (For detailed description with arm movements see Spinning Wheel on page 303.)

- Inhale into your kidneys and widen them. Draw your belly in and squeeze the yoni. Draw qi to the kidney point in the back. Suspend the breath at this point to build kidney energy.
- Exhale into the Sea of Qi point below the navel. Let your belly move outward. Move the qi forward to the navel and down to the dantian. Your hands make a small circle in front of your lower abdomen.

● Engaging the Gates

Your ability to close the gates helps prevent energy leakage. Opening the gates helps you channel energy into whole-body orgasm. Relaxing the muscles helps you receive energy.

- Squeeze the lower gate by the vagina lips to stimulate the kidneys.
- Squeeze the middle gate of the vagina channel to stimulate the liver and spleen.
- Squeeze the upper gate by the cervix to stimulate the lungs and heart.

● Toning the Three Rings

Activate the three rings of muscles in the yoni canal as you sound "oh" and "uuu" (as in "you").

- Make the "oh" sound on a higher tone (mi) and a lower tone (do). Notice how your vagina moves when you sound "oh."
- Contract the upper ring by the cervix as you sound the higher "oh."
- Contract the lower ring—the clitoris and vagina lips—as you sound the

lower "oh." Indicate this internal movement with your hands by touching your wrists and then your fingertips together, making an O shape with your hands. Say "oh, oh!"

- Contract the middle ring of muscles in the vagina channel. Let the left and right sides squeeze together and sound "uuu" as in "youuu." At the same time, clap your hands together in front of your yoni. Imagine your yoni is clapping her hands with joy!

Notice if the left and right sides squeeze equally. If not, try to make them more even. This will help balance any asymmetry in the sides of the body.

● Yoni Elevator

- Squeeze up the lower, middle, and upper muscles of the yoni with three sips (small inhalations): vagina lips, urogenital diaphragm, and deep yoni canal by the cervix.
- Exhale and bear down. Move an imaginary or real jade egg up and down in the yoni canal like an elevator.

● Toning Up the Pumps

- Hum "m-m-m" with rising tones (as in "do-re-mi") to lift the energy up the yoni elevator. Place your fingertips above your pubic bone to feel the lift of yoni muscles and the urogenital diaphragm. Inhale down into your belly while singing "m-m-m."
- Once you have the internal lift, then lift the energy up your sacral, adrenal, and dorsal pumps simultaneously, while continuing to hum "m-m-m" (do-re-mi). Invite someone to press your pumps with their hand to feel the sound vibration in your spine.

● Crystal Bliss Toning

Repeat the previous practice but use the "nng-nng-nng" sound and resonate longer in the skull. Raise the frequency to resonate bliss in the master glands. The "nng" sound lifts vibration above the nose and resonates in the midbrain, the Crystal Palace. Smile as you sing to draw up the sexual energy effortlessly.

Chant "nng-nng-nng" with rising tones (like "do-re-mi") to lift energy up through the sacral, adrenal, and dorsal pumps. Hold out the exhalation for six counts to create empty force, which sucks qi upward.

Inhale and pop open the dantian with wonder and breath.

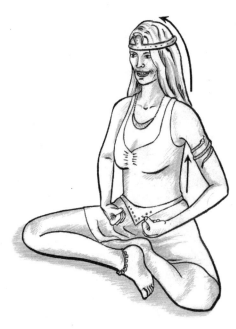

Fig. 5.8. The high priestess raises her serpent power.

● High Priestess

Sublimate your sexual energy to the majestic and mysterious archetype of the priestess. The priestess channels divine light and the natural Shakti power of nature (fig. 5.8).

- Sit tall on your meditation throne.
- Inhale as you lift your hands. Tone "m-m-m" as you catch smiling energy into your eyes and draw your fingers toward your third eye.
- Tone "f-f-f" as you lower your hands and let the energy fall down your Front Channel, like a waterfall of smiling energy. Let go and soften the solar plexus.
- Quickly inhale, sipping up Earth Qi into your perineum.
- Tone "s-s-s" as you shoot energy straight up your spine, making fists and tightening your anus (like in a Power Lock). Hiss like a serpent that is rising and flicking its tongue at the third eye. The snake is a symbol of the sacred feminine and kundalini energy. Feel like a female pharaoh or high priestess wearing a jeweled snake in her headdress. Become confident of your mastery of your Shakti power.
- Inhale with your mouth open in a state of awe, "aaah!"

To enter the kingdom of heaven, become a child again,
with childlike wonder.

CULTIVATING SEXUAL ENERGY

Turning on Your Jade Fountain

The cultivation of sexual energy requires a strong connection with your physical body and with your sources of energy. Let the explorations begin!

What Is Her Name?

Many English names for female genitalia tend to be dark, childish, or scientific—like "down there," "private parts," "pussy," or "vagina." Are you ready for a new name that expresses the meaningful, energetic function?

Yoni, the Sanskrit name for female genitalia, embraces the anatomy, energetic functions, and spiritual dimensions of this vital region. The yoni is the creative power of nature and represents the goddess Shakti, female creative energy. *Lingam* is the Sanskrit name for male genitals. A lingam stone is an upright stone that represents Shiva, and it is usually placed in the yoni stand. The lingam and yoni united represent the indivisible oneness of male and female, passive space and active time, nonduality and limitless potentiality. Their union represents the eternal process of creation and regeneration. In the ancient tantric tradition, Shiva is recognized as the embodiment of pure consciousness, and Shakti as the embodiment of pure energy. Their sacred union manifested spirit into form; thus from the tantric view, creation of the universe in all its manifestations is an act of love.

Jade Fountain is the poetic name that Taoists gave to the female genitalia. This name describes so well the fountain of youth and gushing sensation when you squeeze her jet and a fountain of blissful jade juice rises and overflows in and around the body.

New Name—Fonsli!

Fonsli means "my dear little fountain": *fons* is Latin for "well," "spring," or "fountain," while *li* is an endearment after names in Swiss. In the movement art called Eurythmy, "lll" is a water sound that moves like a fountain; the "eee" sound has an uprising, self-asserting quality. So *fonsli* was born! When I shared this name with people, they laughed because it sounds like "Fonzie," a macho TV character from the 1970s. So we reclaimed the "Fons," this time with a feminine character! One woman said it makes her feel like gently holding and fondling her "fonsli." I have become quite fond of this new name for Her!

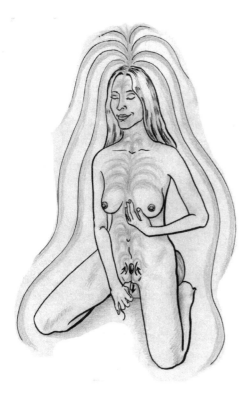

Fig. 5.9. Fonsli, my dear little
fountain, spreads sexual
energy

Wellspring of life,
Mmm, my dear little fountain,
Fonsli, Fonsli, oh my Fonsli!
Gushing, rising, overflowing
Shakti power is ever-growing!

The Yin and Yang of Sexual Energy

Yin and yang are aspects of a dynamic whole. Sexual energy in its yin or cool, passive, unaroused phase is full of potential—like a seed in winter. You can feel it as a steady pulse of life in your ovaries, kidneys, and bones. Moving from yin to yang, the energy awakens, warms up, moves, grows, and builds in excitement. When aroused by the fire of desire and passion it expands into a yang, hot, active, ecstatic, or orgasmic phase of vibrant expression. Then the energy settles back into the yin phase, gathering what is valuable to us, releasing and relaxing. These phases may interchange during lovemaking, or in the cycle of a day, or even within a relationship. As your internal state shifts you can follow the steps for cultivation in a yang or yin way as needed.

Yang Cultivation—Lighting Your Lamp

Yang cultivation activates and mobilizes sexual energy, transforming jing into Jing Qi, which then becomes fluid and available for distribution throughout the body. Yang cultivation is good for addressing problems like frigidity, low desire, cold womb, dampness, candida, states of fear or inhibition, or disconnect between the heart and sexuality. In any case, yang energy will light your passion and get your life steamy and alive!

The yang approach begins with the yang pole, the golden smiling energy, to warm and open the heart and awaken the heart's loving fire. We descend this warmth down to the Ovarian Palace to melt the iceberg of potential, yet frozen, sexual energy. This alchemical process creates steam, which is readily movable and digestible in the body, soul, and spirit. We start pumping this sexual steam with the yoni's squeezing and releasing movement—like a steam piston. This energy, like a warmed-up jet, can be projected to different channels or organs in the body.

To summarize the yang approach, practice Inner Smile, breast massage, ovarian and uterus massage, Yoni Breathing, and Upward Draws. The warmth of the heart melts the icy cold fear in the womb and the pool of inner jing starts to bubble and steam. Move the steam around the Microcosmic Orbit by doing the Crane Neck.

Yin Cultivation—Putting Fuel into Your Lamp

The yin approach nourishes sexual energy with the earth's fertile jing, as well as with the prenatal and ancestral jing stored within the kidneys. You would practice this type of cultivation in the case of low energy, adrenal fatigue, high blood pressure, ungroundedness, disconnection from the earth, lack of will, or stressed-out feelings. The positive intention is that through deep relaxation you allow yourself to fill up. Your energy comes from a place of fullness and giving rather than from neediness. You feel you are supported from deeper resources of vitality.

In this approach we start with the yin pole, bringing yin sources of energy from the earth up through the Bubbling Springs point (KD 1 on the sole of the foot) into the kidneys. This establishes a healthy pipeline that fills the kidneys.

The overflow of this energy will pour over from the kidneys into the ovaries, our potential essence. Imagine how many eggs we are given at birth: every girl is born with over a million immature eggs, or follicles, in her ovaries. With each menstrual cycle, a thousand follicles are lost and only one lucky little follicle will mature into an ovum (egg), which is released into the fallopian tube, kicking off ovulation. Out of thousands of follicles only about four to five hundred will ever mature. We are given so much abundance that can be sublimated up through our chakras for our evolution.

If we need more accessible energy or "cash" to invest in new growth, we withdraw from our "savings account"—our inheritance in the kidneys— the sexual essence given by our ancestors. You need money (Prenatal Jing) to make money (Jing Qi).

To summarize the yin approach, practice Kidney Breathing, ovarian and uterus massage, Yoni Breathing, and Upward Draws.

Yoni Mudra—Locating Your Ovaries

To locate your ovaries, place your hands in a downward triangle, thumbs at the belly button. Where your index fingers touch is where your uterus is, and beneath your pinkie fingers are your ovaries.

✳ Yoni Breathing

Yoni Breathing increases blood and qi circulation, warms up the sexual organs, activates your Shakti power/sexual energy, and tones the lower diaphragms and pelvic floor. It is a good prelude to Ovarian Compression exercises, as well as the Upward Draw and Power Lock. I call these practices Yoni Breathing rather than Ovarian Breathing because we are engaging more than our ovaries in the breathing process.

While practicing Yoni Breathing please remember that *the release is as important as the squeeze.* Tightening and relaxing builds a strong pelvic floor, because a strong muscle is able to both fully contract and fully release. Do not overexert your muscles with mechanical exercise by thinking that more is better. Doing lots of reps of contractions and not fully releasing can cause muscles to become too tight and locked short. Remember to play and feel the whole body move subtly from within, like a jellyfish moves through water.

- Smile down to your ovaries. Rub your hands until they're warm, then rub your ovaries in circles. Spiral the energy in and around the sexual organs. Lift your hand three inches away from the ovaries and feel the aura of the ovaries pulsating.
- Brush down from the ovaries to the uterus and feel the uterus sucking in the ovarian qi.
- Inhale and gently squeeze the vagina as if sucking up and pushing down an imaginary jade egg using the three rings of muscles. (See chapter 6 for more detailed jade egg practices.)
- Blow down internally and lift the pelvic floor at the same time. The belly pushes out. Take notice that when you squeeze your vagina your belly pulls in, and when you exhale down your belly pushes out. This is what is called reverse breathing. On the inhalation, the expansion moves into the lower back and the kidneys; on the exhalation the qi pressure builds in the lower dantian below the navel. By sealing the lower gate we retain and build the energy. This action of up and down pumping will tone the internal muscles and warm up the qi.
- Pump the lower abdomen like a bellows fans a fire with quick forceful exhalations through the nose. This warming breath is called the Breath of Fire. The movement is buoyant, like a golden yo-yo that does not fall to the ground.
- Continue with this Yoni Breathing until a feeling of warmth gathers at the Sexual Palace (between the ovaries, about four finger-widths from the navel).
- Breathe rhythmically, with nine quick breaths and one slow, deep pull upward in between. This trains for shallow and deep thrusting in dual cultivation.

Since I have been practicing Yoni Breathing and jade egg and changed my consciousness about sexuality, I am on a big healing path, liberating a lot of shame and experiencing more joy in relationship with myself. My menstruation is much gentler; I have much less pain in premenstruation and less strong bleeding. Since the teacher training I am sharing these practices and women love it!

SIMONE ESTHER,
GRADUATE OF SACRED FEMININITY

✺ Ovarian Compression

Ovarian Compression builds sexual heat, increases fertility, and stokes the digestive fire. What kind of energy do you want to hold in your sexual organs? Loving energy! By holding smiling energy in the ovaries and uterus we increase internal qi pressure. This pressure kindles passion and burns up the "heavy water" of sluggish stagnation in the lower body, which is a major source of ill health.

Ovarian Compression works like an old-fashioned water pump: you add some priming water and start pumping until the water pumps up by itself. You breathe in smiling energy, compress it into the yoni, and then the pressure uplifts the sexual waters.

Because the womb is a space where women tend to store negativity, it is good to practice Womb Cleansing (see chapter 3) before holding the qi in the sexual organs.

- Breathe in smiling energy. Inhale a golden ball of qi into the third eye. Sip it down to the throat, solar plexus, navel, and Sexual Palace. With each sip the golden ball gets fuller and bigger. Avoid sipping into the heart as this can be too much pressure for the heart.
- Roll the qi ball down. Pull up the vagina to pack the ovaries. Hold the breath. Smile down as you wrap the energy around the ovaries twelve times. Take another sip and draw earth energy into the uterus and wrap inside six times.
- Swallow the charged-up saliva deeply down. This relieves pressure in the head and nurtures the belly.
- Exhale, and feel the pressure rise up the spine. Ding! A red light goes on in the brain, like swinging a sledgehammer in a circus game to ring the "Qigong!" This can feel like a brain orgasm. Let the qi swirl in the brain as your outbreath is suspended. Mix sexual energy with heavenly qi to generate mental and spiritual power.
- Inhale the elixir into the navel center.
- Catch your breath with Yoni Breathing.

✺ Lotus Sublimation

Sublimation is the process of elevating and transmuting sexual desires into the development of the psyche and spiritual experience. The sublimation practices raise energy levels so that the chakras vibrate at higher frequencies. Sublimation is the art of creating sexuality that is a sublime, royal, and golden state.

This practice draws sexual energy up the Core Channel, the Front Channel, and the Back Channel. The soul gestures or mudras express inner realizations that come from within. Channel the enlivened or aroused sexual energy to higher centers and bring down the refined essence and nectar into your center.

● Lotus Bud Breathing

- Feel your feet rooted in the mud and breathe in earth energy through your Bubbling Springs points.
- Form your hands into small downward-pointing lotus buds or beaks in front of your Ovarian/Sexual Palace. Simulate a flower bud opening and closing, pulling your fingers together as you inhale and relaxing your fingers apart as you exhale.
- Notice that when you pulse the buds or beaks, it helps to suction the power of earth energy into the feet and the yoni canal. Sense your yoni breathing like an upside-down bud sucking nectar from the earth. Practice six times before each sublimation.

● Core Power

- Practice Lotus Bud Breathing six times. Exhale down into your yoni.
- Draw energy up the Core Channel into the cauldron at the center of your body. The vitality will naturally spread from this "Grand Central Station" to where it is needed.
- Place your hands in the Yoni Mudra with thumbs at the navel as you hold your breath for a moment (fig. 5.10). Feel a seed of potent energy centered in your core. Exhale down into your lower dantian.

● Heart Blossoming

- Practice Lotus Bud Breathing six times. Exhale down into the yoni.
- Draw energy up the Core Channel to your heart and feel it open like a flower. Sexual waters nourish the heart, where passion grows compassion.
- Place your hands in front of the heart center with the pinkies and thumbs touching, like a flower. Smile into your beautiful, blossoming flower. Suspend your breath for a moment, being in awe, "Aha!"

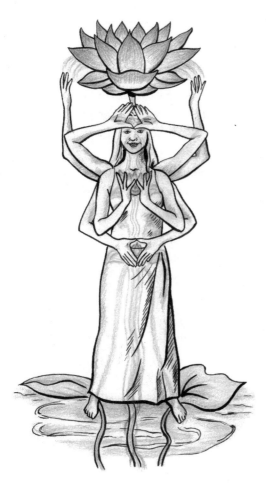

Fig. 5.10. Lotus Sublimation, sublime blossoming of the lotus

- Exhale down into your lower dantian to fill your cauldron with the refined elixir.

● Third Eye Opening

- Practice Lotus Bud Breathing six times. Exhale down into the yoni.
- Draw energy up the Front Channel to your third eye and feel it open like a wisdom eye. Its energy supports the psychic development of intuition and insight.
- As you suspend your breath, hold your hands like a prism in front of your forehead. Form an upward-pointing triangle, with your index fingers together at the apex and your thumbs together forming the base. Exhale down into your lower dantian.

● Crown's Higher Octaves

In this exercise, the hands above your head describe a halo—a satellite dish that picks up higher octaves.

- Practice Lotus Bud Breathing six times. Exhale down into the yoni.
- Draw energy up the spine (the stem of your inner plant) to the crown. Pointing to the spine with the backs of your hands together, draw your hands up over your head.
- Open the crown like a thousand-petal lotus. Begin with your pinkie fingers touching in the back, then circle forward around the ring of your halo so the pinkies touch in the front.

What seems outside of us (palms facing out) becomes inside (palms facing in). Our awareness embraces all. This is another "Aha" moment as we shift from duality to nondual consciousness.

● Return to the Seed

- Practice Lotus Bud Breathing six times. Exhale down into your lower dantian.
- Lower your arms while pulling down the heavens to your navel, returning the seed power to your core. Place your hands over the navel and collect the energy.

In the seed is the whole universe.

❋ Upward Draws

In these exercises, pull energy up your spine in small sips, as though you're sipping up through a straw and holding your finger on the end to suspend the fluid. After each Upward Draw, exhale and bear down into your lower dantian. The compression of your qi ball in your core enhances the opposing upward force.

- Warm up your sexual energy by breathing into your pelvis and rubbing your sacrum. Warm qi naturally rises.
- Inhale and squeeze your yoni and perineum, activating the whole band of pubic to coccygeal muscles (PC pump). With an extra sip (small inhalation), pull up your anus and the "Long Strong" point below the tip of your tailbone, opening the trapdoor into the spine. Your tailbone will tuck in a bit as you draw the qi up to your sacrum.

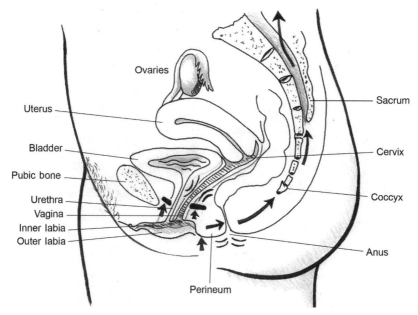

Fig. 5.11. Pulling up qi through the yoni,
perineum, coccyx, and sacrum

- Sip and draw the sexual energy up the spine to the adrenal pump, dorsal pump, and cranial pump with your chin slightly tucked in and your crown lifted.
- Look in and up with your eyes as you sip up to the crown. Spiral the energy there nine times outward counterclockwise and nine times clockwise, funneling heavenly qi into the Crystal Palace. Press your tongue up into the soft back palate, called the Heavenly Pool, to activate the glands of bliss.
- Exhale, bringing any excess pressure or warmth down to cauldron.

● Single Upward Draw

- Using the spine like a straw, inhale with long, smooth draws. Pull energy up to the crown, maintaining contraction below. Suspend at the crown and exhale down. Move energy like a water wheel.
- Use your mind and eyes to direct the energy more. Smile into it. When you smile, your pelvic floor lifts and the sexual energy is effortlessly raised.
- Bring down the Heaven Qi and spiral it into an elixir. Bring this elixir down to the belly and circulate it in the Microcosmic Orbit.

● Several Upward Draws

- Inhale and pull up to the crown three times without exhaling in between. Spiral like a pink tornado, charging up your brain. Exhale down.
- Circulate the refined energy in the Microcosmic Orbit and collect it.

● Seven Pools Breathing

Replenish your yin by filling pools of sexual waters in your body. Sensualize that these pools are connected by seven waterfalls and circle back to the source spring again. Recall the fresh feeling of being in a waterfall.

This exercise is best done sitting, with your back erect.

- Your Inner Smile is like the sunshine sparkling on the water.
- Your tongue is in the Heavenly Pool—the back soft palate.
- Inhale to one pool, hold your breath, and then exhale to the next pool. As you suspend your breath you can spin the energy like water rolling over a round rock. Make an affirmation about becoming full of life, like "I am luscious" or "I am juicy."
- Begin with the Bubbling Springs point, and continue inhaling and exhaling through each of the seven pools below.

1. Bubbling Springs. Deep springs in the earth bubble up through the soles of the feet.
2. Kidneys. Hold your hands over your kidneys.
3. Ovaries. Place your hands over your ovaries.
4. Uterus. Many rivers originate in this tidal pool, which empties and fills with the phases of the moon.
5. Perineum. This is the Hui Yin point ("Meeting of Yin"), which connects us with sources of yin from the earth.
6. Brain/Sea of Marrow. Exhale, squeeze your anus, and thrust a jet or geyser up to the brain.
7. Sea of Qi. This point is two finger-widths below the navel. After holding the qi here, exhale and compress it into a blue pearl of water essence. Affirm in your pearl your ability to peacefully fill your pools of jing.

● Jing Express

This practice awakens and activates the body, stimulates more yang, and warms you up. Distribute the gems of jing from the kidneys into the body for whole-body radiance!

- Sit up with a tall spine, chin lightly tucked in so the base of your skull is open.
- Smile as you breathe. The tongue is in the fire position behind the teeth.
- Sip to each energy center like sipping nectar: kidneys, ovaries, uterus, and perineum.
- Exhale and thrust energy up the spine to the crown with Empty Force Breathing. Suspend the breath for three counts as you smile to universal qi.
- Inhale back into the cauldron at the dantian.
- Exhale, compressing the qi into a golden pink pearl.
- Affirm in your pearl your ability to awaken your vibrant jing.

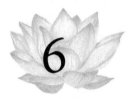

6

Jade Egg Practices

The jade egg practices were initially developed long ago by the three female advisors of the Yellow Emperor. In modern times there has been a renaissance of using yoni eggs to cultivate the female sexual energy. Many of the practices presented in this book have been created through the sharing of my personal practice with other women.

Jade egg practices strengthen the pelvic floor; warm, circulate, and activate the sexual energy; articulate the vagina as an instrument of love; and open portals for endless dimensions of orgasm. In these practices, the jade egg is placed inside the vagina and moved in such a way that it massages the reflexology zones of the vital organs. The practices have the result of lessening blood loss and discomfort during menstruation. The blood is transformed into qi and circulated through the body to nourish the soul and spirit. The integration of awareness, touch, movement, sound, and breath leads us into endless discovery of ourselves as creative, sexual beings.

Jade is an ancient stone that has historically been used to attract love. The Chinese have always valued this stone more than gold because of its balanced energy. Jade is the sacred crystal of the wood element, which activates the liver and the uprising movement of qi. This element moves the sexual energy and is the power behind arousal and erection. It enhances creativity. Jade was considered to be hardened dragon sperm!

Jade eggs have a high vibration. Exercises with a real or imaginary jade egg inserted into the yoni, with a real or imaginary weight attached, build internal strength. They increase tone in your pelvic floor and bladder like a form of internal Pilates. A strong pelvic floor is vital for preventing prolapsed organs and energy leakage. Developing a springy trampoline quality in the pelvic floor enhances our ability to raise energy to higher centers.

In addition to strengthening the pelvic floor, regular practice with a jade egg also has the following benefits:

- Activates strong and vital hormones. (Squeezing the jade egg surges energy up through the glands.)
- Helps relieve PMS.
- Massages the whole body from within (by massaging the reflexology zones of the vital organs within the yoni).
- Lifts the uterus up off the bladder to prevent incontinence.
- Tones the facial skin (a natural consequence of toning the uterus).
- Tones the vaginal canal and G-spot, enhancing sexual satisfaction for both partners.

It's hard to find words to express how working with the jade egg has changed my life. From healing old deep emotional and sexual wounds and traumas to experiencing pleasure on a whole new level, I am not the same person I was seven years ago, when Minke introduced me to the jade egg practices. Not only did I change inside, I also changed my whole lifestyle, making me feel alive again, nourished, and most of all loved to the core of my being!

It brought to my attention a conscious choice of having this reflected to me in relationship as well. Once I opened up my channels and let love pour through me, there was no going back to an old habitual way, even if it felt like it for periods of time. I attracted a partner also cultivating sexual energy and so we are able to generate a lot more energy together than on our own.

The jade egg practices help me to stay connected to a divine love and to myself. It's like having my own love affair with myself, which then translates to a much more vital, healthy, and vibrant body and an extremely fulfilling sex life! Miracles happen on a daily basis; an abundance of energy and love and manifesting becomes second nature after a while.

LENKA, UNIVERSAL HEALING TAO INSTRUCTOR
AND SACRED FEMININITY FACILITATOR

CHOOSING YOUR JADE EGG

Yoni eggs can be purchased in several sizes and materials. Jade is preferable because it is sturdy, smooth, and nonporous. Jade can also be drilled, so that a string can be attached for resistance training and easy removal. If possible, find an egg with the hole drilled across the small end, so there is less string on the egg (fig. 6.1).

Medium-sized eggs are most commonly used for these practices. Medium is a good size for gripping and for toning your yoni. If the egg falls out when you stand up, you could consider using a larger egg. A larger egg is also helpful if a woman's yoni has been stretched from childbirth. I like using a larger one as an internal anchor in Bathtub Bliss practice. A large egg has more weight for walking and moving around. The small eggs can be used if a woman's yoni muscles have shrunk from lack of use. Playing with two smaller eggs inside can be fun! You could gradually build up to a medium one.

Jade comes in many colorful tones ranging from light to dark green, lavender, gray, white, and yellow. The dark green is nephrite jade and has the properties of deep yin vitality.

Other crystals can be explored for subtle shifts in your healing and empowering experiences. Your yoni will amplify the healing effect of the crystal. You may choose a crystal that attracts you or a crystal that will have an alchemical effect—like a red-colored egg to warm the water element. You may also choose a crystal to attune with the moon's phases—obsidian at the new moon, rose quartz at the full moon, and jade at any time. Here are some examples:

* Black obsidian, glassy lava, is a powerful psychic cleanser that protects you from negativity and grounds you to Gaia's core. This crystal is a catalyst for releasing from abuse or attachment. It also helps to clear bacterial or viral infections.
* Rose quartz, with its pink color, can enhance self-love. This crystal has planes inside, which can break, so handle with care. I recommend low-impact practice with this crystal: meditation, Heart/Yoni Breathing, and sleeping with your egg.
* Green aventurine's color resonates with the heart chakra and thus enhances emotional balance.

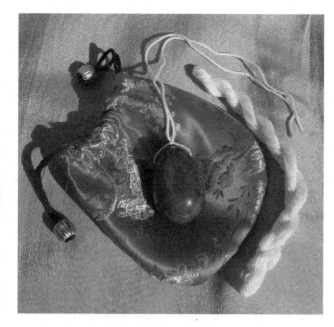

Fig. 6.1. Jade egg with silk string and brocade bag (Photo by Minke de Vos)

Be careful when buying your egg that it was not treated with dye, chemicals, polishes, or radiation for color enhancement. You can buy certified nephrite jade, obsidian, and rose quartz yoni eggs at taotantricarts .com and femininetreasures.com.

Threading the String

Silk cord is strong and long-lasting; cord that is smooth and tightly spun is ideal. It is more comfortable for pulling the string in the practices.

Cut a single string about twenty inches or fifty centimeters, long enough that you can tie a bag of weights. If your jade egg is horizontally drilled it will be easy to thread. If your egg is vertically drilled, you can ease insertion by threading it with a floss threader (a blue loop you can buy at a pharmacy). Tie a double knot close to the egg, at the small end, like you are tying a shoe two times.

Replace the string as needed. If you prefer throwing away your string after use, ribbon dental floss (like Glide) lies flat on the egg.

Caring for Your Jade Egg

Before the first use you can sterilize your egg by pouring boiling water into a cup and submerging the egg in this hot water for five minutes. Do not boil the egg directly, as this can damage the subtle vibration of the crystal.

Jade is a very strong stone but other stones can be more fragile. This treatment will also remove any wax that may have been used to polish the egg. For regular use, cleanse your egg with hot water and a few drops of tea tree oil soap. You can also use a few drops of highly diluted tea tree or lavender essential oil, or apple cider vinegar. Use of soap depends on your sensitivity to the ingredients in the soap; Dr. Bronner's tea tree castile soap is a mild natural soap that is generally nonirritating.

You can clean the cord along with your egg in hot water and tea tree oil soap. Carefully wash through the drilled hole and move the string as if you were flossing teeth. Rinse well with lots of running water, and dry thoroughly. Let it cool off before use!

Place your jade egg on your altar so it does not hide in your drawer! You can give your jade egg a name but do not tell anyone, as it is like the genie in the bottle! Bathe your jade egg in the sun or moonlight to charge it up with cosmic energy.

SELF-HEALING WITH JADE EGG PRACTICES

In conditions of excess, blockage, and stagnation—like endometriosis, fibroids, and cysts—women should follow the complete protocol of Inner Smile, Three Fires Transformation, Opening Channels, and Healing the Womb before practicing with a jade egg. The jade egg practices will bring awareness to open this area, which could have been closed in some way. Use your intention to cleanse the area of blocked energy. The energy is circulated so if the river is dammed up and too full in an area we get the river to flow again! If a woman has cancer in the sexual organs I would recommend energetic massage, not even touching the skin.

Avoid forcing and pushing yourself, which will make practice another "I should do it" task, which can then become mechanical. Jade egg practice is not just push-ups with the vagina! If you are restoring your pelvic floor and sexual organs, you may wish to practice daily. I recommend a relaxing and an empowering practice on a weekly basis.

Self-Love Challenge

Have a date with yourself. Move and caress your body as you practice breast massage and jade egg. Your pleasure is your medicine. I recommend committing yourself to a twenty-one-day challenge to make time for practicing self-love. In this way you take responsibility for what arises and for enjoying your life.

Healing Tip for Yeast Infections

This is based on the natural remedy of putting yogurt into your vagina so the probiotics can clear the excess yeast. Coat your jade egg well with plain unsweetened yogurt. This practice can be done in the shower. Squat or bring one leg up. Massage the opening of your vagina and pop in the jade egg.

Use the kidneys' healing sound, "choo-oo-oo-oo," to energetically blow out excess yeast. Then speak to the cells in your vagina, "May my vagina return back to normal function."

PLAYING WITH YOUR JADE EGG

At first, practice with the jade egg while you lie on the floor, on your bed, or in the bathtub so you can relax into your body. You will build up skill and tone. Then start to sit, stand, and dance with your jade egg inside. When your jade egg stays in with these practices, you can empower yourself by attaching a small weight (see Qi Weight Lifting on page 250).

When you are able to retain the yoni egg in standing and walking positions, you can keep your egg inside you as you move around the house or when you are exercising, doing yoga, or dancing. Remind yourself to "pull up" the energy from time to time, and remember to take the egg out before you pee. Formulate a self-sustaining intention as you wear it, such as "Make me strong, vital, and beautiful."

Wait until your period is over to practice with the jade egg as it will increase the blood flow otherwise.

Sleeping with Your Jade Egg Inside

Do not sleep with the egg inside your yoni every night, as it can put too much pressure in one place in the vagina—especially if you sleep on your side. If you would like to receive spiritual guidance while you sleep, however, you can sleep with your egg. Program your question into the egg by rubbing it in, then "sleep on it." Notice any messages from your inner voice when you awake.

During naps with your jade egg you can make an affirmation like "I attract abundant, balanced energy as I rest." You can also invite lucid and profound dreams by saying, "Allow me to recognize that I am dreaming."

Preparing for Your Jade Egg Practice

Create a bubble of sacred light around you. Ask your body if you have permission to do this practice. Trust your inner guidance above all else.

When you are ready to proceed, begin with the self-massage and other preparation practices described below. The body needs to be prepared for the jade egg, just as it is important to prepare soil before planting. Through self-massage the lower body becomes soft and receptive and is embraced by awareness. The Taoists call this self-foreplay "warming the waters."

✸ Warming the Ovarian Palace

Massaging your ovaries and the surrounding area increases blood and qi circulation, thereby preventing the stagnation that can build up and form fibroids or cysts. By regularly warming the ovaries through massage, you can prevent menstrual cramps due to excess coldness and water retention. The gentle touch of self-massage can also dissolve the armoring that many women develop from having been entered before they were ready.

- Rub and warm your hands. With your palms, massage your Ovarian Palace like a fountain—stroking up the midline over the uterus and washing back down over the ovaries. Massage with small circles around the ovaries, then reverse direction. Enjoy the pleasant warmth and how much your ovaries love being massaged!
- Lightly and quickly tap your ovaries with your fingertips to wake up the qi there.
- Rub the hip crease between the pubic bone and your thighs to open the Rushing Gates.
- Rub your inner thighs toward you to move the qi in the yin channels.
- Rub your kidneys. When your kidneys are warm there is less fear and tightness in the opening of the vagina, and the jade egg will be easier to insert.
- Rub your sacrum with your knuckles to activate the back of your sexual chakra.

✳ Opening Gaia's Belly

The belly lies between our heart and our sexual organs. When we relax this area the flow of communication between the heart and sexual energy is greatly enhanced.

These belly massages, done with your jade egg, release built-up tensions in the belly, free up energy from the core, and help us get in touch with our gut's intuition.

- Warm the jade egg in your navel. Then you can use its big end as a massage tool.
- Relax your heart by rubbing the tip of your egg on your nose, which is the reflexology zone on the face for your heart.

● Navel Wind Gates

The wind gates around the navel allow qi from your core—your original umbilical cord—to radiate out to the organs.

For the steps below, massage around your navel with your egg, pressing the energy gates about a finger-width from the rim of the navel. Massage each point with a small clockwise spiral, the direction of digestion and elimination. See the detailed discussions of the wind gates and self-acupressure points in chapter 2.

- Exhale and press your egg as deeply into the point as you can relax into. Then pause and melt, waiting for the release. Your belly will pop open by itself as you inhale. The order for the massage is an unwinding, counterclockwise circle around the navel: left side, upper left, top, upper right, right, lower right, below, lower left (fig. 6.2).

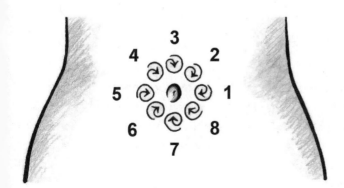

Fig. 6.2. Unwind the navel wind gates in a counterclockwise circle starting on the left side of your belly.

● Lower Belly Points

After the wind gates, continue your belly massage with the following points. For more details on these points see self-acupressure in chapter 2.

Sea of Qi. Press your egg or your fingertips into the Sea of Qi point, two finger-widths below the navel. Exhale with the heart sound, "ha-a-a-a-a-w", sending in a hot wind to stoke up your stove and evaporate any cold, sick winds.

Guan Yuan. Press this point four finger-widths below the navel.

B Spot. Massage just above the pubic bone and breathe deeply.

Mound of Venus. Massage all around and on top of the pubic bone. This helps prevent stagnation and masses from forming there.

Rushing Gate. Massage the hip creases to increase qi and blood circulation.

✺ Empowering Your Jade Egg

- Hold the crystal egg in prayer hands and blow loving warmth into your egg with the "ha-a-a-a-a-w" sound.
- Warm the jade egg by rubbing it in your hands. As you rub your egg, invoke the magical spirit of a mythical genie who can fulfill your inner wishes. Affirm in your egg all the good things that you want to cultivate in your life: "Fill my creative center with love, strength, . . ." and so on.
- Put into your egg all the ingredients of a creative project. Sense that you are giving birth at the end of your practice to your initiative as a complete energy.
- Penetrate into the egg the qualities you long for in a partner, like integrity, good humor, chivalry, and so on. This attraction is multiplied by the magnetism of your yoni.
- Hold your egg on your heart center to absorb the qi of self-love.

✺ Putting in Your Jade Egg

Lubrication (jade juice). Prepare to lubricate your egg with "jade juice"—an elixir made up of energized saliva. Pull up your sexual energy from your Jade Fountain and mix it into your saliva. Swirl your tongue in your mouth and suck a "qi candy" to gather qi in your saliva. Put your saliva in your palm and coat the big end of the egg. Alternatively, you can suck your egg or swirl your tongue around the egg until it is wet. You can also use a natural lubricant, like aloe vera.

If your yoni becomes chafed from the egg exercise I would suggest a longer breast massage practice and putting more saliva or healthy lubricant on the egg before insertion. Frequently practice breast massage and saliva sucking in your mouth, and call more water element energy into your Jade Fountain.

Positions for entry. Lie flat with your knees bent and your feet apart on the floor. Alternative insertion methods are to squat, kneel, or lift one leg.

Entering your sacred temple. Relax and do not force anything. Smile down. Enter the jade gate to your sacred temple with reverence and gentleness. The opening of the vagina opens when your heart opens with loving acceptance.

- Massage up and down the vaginal lips.
- Spiral the egg, large end first, into the yoni. As you spiral, circle your hips clockwise, up the right and down the left in the "pelvic clock." You can also circle your tongue in the same direction on the inside of your mouth.
- As you spiral, open your mouth by sounding a deep, relaxing, sighing "a-a-a-a-a-ah" and vaginal lips by sounding the heart sound, "ha-a-a-a-a-w."
- Suck up your egg with a loud slurpy sound as if you are sucking something delicious up a straw.
- If the egg starts to slip out, use your middle finger to push it up into the vagina. If the egg slips out, lift your knees or squat and push it deeply inside or suck it up.
- Rest. When you rest you can feel the qi building up in your whole pelvic region. Notice qi flows and bodily sensations. This is the yin phase of practice.

TAO YONI YOGA

In between jade egg practices, massage your breasts and circulate the Microcosmic Orbit to spread the warmed energy in the body.

❈ Journey through the Yoni Channel

We can hold hurtful feelings in the Sexual Palace, which can obstruct deeper vaginal orgasms. In the journey below, you'll activate the reflexology zones of the vagina with their corresponding healing sounds to release trapped negative feelings—as dark, murky, sticky energy—into the egg to be transformed by compassion.

- Spiral the egg into the vaginal lips with the heart sound, "ha-a-a-a-a-w," accepting the egg with an inner smile.
- Squeeze the egg with your PC muscle while making the kidney sound, "choo-oo-oo-oo." Sounding subvocally has a deeper effect. Release any fear into the egg. Fill your yoni with calm blue light.
- Squeeze the egg just inside the PC muscle, which is the liver zone, and sound "sh-h-h-h-h-h." Release any anger into the egg. Fill your yoni with the green light of kindness.
- Move the egg about halfway up your yoni canal, into the spleen zone, and sound a guttural "who-o-o-o-o-o." Release any worry into the egg. Fill your yoni with the yellow light of openness.
- Suck the egg deep inside and make the lung sound, "ss-s-s-s-s-s." Release any sadness. Fill your yoni with the white light of courage.
- Move the egg up toward your cervix—to the heart zone—and sound "ha-a-a-a-a-w." Release any impatience you may have with your sexuality into the egg. Fill your yoni with the red light of joy.
- Breathe out anything you are ready to let go of and sound "he-e-e-e-e-e." Fill your yoni with clear light.
- Mix all the virtues into the golden glow of compassion. Fill your yoni and the egg with golden light.
- Lay your "golden egg" with gratitude and wash it afterward.

✸ Emotional Cleansing from the Organs and Uterus

Women tend to hold negativity in the uterus, like a dark cave in the bottom of the torso. Difficult feelings can get swept into an underworld and suppressed there. Negative thoughts or emotions from our partners can also accumulate in the uterus and we may not be able to transform this "gray sperm" without special attention.

It is very important to cleanse the uterus to make room for higher frequencies to grow there.

● Preparation

- Create safe and sacred space to practice this powerful cleansing ritual.
- Connect with your guides, guardians, and angels and allow divine light to make you a vessel for self-healing.

- Start this practice with the Inner Smile, melting the warm golden light of unconditional love down the front, back, and center of your body.
- Set up a clockwise vortex underneath you to wash any murky energy into the earth to be transformed.

● Clearing Out Murky Waters and Refreshing the Uterus

Clear out anything that is not serving your evolution, then reprogram with high-frequency energy. This is like squeezing dirty water out of a sponge and then filling up with fresh water.

For each element, you will make three healing sounds, squeezing out of the organ with the first sound, squeezing out of your uterus with the second sound, then squeezing into the jade egg with a third sound. Pull your string gently with each healing sound. Then breathe in from below upward, filling pure colored light into your jade egg, uterus, and organs. Reprogram with the virtues that you would like to attract in your life.

Metal element: Clear sadness out of the lungs while saying "ss-s-s-s-s-s." Squeeze out of your uterus with another "ss-s-s-s-s-s," then squeeze into the jade egg with a third "ss-s-s-s-s-s." Pull your string gently with each healing sound. Breathe the pure white light of inner strength into your jade egg, uterus, and lungs.

Water element: Clear fear from your kidneys while saying "choo-oo-oo-oo." Squeeze out of your uterus with another "choo-oo-oo-oo," then squeeze into the jade egg with a third "choo-oo-oo-oo." Pull your string gently with each healing sound. Breathe the pure blue light of peace into your jade egg, uterus, and kidneys.

Wood element: Clear anger out of the liver while saying "sh-h-h-h-h-h." Squeeze out of your uterus with another "sh-h-h-h-h-h," then squeeze into the jade egg with a third "sh-h-h-h-h-h." Breathe the pure green light of kindness into your jade egg, uterus, and liver.

Fire element: Clear separation out of the heart while saying "ha-a-a-a-a-w," squeeze out of your uterus with another "ha-a-a-a-a-w," then squeeze into the jade egg with a third "ha-a-a-a-a-w." Breathe the pure red light of love into your jade egg, uterus, and heart.

Earth element: Clear worry out of the spleen while saying "who-o-o-o-o-o." Squeeze out of your uterus with another "who-o-o-o-o-o," then squeeze into the jade egg with a third "who-o-o-o-o-o." Breathe the pure yellow light of openness into your jade egg, uterus, and spleen.

Fill your jade egg with the golden light of unconditional love and compassion. Lay your "golden egg" with gratitude and wash it afterward.

❁ Tug of Love

One playful way of using your jade egg is the Tug of Love exercise. When you pull the string your muscles will naturally grip around the egg with an extra squeeze. Using the law of opposing force, there will be an equal force rising into your body as you are pulling the egg away from your body (fig. 6.3).

- Lie down with your knees up and your feet and back pressing into the ground. Hum and pull the string three times. Start tugging gently so you do not pull out the egg! Feel the opposing force ripple up your body.
- Pull the sexual power up inside with the strength of the energy channels, organs, and glands. Deeply penetrate the rejuvenating sexual energy by humming a warm, smiling, merging "mmmm"—the sound we make when we taste something delicious! Be rhythmical and playful. Hum at the tone you feel vibrating in the organ. The sound vibration heals and strengthens your body.
- Pull the string attached to the jade egg in different directions. Pull in opposition to the organs that you wish to activate and in opposition to the Left and Right Thrusting Channels. Pulling the egg's string in different directions gently stimulates the reflexology zones for the whole body. Place one hand over the area to feel the resonance penetrate it. Press the activated area into the ground.
- Hold out your exhalation. The empty force sucks up the sexual energy and builds qi compression like a spring loading. Press your tongue to the roof of your mouth.
- Inhale and expand your Sexual Palace with qi.
- Pull up qi to the three dantians with the rising tones: do re mi.

● Tugging to Activate the Organs and Glands

- Pull the string slightly to the front to activate the kidneys/adrenal pump, the C7/dorsal pump, and the cranial pump at the back of the head.
- Pull the string slightly to the left to activate the liver, right lung, and right brain.

- Pull the string slightly to the right to activate the spleen, heart, and left brain.
- Pull the string straight down toward your feet to activate the pancreas, thymus, and master glands.
- Pull the string straight down toward your feet, sounding "ee-ee-ee" as in "me," to empower your Central or Core Channel. Sense the pillar of light that holds you up energetically.

● Tugging to Pack the Organs

Use the powerful suction of the organs to pull against the string. Inhale and suck with virtue energy. Packing is inhaling into a specific area and holding the breath there so the nourishing Sexual Qi can be absorbed. The wrapping spirals qi in and around the organ. Hug your organ with one hand to feel the fullness gather there. If you have a weak or achy organ you could pack and tonify that one area until you feel a shift.

- Pull the string to the right, which will pull up the left side of your anus to pump up energy to the left kidney. The left and right sides of the anus act as pumps to thrust energy up the left and right sides of the body. Place your left hand on the left kidney. Pack and wrap qi around the organ as you gently hold your breath. Smile down to the left kidney. You can use the corresponding healing sound as you exhale to relax the organ.

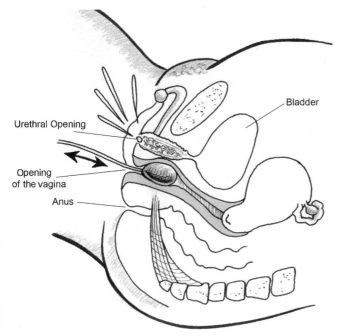

Urethral Opening

Bladder

Opening of the vagina

Anus

Fig. 6.3. Tug of Love awakens female ejaculation.

- Continue to pack the spleen, heart, throat, left brain, and whole left side, while continuing to pull the string to the right. Exhale between each organ with a long, deep sigh.
- Compare the two sides to notice the how much fuller and alive the left side is. Repeat on the right side, pulling the string to the left. Pack into the right kidney, liver, right side of the brain, and whole right side. Exhale between each organ and relax.
- Hug yourself and put your knees together. Relax and absorb the qi.

✸ Tiered Fountain

The fountain motion scoops up sexual energy from your yoni—your Fountain of Youth—to rejuvenate the inner body. Multi-spot stimulation gets the sexual energy warmed up, particularly in women, whose bodies are multi-erogenous. Imagine you are a luscious fountain with four tiers of flowing water rising through your core and washing down your body. This whole-body flow paves the way for expanding multiorgasmic experiences.

- Lie on your back with your legs extended.
- Initiate subtle squeezing and releasing movements in the yoni by rotating your feet (fig. 6.4).
- Exhale. Rotate your legs outward, with feet flexed out.
- Inhale. Rotate your legs inward. Point your toes and pull your big toes up together. This activates the yin meridians that flow up the inner legs and through the Ovarian Palace. Notice when your yoni and buttocks squeeze. This action hugs your egg and tonifies your vagina, which increases the possibility of having a G-spot orgasm.
- You can sound the water sound "l-l-l," as in "lifting, licking, or lapping." Wash and nourish the lotus flowers in your body.

First tier, deep earth fountain: Breathe in earth energy through the Bubbling Springs points in the soles of your feet.

Second tier, jade fountain: Move your hands like a fountain in front of your womb, rubbing your ovaries in circles, up the middle and down the outside of the ovaries.

Third tier, fountain of love: Massage your breasts in circles, up the middle and down the outside of the breasts.

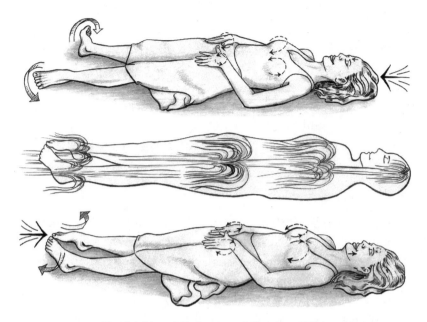

Fig. 6.4. Tiered Fountain and Shower of Bliss

Fourth tier, fountain of bliss: Pulse your tongue on your soft palate, the Heavenly Pool, in rhythm with your upward massage. You can lightly massage the third eye with your middle fingers, up the middle and down the outside. Sensualize a little fountain in the "glands of bliss," the master glands in the center of your head. Keep the movement of all four tiers pulsing together.

Shower of Bliss: Lift your hands above your head and pull the heavenly qi down your Core Channel. Reverse the movement and shower the refined energy back down. Massage your breasts and ovaries down the middle and up the outside to gather bliss, love, and creativity. Hum with a descending "mmm" sound to melt through tension and merge smiling, loving energy down through the body. Taste your essence, like we say "mmm" when we taste delicious nectar!

PELVIC MOTION, THE INTERNAL DANCE

The following exercises are grouped into four different series, each of which focuses on a different type of movement.

Rock My World

The pelvic motion exercises in this series are all performed on the floor, lying on your back with your palms down by your sides, knees up, and feet flat on the floor. Pelvic movements done in this position with the jade egg help open the hips and activate the pumps along the spine. This is a natural posture for lovemaking, as the pelvis can rock with the rising energy. The sacrum, the back of the Sexual Palace, is loosened up to move energy. The feet keep a good grounding and connection with the earth. When you press the feet the tendon lines into the pelvis are engaged.

❊ Spinal Pelvic Rock

This is a great practice to get your breath, qi, and body in motion. It is a good choice to start off your Jade Egg practice. The natural motion of the pelvis moves sexual energy by activating the sacral, adrenal, dorsal, and cranial pumps along the spine. Circulate the sexual energy in the Microcosmic Orbit with continuous deep breathing and a whole-body wave.

The rocking of your pelvis is initiated by pushing and pulling your hands and feet in a kneading motion. Claw and curl your fingers and toes as you inhale, and stretch them as you exhale. Suck the nourishing energy from the earth like a baby suckles from its mother's breast, with its fingers and toes kneading. Watch a cat in pleasure, clawing and purring.

- With each inhalation, your back arches as you claw the hands and feet. With each exhalation, press your middle back down as you push the heels of your hands and feet into the ground (fig. 6.5).
- Pump energy up through the arms, legs, and groin, allowing your pelvis and spine to move in a sensual, undulating wave, like an orgasmic wave.
- You can also rev up your motors by turning the "water wheels"—spinning qi around the ovaries and rolling qi around your eyes.

❊ Empowering the Three Dantians

- Continue the Spinal Pelvic Rock. Place your right sending hand over the Sexual Palace. Press, palpate, or spiral at the perineum, then pull the jade egg's string on the exhalation as you press your feet into the ground. Relax on the inhalation.
- Put your left hand over the navel, empowering the strength of willpower. Rhythmically pump up sexual energy with your breath to the left receptive hand. Smile into it.
- Move your left hand to the heart center, empowering the warmth of love.

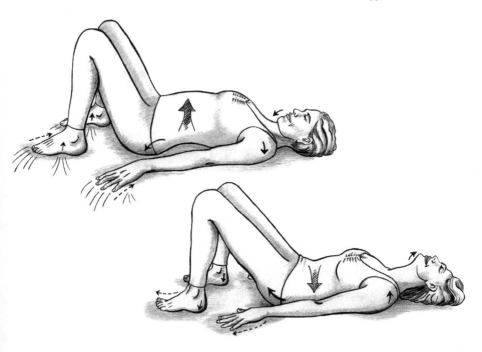

Fig. 6.5. Spinal Pelvic Rock: arch on the inhale, and press on the exhale

- Shift your left hand to the third eye, empowering the light of wisdom.
- Lower your left hand back to the heart, so your thinking integrates with the warmth of feeling.
- Bring it down to the navel so you can manifest and act with clarity, love, and compassion. Allow direction and love to flow into your actions, so you do not become a victim of wild desires.
- Rest and feel all three areas integrate harmoniously together.

✳ Empowering the Microcosmic Orbit

Continue in the same position as the Spinal Pelvic Rock.

The water cycle with relaxed breathing is a fluid way to move energy through the Orbit, generating a soft and continuous flow like water.

- Inhale up the Front Channel, sucking the energy up to the third eye. The back will arch and the chin will tuck in.
- Exhale and press the lower back and feet downward and pull the string. Wash over the crown and a waterfall of qi cascades down the back to your heels as you pull the string. Water flows to the earth.

The fire cycle with reverse breathing is a powerful way to surge energy through the Orbit, generating power.

- Pull the string as you inhale up the pumps along the spine, sucking energy to the crown. Press your feet, feel your lower back pressing downward, and pull the string.
- Exhale as you blow warm qi down the Front Channel into the dantian. The belly expands upward and the back arches.

✳ Ripple Rock

Continue in the same position as the Spinal Pelvic Rock. Loosely rock and ripple the body by tapping toes and heels. Press your toes (lift your heels) and press your heels (lift your toes). Notice how your pelvis and head rock. Speed it up. Surrender to this natural rocking motion and the vibration it creates.

✳ Spinal Pelvic Clock

This circular pelvic movement loosens and lubricates the lower back. It creates a "screwing" motion in the sacrum and massages acupuncture points around the sacrum, behind the Sexual Palace.

- Continue in the same position as the Spinal Pelvic Rock.
- Imagine that you have a clock around your sacrum. 12 o'clock is at Mingmen, 3 o'clock is below and to the left of Mingmen, 6 o'clock is at the tailbone, and 9 is on the right, midway between the tailbone and Mingmen.
- Push your feet into the floor to "kick-start" the circle. Lean and roll into it like the edge of a lid or Frisbee. Roll around the clock counterclockwise, up the left and down the right, then reverse the direction.
- Make a small circle with your nose, which will set the cranial pump into a circular motion. Move at the same pace as your sacral circle. This links up your cranial and sacral pumps like two wheels on the same axis.
- Your body makes a circle around the jade egg. Gently pull the string and feel a spiraling massage of the organ reflex zones inside your yoni canal. This particularly massages the liver and spleen zones.

❀ Pelvic Tilt

The tilt is great for bringing the jade egg deeper inside before standing practices.

- Continue in the same position as the Spinal Pelvic Rock. Press your feet and lower back into the floor as you lift your yoni toward the sky.
- Bear down on the qi ball in your dantian, pressing it into the Mingmen to jack up your pelvis into a steep tilt.
- Grip the egg as you pull the string, sounding "h-u-u-u-m-m." As you relax, open your yoni and loosen the string, allowing the jade egg to drop deeper into the yoni toward your cervix.
- Let your legs open slightly. Open your mouth and jaw, sounding "m-a-a-a," maintaining the pelvic tilt.

Raising the Mound of Venus

In this series, we position ourselves so that the sexual organs are higher than the head. In this way, the sexual waters are moved by gravity to the higher centers. The inverted position prevents and helps restore prolapsed organs. When you pull on the string, an equal force will rise up through your body. This is very energizing for the glands and chakras.

❀ Raise the Mountain

- Press your feet into the ground to lift your hips and spine up (see fig. 6.6 on page 228). Tuck your chin in; this gentle tuck squeezes the throat and massages the thyroid gland.
- Sound "hoo" (as in "who") as you pull the string. "Hu" is a name for divine breath; you are calling out to the Divine with your yoni. Making this sound with your lips will naturally squeeze your jade egg, yoni, and buttocks. Make nine quick "hoo" sounds followed by a slow sound. Imagine that you are howling to the moon!
- Relax and roll your spine back down. Feel your sacrum widen and melt into the earth. The roll up and down increases the flow in the spine and allows the egg to drop deeper toward your cervix.

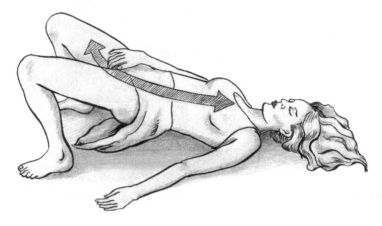

Fig. 6.6. Raise the Mountain, sounding "hoo."

✳ Alternate Hip Thrusting

Now for some belly dancing moves! When your pelvis is up in the air, thrust up one hip and then the other, alternately squeezing your left and right buttocks. Your pelvis will swivel. Squeezing energizes the left and right sides of your yoni and the two Thrusting Channels, which extend up to the brain.

Make a quick "hoo" sound nine times for each hip: right-left-right-left (for a total of nine cycles), followed by one slow one in the middle. Slowly roll down and relax. Start with the right hip up, then repeat the set starting with the left hip up.

✳ Fan Your Fire

Keep your pelvis raised and support your lower back with your hands. Fan the dantian fire with bellows breathing or Breath of Fire—take a long deep breath in and exhale with a series of short forceful breaths through your nose. Breathe nine times and slowly roll down as you exhale. Hug your knees and rock your lower back.

✳ Spinal Skipping Rope

Raise the mountain and circle your hips in the lifted position, moving your spine like a skipping rope. Inhale at the top of the circle, pulling the string, and exhale down. Let the jade egg massage in a spiraling motion inside your yoni.

❀ Swimming Snake

Suspend your pelvis up a few finger-widths from the floor, supported by your legs and shoulders. Keep your legs parallel. Imagine that your hand pulling the string is the head of a snake and your spine is the tail. Pull the string to the left and right and allow your hips, spine, and head to follow in a snaky wave. Surrender to the waving impulse from below. Slowly come down and relax your spine. Feel the serpent power move inside of you.

❀ Rap and Shimmy

Lightly lift and drop the sacrum, sending vibrations through your pelvis. Make a releasing sound "aaahh" as you break up holding patterns in your lower body.

Shimmy your hips sideways like you are wagging your tail. Make a pleasurable sound "oo-oo-oo." (as in "moo"). This shakes off tension and stimulates vibration like ringing a bell.

Emerging Butterfly

This series of movements explores how you can stretch and practice yoga with your jade egg. These floor exercises provide some effective ways of opening the hips and lower back. They are great stress relievers! Move your body in opposition to the pulling of the string to create strengthening resistance and warm up the qi. Move rhythmically with your breath.

❀ Kidney-Bladder Rock

- Lie down with your knees bent and feet on the ground. Cross your right leg over the left leg and bring your right knee to your chest.
- Rock your lower body, inhaling as you rock up and exhaling as you rock down. Your left foot will bounce up and down.
- Extend your left leg if you want more stretch in your hamstrings and the Urinary Bladder channels on the backs of your legs. The bladder is lifted above the uterus. Let the rocking gently massage your kidneys.
- Hold the string between your legs and pull it downward as your legs rock upward. This stimulates the upper zones of the yoni.
- Inhale up the spine and exhale down the Front Channel. Repeat on the other side.

❀ Yoni Whirlpool

Hold your knees to your chest and make a circle with them. Circle your sacrum around the pelvic clock. Imagine qi spiraling clockwise down into the lung and heart zones, deep in the yoni canal. Move counterclockwise and imagine water swirling like a whirlpool in your yoni.

❀ Side Rocking

- Roll onto your side. Rub your knees together to stimulate the yin meridians, particularly the Spleen meridian, which puts blood in the proper place.
- Hold on to the string between your legs. Exhale and pull your hips back slowly as you pull the string forward.
- Inhale and gently rock back to a neutral position. Imagine making love with your lover behind you. Rocking in slow motion deeply relaxes the body-mind.

❀ Opening the Rushing Gates

- Stay lying down with your legs extended. Hold your left knee and squeeze it toward your chest as you pull the string slightly down to the right.
- Exhale as your knee circles out and away from your chest, rotating the hip in its ball-and-socket joint. This opens the Rushing Gate, the crease in your hip joint.
- Rotate your knee in the opposite direction, then fold it toward the right side in a spinal twist. Face your head to the left.
- Exhale, pressing the left knee down as you pull the string with your right hand behind you.
- Inhale, releasing back in a gentle sideways rocking motion.
- Repeat with the right knee up.

  This exercise opens the "sex points" in the lower back.

❀ Butterfly Opens Its Wings

- Lie on the floor with your knees up and your feet together. Open your knees and sound a relaxing "aaahh." Open your yoni with a feeling of "Yes!" as you make love to the universe.

- Squeeze your thighs slowly together as you grip the egg, pull the string, and sound a pleasurable "oo-oo-oo."
- Suck up your egg as if you were pulling on a Jade Stalk. This tones your love muscles to get ready for great lovemaking! The opening and closing of your mouth and yoni move together as one.

❀ Butterfly Rock

This feels like a birthing movement and gives a lot of freedom for your spine and pelvis to move.

- Continue in the same position as the Butterfly with your knees open and feet together. Sit up a bit and lean on your elbows.
- Rock your pelvis. Inhale as you rock forward and your belly comes up. Exhale as you rock backward, letting your belly come down and your feet press away from you. Come slowly down into the Butterfly Hug.

❀ Butterfly Hug

- Continue the same position as the Butterfly with your knees open and feet together.
- Cross your arms at your chest and hug yourself. Smile to your heart. Make a soft heart sound, "ha-a-a-a-w." Imagine sunlight or moonlight shining into your yoni. Love your Self!

❀ Birthing Butterfly

- Sit with your knees hip-width apart and hug your knees, clasping your wrists. Rotate your torso, inhaling as you come forward and exhaling as you go back. Stir your creative energy in and around your womb. Imagine you are a butterfly emerging out of a cocoon.
- Lie flat and relax totally. Place your hands over your navel to collect the energy.

Internal Dance

This series of practices plays with rhythmical pulsations and subtle movements in the yoni. The exercises can be done lying down, sitting, or standing. Your qi body loves a good steady rhythm. Explore ways to spontaneously dance with the qi!

❀ Playing the String

Tilt your pelvis upward. Pull the string taut and play it with your fingers, sending delightful vibrations up through your body. Imagine that you are playing a valuable violin! Smile and pulse your tongue on your soft palate. Then relax down and pluck your nipples.

❀ Riding the Pulsations

- Squeeze below your egg, squeeze above your egg, then squeeze the middle of your egg.
- Hold your breath for six counts and move your egg up and down using lower, middle, and upper muscles of the vaginal canal. Exhale and relax.
- Move with slow and fast rhythms. Practice with music! You can do three quick pulsations (up and down movements) as you inhale, three as you hold/suspend the breath, and three as you exhale and pause. Hold the string to feel the pulsations inside.

❀ Dancing with Your Jade Egg

Rhythmically dance or "make love" with the egg by moving the string in different directions while swinging and bouncing your hips. Put on some lively music!

❀ Butterfly Wings

- Squeeze and relax your vagina muscles in a series of quick, pulsating contractions. Imagine the side walls of your vagina fluttering like the wings of a butterfly! These vaginal tremors are similar to the vibrations that happen spontaneously during orgasm.
- Practice slow contractions by squeezing the lower, middle, and upper rings of muscles as you inhale, and slowly releasing the upper, middle, and lower muscles as you exhale.
- Create quick musical impulses by making six little contractions as you inhale and six gradual releases as you exhale. Make your practice musical by alternating slow and fast rhythms.

✺ Orgasmic Impulses

Move the jade egg up and down in the vagina. Suck it up as you inhale. As you exhale, pull the string to move it back down. Allow vaginal contractions to gradually move on their own. Feel the contractions of your uterus inside your brain.

TRIPLE CHANNELS
Alternate-Channel Breathing

Ancient yogis developed an effective way to support the process of internal alchemy. Known in yoga practice as alternate-nostril breathing, this exercise readily lends itself to Taoist practice as well. Alternate-Channel Breathing clears the Thrusting Channels of psychic toxins and empowers their potential qualities. This exercise is similar to the Tibetan "Three Poison Exercise," which overcomes the three poisons of anger, clinging, and ignorance that are deep inner causes of our suffering.

Many practitioners believe that the right nostril stimulates the arousal-producing sympathetic nervous system, while the left nostril activates the relaxation-promoting parasympathetic system. Alternating the flow of air thus creates equilibrium in the autonomic nervous system between excitation and relaxation. The pulsing synchronicity between the two hemispheres of the brain awakens extraordinary faculties. Apparently by holding the breath for 144 seconds levitation is possible!

These channels naturally shift about every ninety minutes. If they do not, then some imbalance or ill health is developing. When the channels are clogged it is important to clear them to prevent deeper imbalance.

The Left and Right Channels

Shifting between the Left and Right Thrusting Channels balances the masculine and feminine energies and grows the potential of unity in the Central or Core Channel. When the male and female energies dance, exchange, and make love within, the potential neutral force—True Qi or the Immortal Child—can be born.

The internal channels are the opposite energetic polarity to the physical sides of the body. In the Tai Chi symbol there is a white dot in the black lobe, yang within yin and a black dot in the white lobe, yin within yang. The left channel is red and yang; the right channel is blue and yin; the central channel is white gold. (See Fig. 6.7.)

The channels can become tainted by the emotional environment they move through, like a river flowing through polluted fields. As a pure river flushes through the field, it becomes purified. Flush excess murky qi out the opposite side using the power of virtue. Transform negative emotions with the power of bright virtue energy.

Left Side

The left side of the body has more feminine, magnetic, receptive qualities. The imbalanced emotions of the spleen—like anxiety and attachment—can be cleared from this side by visualizing murky colors leaving or recycling into pure light.

Kindness and generosity from the right side (liver qualities) will move through and sweep the murky spleen energy out.

Right Side

The right side of the body is associated with more masculine, electric qualities of initiative and aggression. The imbalanced emotions of the liver—like anger—can be cleared from this side.

Openness and trust from the left side (spleen qualities) will move through and sweep the murky liver qualities out.

Central Channel

The Central Channel of the body is considered the carrier of illumination and fulfillment. Its shadow side is ignorance.

Switching Tracks with Head, Hips, and Feet

Our channels start and end in the feet and head, so we can shift tracks at either end.

Triggering with the Feet

By pointing the toes and breathing into the big toe especially, we induce energy to flow up the yin channels, along the inner aspect of the legs. Pointing the toes of the left foot and pulling up the left side of the perineum and anus will thrust energy up the Left Thrusting Channel. Pointing the toes of the right foot and pulling up the right side of the perineum and anus will thrust energy up the Right Thrusting Channel.

When we flex the feet (toes up), we stretch the backs of the legs and bring energy down the yang channels.

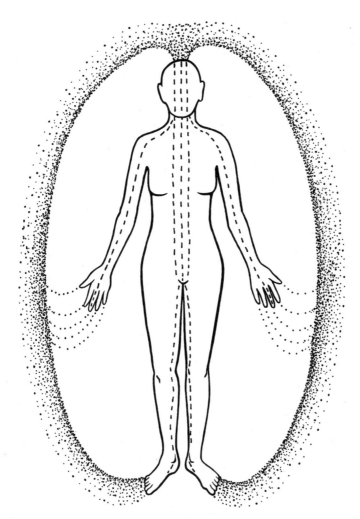

Fig. 6.7. Three Thrusting Channels:
right/red, central/white gold, left/blue

Triggering with the Head

Turning the head activates a switch at the neck that effectively closes one channel and opens the other. When we turn our head to the left we close off the left channel and open the right channel. Turning to the right closes the right channel and opens the left.

Bring your head to a neutral central position as you hold your breath. Turn your head as you exhale and keep your head there as you inhale into that side.

✸ Pulleys from the Hip

In a lying-down position, explore how your head moves when you swivel your hips. The hip crease acts like a pulley: as one hip pulls upward toward the head, the other hip extends downward toward the feet.

Imagine a string connecting your chin to your hip crease. As your right hip pulls up, your head is pulled to the right. Then the left hip starts to pull up and your head comes back through the neutral center position. Moving with this awareness allows for effortless flow as you breathe with the head and feet triggers.

✸ Triple Purification

Without using your fingers, movements, or grimaces, open your nostrils mentally by following the breath up and down the Left and Right Thrusting Channels with your inner eye. You can visualize the colors of the channels like colored lights moving up and down a thermometer or a glowing pearl in a fiber-optic tube. A gentle chin tuck (chin lock) and tongue press will also cue the holding of the breath, sealed in the vessel of the body.

● Clearing the Left Channel

Negative qualities associated with the left channel include attachment, addiction, seduction, worry, anxiety, scarcity, compulsion, obsession, neediness, stickiness, clinginess, resistance to change, sentimentality, stuckness, sloth, and distrust. When this channel is deficient, you might notice a lack of nourishment, fickleness, or an uncentered, distracted monkey mind.

- Clear out the negative energies of the Left Thrusting Channel as a blackened, burgundy red color. Exhale any disturbing qualities through your left nostril, fingertips, toes, and skin, or send them into the cauldron to be fused and transformed. If no coarse or murky emotions arise, polish and illuminate the virtues with your breath and mind into gem-like colors.
- Cleanse to ruby red. Inhale and hold the breath to empower inherent ennobling qualities, including femininity, receptivity, openness, sensitivity, inspiration, and magnetic attraction.

● Clearing the Right Channel

Negative qualities associated with the right channel include aggression, struggling, fighting, intimidation, defensiveness, aversion, anger, agitation, frustration, dominance, manipulativeness, and cold intellectualism. Deficient qualities include indecisiveness, laziness, and lack of higher motivation.

- Clear out the negative energies of the Right Thrusting Channel as a darkened, smoky navy blue color. Exhale any disturbing qualities out of the right nostril, fingertips, toes, and skin, or send them into the cauldron to be fused and transformed.
- Cleanse to sapphire blue. Inhale and hold the breath to empower inherent ennobling qualities, including masculinity, initiative, force of change, organizing, and electrifying motivation.

● Clearing the Core/Central Channel

Negative qualities of the Central Channel include ignorance, delusion, self-righteousness, pride, judgment, blame, avoidance, indifference, and egoism.

- Clear obstructions from the Central Channel as cloudy gray smoke. Exhale any disturbing qualities from your nostrils, fingertips, toes, and skin, or send them into the cauldron to be fused and transformed.
- Cleanse to radiant gold or white. Inhale and hold the breath to empower the inherent ennobling qualities of illumination, fulfillment, integration, wisdom, and electromagnetic power.

❋ Alternating Channels with the Jade Egg

- Make an energetic bow that stretches between your string and the top of your head. Trace with one hand the route of the qi rising up one side and down the other side. Breathe slowly and smoothly.
- Pull the string to the left with your left hand when you breathe up the Right Thrusting Channel. Turn your head to the left to shut off the left channel and open the right channel. This will open the right nostril. Trace up with your right middle finger from the right ovary to the right nipple. Pull your nipple and look up internally with your eyes to the crown. Pump up the sexual vitality through the right ovary, right kidney, right breast, and right hemisphere of the brain.
- Turn your head back to the center, let go of the string, and touch your

right hand to your heart center. Hold the breath and smile down the Central Channel.

- Exhale down the left channel as you turn your head slowly to the right. Trace with your right middle finger from the left nipple down to the left ovary. Flex your left foot to breathe down the yang meridians, down the back of the leg to the Bubbling Springs point on the bottom of your foot.
- Start inhaling by pointing your left toe to breathe up the yin meridians that run up the inside of the leg. Change hands. Pull the string with your right hand to the right. Trace up with your left middle finger from the left ovary to the left nipple. Pull your nipple and look up internally with your eyes to the crown. Pump up the sexual vitality through the left ovary, left kidney, left breast, and left hemisphere of the brain.
- Turn your head back to the center, let go of the string, and touch your left hand to your heart center. Hold the breath and smile down the Central Channel.
- Exhale down the right channel as you turn your head gently to the left. Flex your right foot to breathe down the yang meridians, down the back of the leg to the Bubbling Springs. Trace your left hand back to the right ovary.

✸ Alternating Channels with Breast Massage

This is one of my favorite regular practices, as I feel very balanced and full of qi afterward. My whole body-mind, breath, and inner channels feel well integrated from head to heart to toes. Use the same feet and head triggers as in the previous exercise.

- Place your hands over your breasts with your fingertips pointing to your heart center (fig. 6.8).
- To guide the rising energy up the right side, massage your right breast up the inside and down the outside, like a fountain. Breathe up the body as you massage six spirals around the breast.
- Hold for a count of six as you smile down the Central Channel. Especially smile to your thymus gland to boost your immune system. Smile down to all the glands to promote hormonal balance. Do not hold the energy in your head or heart as you do not want to overheat these organs. It is best to bring your awareness down to the lower dantian, where you need heat to digest your food and warm up your will and passion for life. Relax into your fullness as you hold the breath.

- To guide the descending energy down the left side, massage the left breast down the inside and up the outside. Exhale down the body as you massage around the breast with six spirals.
- Let go at the end of the exhalation to surrender into the emptiness.
- Continue to alternate sides.

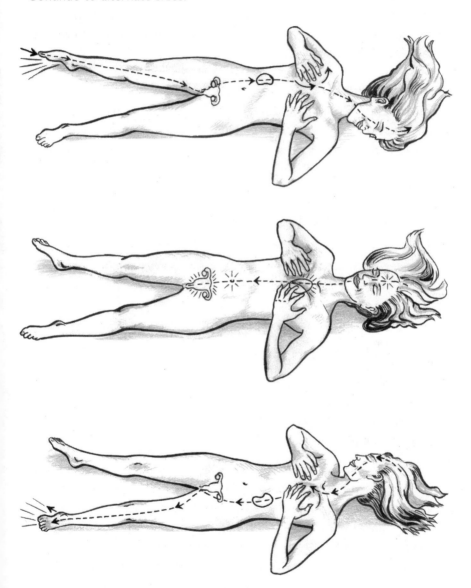

Fig. 6.8. Breast massage guides the flow
in three channels.

❀ All Three Channels

- Breathe up all three channels with your head in the neutral position. Point both toes. Massage your breasts up the inside and down the outside with six spirals. Move the qi like a fountain.
- Reverse direction on the exhalation, flexing both heels. Massage your breasts down the inside and up the outside with six spirals. Move the qi like a waterfall cascading down your body.

Riding the Wave

In this series of Thrusting Channel practices we sit up in a kneeling position or sit at the edge of a chair. The uprightness encourages the raising of the energy from earth to heaven and induces the sublimation of ecstasy. Rock your sacrum freely as if you were riding a wave or a dolphin.

❀ Playing the Thrusting Channel

Pluck your left nipple with your left hand, like you are playing an instrument. At the same time, use your right hand to milk your string downward, pulling rhythmically. This will open the left channel beautifully! Then repeat on the other side.

❀ Dragon Stretches Her Tail

This exercise stretches the Left and Right Thrusting Channels and surges sexual energy to clear these channels. It flushes out the lymphatic system, opens and connects the throat with the rest of the body, and also opens the *kua*—the fold in the front of the hip.

- Sit on your heels in a kneeling position with your left hand behind you on the floor. As you exhale, pull the string with your right hand, thrust the right hip up, and twist to the left in a progressive spiral from the lower spine through the middle and upper spine to the neck. Stretch your eyes to look behind you. Stretch the whole Right Thrusting Channel from the groin up to the chest, neck, and right hemisphere of the brain.
- As you inhale, sit back down on both heels and return to a neutral position looking forward.
- Repeat three times before changing to the other side.

❋ Toning the Taiji Pole

Raise the sound vibrations up your Core Channel as you pull the string downward. This will create amazing suction power, especially with sound!

- Kneel, sitting on your heels, and hold the string between your legs.
- Elongate your body upward as you exhale. Soften your belly and spine as you inhale.
- Exhale, chanting "Ill-aaa-uuu-mmm," and follow the sound up the three dantians with your free hand, palm up. Inhale and lower your hand, palm down.

  With your hand at your yoni, chant "Ill" as in "lift" and "luscious."

  Hand at your lower dantian, chant "aaa" as in "alpha."

  Hand at your middle dantian, chant "uuu" as in "tune."

  Hand at your upper dantian, chant "mmm." Smile up to your crown and
merge your awareness with the humming sound.

❋ Riding the Horse

The rocking motion of this exercise is like being on top of your lover. Sexual energy is our horsepower and in this position you can ride the waves of bliss like a cowgirl!

- Sit on your heels in a kneeling posture. Rock your pelvis back with the Crane Neck—reaching your chin out as you exhale downward. Tuck your pelvis under as you roll up with the chin tucked in.
- Circulate energy in the Microcosmic Orbit. Pull the string as you roll upward, inhaling the qi up your Back Channel to the crown. You can also reverse this, circulating qi in the water cycle (up the front and down the back) as you do the Turtle Neck.

❋ Squatting and Shaking

In a squatting posture, shake your sacrum forward and back and your hips from side to side. Feel your whole spine move like a snake. You can also rotate your hips to move the qi in the Belt Channels.

❋ Raising Ecstasy

- Kneel, sitting on your heels. Hold a spinning qi ball in your hands. Circulate energy up the three dantians in an undulating wave. Gradually raise the energy until your hands are up in the air and the ecstasy is effortlessly shimmering through you. You can breathe with your mouth, making the heart sound, "ha-a-a-a-a-w." The sound will rise in pitch as you move the qi ball upward.

• Bring the ecstatic qi back down with the water cycle, rolling it down your spine. Receive the high, refined qi into your cells, smiling with the bliss of the body.

❀ Centering

Always close with the Microcosmic Orbit and collect the energy at the navel (see chapter 2).

Goddess Rebirthing

This primal sequence induces an empowering process of giving birth to the goddess within yourself. I would suggest listening to shamanic music like drum and didgeridoo sounds as you raise the energy, and listening to lyrical music as you soar and come back down.

❀ Rebirthing the Goddess Within

Consecration: Sit up and lift your hands up to the heavens. Connect to Higher Guidance to liberate your body, heart, and mind, allowing orgasmic freedom. Say, "May the Divine Feminine be reborn with grace, for the awakening of all beings."

Continuous circular breathing: Lie down with your knees up and feet on the floor. Breathe in with your nose, filling your torso. Breathe in all the energy you need to ride the waves into ecstasy. Exhale effortlessly with an open mouth, letting go of control, keeping your jaw relaxed, and making a soft "ha-a-a-a-a-w" sound. Remind yourself, "It is safe to trust the breath and qi."

Building up rhythm: Thump your sacrum by lifting and dropping it on the ground. Shake out any old holding patterns and ground. Build a strong rhythm. As the waves get stormy, become aware of the middle of your yoni, squeezing and releasing the egg.

Water cycle: Practice the Spinal Pelvic Rock with your tongue up on the roof of your mouth. Inhale and fill yourself with qi as you arch your back and

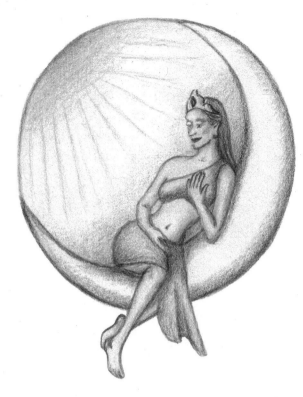

Fig. 6.9. Goddess
Rebirthing

expand your belly, like you are pregnant. Exhale and press your feet into the floor as you pull the string and bear down.

Raising the Mountain: Waves ripple up and down your spine as you lift your pelvis up in the air and roll it back down.

Butterfly Rock with knees open and the soles of your feet together. Lean on your elbows and rock your pelvis.

Opening the heart: Kneel and sit on your heels. Lean back on your hands, arch the front of your body, and open your heart. Become aware of your cervix pulsating with your heart.

Raising energy: Kneel upright on your knees. Allow energy to roll up and down in undulating waves, circulating qi in the lower, middle, and upper dantians. Raise the energy up the middle and down the outside of your aura in fountains. Rotate your torso with the Belt Channels.

Spreading qi: Let the orgasmic vibrations roll, flow, and grow. Begin in cat position on all fours, then rise into standing and free-flow ecstatic dancing.

Generate life, love, and light in the glands of bliss as the third eye, heart, and uterus pulsate together. Become aware of every cell and every strand of DNA making love. Feel the subtle qi sensations spreading everywhere, even into your auric field.

Surrender: The waves of qi become gentle and spontaneous. Allow the qi to move you like a bird soaring through blissful clouds. Opening in sweet surrender to the Divine, say, "Take me!"

Spoon as if you were a newborn child. Hug yourself as you rest. Lie flat with your hands over your navel to center. Say, "I am whole, full, and satisfied. I am an orgasmic, creative being."

Love Ball Entwines

Miracles and majesty expand within me
Breathing and seeing deeply within me
Heaven and earth coupling within me.

Love ball of fingers entwining
Love ball of legs spooning
Love ball of light whirling.

Swirl while breathing
Spiral, rebirthing
Wet cheeks, softly releasing.

Miracles of breathing
Majesty of feeling
Entwining of love threads
Weaving within me.

BATHTUB BLISS

A lot of this book was birthed in the bathtub! In the state of deep surrender, I listen with my whole being to the creative muses.

In the bathtub you can relax and easily put in your jade egg. It's nice to put some pleasant essential oils in the water. Your body can float so you can immerse yourself in the feminine flow. I like to use a large jade egg in the bathtub as it makes a good anchor inside for the fluid movement in and around the body.

Bathtub bliss
Whole body kiss
Swirling and sliding
Floating and gliding
Waving seas deep inside me.

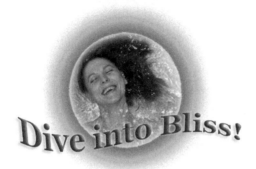

Dive into Bliss!

❋ Coconut Oil Massage

Before bathing or showering it feels wonderful to massage your whole body with coconut oil. It will soak into your skin and scalp to moisturize your skin and prevent drying.

Massage:

- Your scalp, face, neck, shoulders
- Your hands and up your arms to encourage lymph drainage
- Down your back, kidneys, and sacrum
- Your buttocks, arching and curling your back
- Your feet and up your legs
- Around your belly clockwise

❋ Warm Stone Stroking

Once you are in the tub or shower, you can perform the sensual jade egg massage below as a preparation for inserting your egg.

- Dangle the egg from the string and lightly stroke your skin. Gently spiral the egg around your navel 9 times counterclockwise and 9 times clockwise.

- Stroke with the egg around both breasts in figure eights, 6 to 12 times each way.
- Stroke around both ovaries and the Rushing Gates—the lymph nodes inside of your hip bones—in figure eights, 6 to 12 times each way.
- Lightly swing the egg and tap the opening to your Jade Fountain and clitoris 6 to 12 times.
- Slide the jade egg up and down your centerline to your heart 3 to 6 times.
- Lightly swing the egg and tap your nipples 6 to 12 times.
- Rub the egg up and down the vagina opening and slide in your egg.

❁ Shower Practice

The shower is a great place to massage your breasts and body with soap or yogurt (Indian moisturizer). Work your string in the shower. Give resistance with the string as you inhale, pulling the energy up your spine. Exhale to bring the energy down the Front Channel.

Shores of Dreaming

Soft pink clouds give way
To the rising golden sun.

Fingers touch the silky surface
Of skin, familiar yet mystical.

Breathing in musical intervals
in and out of blissful dream.

Shall I dive into the ocean?
How deep are the blue waters?

Washing up on the white shore
riding the sweat of my lover's back

We are a dream to live fully
on endless shores of reality.

❁ Bathing Bliss with Your Jade Egg

You can do any or all of the following exercises whenever you are in the bath.

● Flying Fish

Plant your feet on the rim of the tub, keeping your knees bent. Open your knees outward as you inhale.

Squeeze your thighs together as you exhale, and suck the egg up and pull the string. Feel like a flying fish propelling through the water!

● Spiral Your Tail

Rest your buttocks on the bottom of the tub. Circle your waist. Exhale, pulling your spine back. Suck up with your egg and pull the string. Inhale, arching your back and expanding your belly upward. The egg will spiral and massage inside your yoni. The water will follow you across your belly and your arched back.

● Waving Seaweed

Pull the string to the right as you make a C curve with your body and tilt your head to the right. Massage your left breast. Repeat on the other side.

● Swimming Snake

Place your feet at the end of the tub. Pull the string and allow your body to move in sideways curves (fig. 6.10). Feel your spine as a snake and your hand as the head of the snake. Float like pulling a boat. Relax your jaw and hips and joints. Let your hair wave like a mermaid's.

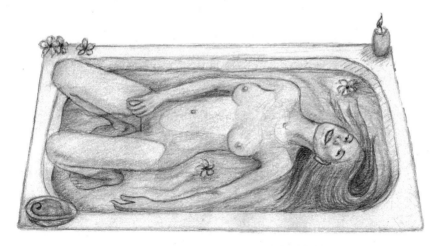

Fig. 6.10. Swimming Snake in the bathtub

● Riding the Sea Horse

Ask your partner or a friend to pull the string sideways and follow it with your body. Surrender to your friend's impulses. Your partner can massage your breasts at the same time or hold on to your pubic bone, your mound of Venus, and move you sideways or in circular waves, like mini Microcosmic Orbits. This feels like riding a seahorse!

● Playing the Bow

Pluck the string like playing a harp. Feel the vibrations inside! When you pluck the string close to your body the water will wave up your clitoris. Play a love song for yourself!

● Walking on Water

Sit in your tub and float your arms and legs. Squeeze the right side of your jade egg to draw up and shorten your right leg. Exhale and relax and your leg will extend.

Alternate sides, taking one full breath on each side. Move your legs from inside your yoni! Pull the yin qi up to the left and right ovaries, then to the left and right kidneys, like pulleys from your organs.

● Wave Rock

Plant your feet on the end of the tub. Allow your head and body to float. Push your feet down. Inhale and suck up the egg in your yoni. Suck your tongue into the Heavenly Pool, the soft palate. Draw the energy up your spine to the crown. The water will wave down your front. Feel how the water follows after you.

Exhale, pulling the string down, and the water will wash up your back. Allow your body to rock up to the crown and down to the perineum, like a pogo stick. Allow the Microcosmic Orbit to be stroked by the water as it follows your movement. Out of water you can do the same exercise by slightly suspending your buttocks off the ground. Rub your back up and down.

● Tiered Fountain

- Push your feet into the end of the tub to set off your yoni squeezes.
- Massage your ovaries in circles.
- Massage your breasts in circles.

- Press your tongue on the roof of your mouth and feel a fountain rising up your Central Channel and gushing in your master glands.
- Massage your scalp, "aaahhhh!"

● Merging Bliss and Emptiness

- Inhale up the Front Channel as you pull the string and stroke up from your yoni to the navel. Exhale and relax the flow down your spine as you return your hand to your yoni. Pause at the end of the exhalation, becoming aware of the silence, the vast emptiness.
- Inhale as you pull the string and stroke up from your yoni to the third eye.
- Fill up with qi to your crown. Pause at the end of the inhalation and be aware of the silence, the bliss of the body. Exhale and relax the flow down your spine as you return your hand to your yoni.

As you breathe, bliss and emptiness merge into a continuous stream of awareness.

● Warm the Kidneys

Rest your knees on the sides of the tub. Pull the string as you inhale and pack qi into the kidneys. Press your lumbar down. Hold and spiral 6 to 12 times in and around the kidneys. Exhale a warm wave of love from your heart down to your kidneys.

● Collect Qi

Spiral energy into your Sea of Qi, two finger-widths below your navel, whirling into a vortex. Rest in the peacefulness of your center.

❀ Turtle Rises from the Water

This exercise is good for strengthening the kidneys and bladder. Regular squatting will tone the gluteus muscles in your buttocks, strengthen the pelvic floor, and help the muscles and joints shift tension patterns. It nourishes the yin reserves in the kidneys.

- Squat in a "birthing position" with open hips. Imagine tribal women and your own ancestors who squatted to give birth. Place your free hand on the tub or floor in front of you.
- Pull the string and pull up with the kidneys, making your back round like

a turtle shell. Make the kidney sound, "choo-oo-oo-oo," as you inhale to draw up water energy.
• Exhale and rock back.

Push and gently pull out the egg and wash it.

Remember to massage your breasts before or after the bath
with some essential oils!

QI WEIGHT LIFTING

Qi Weight Lifting is done by attaching a small weighted bag to the string of your jade egg. You lift the weight with the internal power of your whole body, not just your urogenital muscles. The standing exercises performed with these weights are challenging, strengthening, and energizing for your whole system. They can be practiced with a real weight or an imaginary one. A real weight, though, will give you feedback and build internal power. Once you understand the principles, be creative with your movements!

The stronger the downward pull, the more strongly the upward opposing force will pull qi to your higher centers. You can increase the challenge with more weight or more movement while gripping the egg and weight. If you don't usually feel the egg inside you, the pull of the weight and the swinging vibrations will make the egg's presence more vivid.

After my first jade egg weight-lifting session I took out the egg and was lying flat on the ground. My whole yoni felt so full of energy. One of the first interpretations of this energy I had was "oh my god my yoni feels like she's on psychedelics!" I could energetically feel the string and the egg after taking it out, and there was a palpable vibration inside that felt like a combination of Tibetan singing bowls and a didgeridoo! What a beautiful experience!

HILARY KIMBALL, YOGA TEACHER

Creating a Weight-Swinging Bag

Weight is added to the jade egg in a bag that you tie to your jade egg's string. A drawstring bag about the size of your palm will work. Weight-swinging bags, made in Thailand, with a long drawstring can be purchased at femininetreasures.com.

You can use small "treasures" in your bag, like marbles or polished stones. Dried chickpeas, lentils, or rice make soft weights, so if the bag hits your leg it makes a softer impact. Start with a few tablespoons of beans and gradually add more weight as you progress.

Attach a long string to your bag so the weighted bag hangs just below your knees. If you want to wear something, make it short, as a long skirt will obstruct the swinging of the weight.

Preparing for Qi Weight Lifting

Begin your standing practice with breast massage and floor exercises, then tie on your swing bag. After inserting your egg, sit and attach the bag to your jade egg's cord. Attach the two strings together like you would tie a shoe or a sash with a single loop: twist the bag's cord around the egg's cord, make a circle with the bag's cord and pull a loop through it with the egg's cord. Then pull it tight. You can also make a double knot.

✹ Hook-up from Your Core

- Create an energetic "hook up" in your core by squeezing a qi ball in your abdomen, bearing down your diaphragm and lifting your pelvic floor (see fig. 6.11 on page 252). If it is your first time, hold on to the string as you rise up. Hook up the weight from the internal power or qi pressure rather than just your yoni muscles. When this is established, release your hand from the string.
- To swing the weight, the internal gesture is concentrated—like swinging a pendulum with your fingertips. It is the squeezing and releasing of your yoni that will swing the weight forward and backward, rather than big pelvic thrusting.

It is challenging for women to lift a lot of weight because it is a slippery affair! Instead of tensing your body to hold up the egg, keep your core strong and the body fluid. Your lower-body strength will give the upper body freedom of movement—like a well-rooted plant that can sway in the wind. Ground your legs to create an opposing force of lightness.

Grounding

Uplifting your weight demands being well rooted in the earth. The earthy ability to hold and contain one's energy becomes empowered. The more

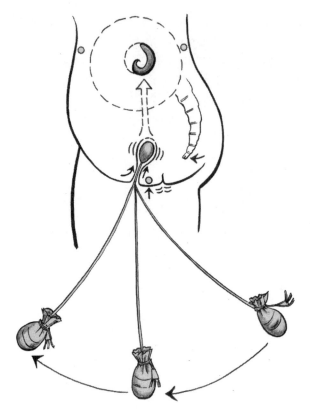

Fig. 6.11. Hook up the weight from your core.

you ground, the easier it is to hold the weight for a longer time. Grounding builds the foundation for spiritual practice: "The deeper you go, the higher you can rise."

A simple way to ground is to sensualize that you are a tree with wide and deep roots, solidly rooted in the earth. Your trunk is erect and your branches are reaching to the heavens. Relax, soften your knees, and drop your center of gravity. The key to grounding is conscious breathing, centered in your belly and embracing the whole body. Your center is the magnetic core of the earth in your body. Sense all the muscles and tendons at work in your body as you practice. Be aware of your energy and make subtle adjustments from moment to moment.

For greater uplift in your muscle power, smile! To test the uplifting power of a smile, hold out your arm and have someone press down on it. When you frown the arm is weak, and when you smile your arm is strong.

Build your grounding by practicing Qigong with your jade egg and swing bag. The weight enhances the penetration of qi into your physical structure. Your creative energy becomes manifest. After using the weight, complete your practice with Bone Breathing, Bone Toning, Tapping, and circulating qi in the Microcosmic Orbit. Collect the generated qi in your center.

Playing with Your Swing Bag

After centering and making sure your egg is well inside, practice the following exercises to get comfortable with the weight. It feels like you have a long testicle dangling between your legs! Better get your laughter out of way before you start because it can push out the egg! Make it fun with some sexy music.

When we allow the qi to move us, a natural grace comes out. Play music that moves you as you practice; it will allow your creative juices to flow. High-quality music can uplift the soul and channel sexual energy into liberating experiences. Smile and breathe into your body. Let every cell vibrate and dance with joy!

Belly dancing is Qigong to music!

✸ Dancing with Your Swing Bag

Start subtly moving your sacrum. Allow the qi to dance as it will while you uphold the weight. Squeeze and release your yoni rhythmically and move the creative qi into all aspects of yourself. Your dance partner in the little bag will not step on your toes, so be playful!

✸ Grinding

Stand in a wide stance and rotate your sacrum in small, sexy circles. This will move your swinging weight in a circle between your knees!

✸ Drawing from a Bottomless Well

Imagine that you are drawing a bucket of water from a bottomless well of abundance by clenching your right hand as you inhale. Squeeze the right side of your yoni and roll your right shoulder down the back. This pulls qi up your Right Thrusting Channel. Alternate left and right sides.

❋ Wagging Your Tail

Stand in a wide stance and bend your knees. With your hands on your knees, wag your sacrum sideways, swinging your weight like a tail.

❋ Stroking Channels

Caress your body like you are peeling off old skin, then toss it away like a striptease dancer!

- Stroke the qi up the insides of your legs. Cross your arms at your solar plexus, then caress over your breasts and down the insides of your arms. Toss the old qi out through your fingers.
- Stroke up the outsides of your arms, wash over your head, down the neck, over the shoulders, and all the way down the backs of your legs. Toss the old qi into the earth.

Feeling the Power of Qi Weight Lifting

Adding weight lifting to your Qigong workout will help build your bones, muscles, and tendon power. It will challenge your grounding, breathing, and ability to raise energy upward. Most moves work really well if you stand in a wide Horse Stance.

Balance your practice of regulated Qigong with wild, free-flow movement.

Dedicate your practice to living your highest potential. Explore your edge with the following practices!

❋ Power Lock

Sometimes called the "Orgasmic Upward Draw," this practice prevents the loss of sexual energy (whether aroused or nonaroused) by drawing it to higher centers. The use of muscular pumps will activate the lymph system and improve qi and blood circulation. The lifting of sexual waters works like the locks of a canal, lifting boats to a higher level. This practice is similar to the "bandhas" of the yogic tradition.

- Breathe in, sucking qi in through the six gates: perineum/yoni, palms and soles of the feet, and your crown (fig. 6.12).

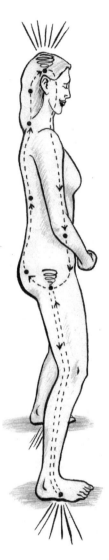

Fig. 6.12. Power Lock
circulates sexual energy.

- Breathe out, pushing your belly out (reverse breathing). Nine quick breaths fan your inner fire.
- Exhale and push the qi ball down by compressing your Sexual Palace.
- Inhale, pulling up your yoni and drawing earth energy up to the perineum. Combine this energy with your sexual energy.
- Lift your anus and sip the energy up to the pumps along your spine. At the same time, squeeze up the muscular pumps: squeeze your yoni, perineum, and anus, claw your feet, clench your legs and buttocks, and make fists at the groin with your elbows to the side.

- Sip up the pumps: sacral, adrenal, dorsal, and cranial. Breathe up the back with your chest relaxed and chin tucked in. Press your tongue up to the Heavenly Pool (soft palate). Clench your teeth, smile up, and look in and up to your crown.
- Spiral energy in your head by rotating your (closed) eyes to the left in a counterclockwise, expanding spiral. Spiral 6 to 9 times. This grows mental and spiritual power in the brain.
- Look to the right and spiral clockwise 6 to 9 times to draw in and condense heavenly energy in the master glands. Swallow down when saliva fills your mouth—especially after the last Power Lock. Exhale downward to fill the elixir into the cauldron.
- Exhale again, releasing your fists, and ground by feeling the qi flow down your legs and into the earth.

✺ Swing Ups

Swing your weight using the power of your pumps and the Microcosmic Orbit. The tendon lines connecting the yoni to the tongue are also activated.

- Inhale, squeeze the egg, and pull up the perineum and anus. Engage your legs and buttocks. Press your tongue up. As the weight swings forward, make fists in front of the ovaries.
- Exhale to swing the weight back. Smile to keep the upward pressure with your pelvic floor while bearing down into your qi ball. Your arms swing slightly backward as you open your palms.
- Tread water by the hips, swinging forward and back with the weight.

Your sacrum will rock slightly forward and back, but keep the external swinging of your hips to a minimum. This helps maintain a stronger fulcrum for lifting heavier weights. Concentration keeps the energy high!

● Pumping Power

Swing up the counterforce of the weight with the power of each pump. Swing up 6 times to each pump: sacral, adrenal, dorsal, and cranial pumps. Swing all the way up to the crown making a fist. Swing down into the navel, releasing the fist.

● Undulating Wave

Surge the energy in a wave from below. Press your feet into the floor, tuck your sacrum, and ripple up through the spine. Allow your arms to be carried by the waves spontaneously.

✳ Tree of Light

Stand tall like a tree. Uplift sexual energy and the weight of your swing bag with the power of the virtues and your higher purpose. The power of compassion and positivity has the ability to alleviate the weight of suffering.

Affirm your higher purpose for cultivating sexual energy in your personal star above your crown. Feel the light of your star hook up your energy from above like a divine lift (elevator).

- Practice Yoni Breathing three times to warm up the sexual energy and exhale down to feel the ground.
- Sip energy from the earth and perineum to the yoni. At the same time, scoop the energy with your hands, palms up, and point your fingers to the Sexual Palace.
- Sip and squeeze your yoni and draw the sexual energy up to the kidneys. At the same time, scoop the energy with your hands up your sides and point your fingers to the kidneys. Light up the kidneys like gems of sapphire blue color. Uphold the weight with the power of peace. Do not force the holding of the breath and smile with ease.
- Turn your palms down, lower your hands, and exhale. Bear down and compress a qi ball in the dantian. The stronger the compression, the more the opposing uplifting force will be like a hydraulic jack. Press your feet into the ground and grow tall.
- Repeat the above steps for the liver, spleen, lungs, and heart.
    Liver: Light up like green emeralds. Uphold the weight with the power of kindness.
    Spleen: Light up like citron gemstones. Uphold the weight with the power of openness.
    Lungs: Light up like white quartz. Uphold the weight with the power of courage.
    Heart: Light up like red rubies. Uphold the weight with the power of love.

- Repeat the above steps for the ovaries, then the pancreas, thymus, thyroid, pituitary, and pineal glands.

   Ovaries: Light up like pink quartz gems. Uphold the weight with the power of creativity.

   Pancreas: Light up like an amber gem. Uphold the weight with the power of centeredness.

   Thymus: Light up like a golden gem. Uphold the weight with the power of healing.

   Thyroid: Light up like a turquoise gem. Uphold the weight with creative expression and the power of your dreams.

   Pituitary: Light up like an indigo gem. Uphold the weight with the power of insight.

   Pineal: Light up like an amethyst. Uphold the weight with the power of direction.

- Sip up to your personal star, sparkling with clear light. Uphold the weight with the power of higher guidance. Hold your hands above your head in prayer posture. Channel vast consciousness through your personal star to empower your higher purpose.

- Bring your hands slowly down as you pull down divine light, showering rainbow light through every cell. Download the virtue energy into the body to manifest high frequencies into your actions.

✳ Removing Your Jade Egg

At the conclusion of your jade egg practice, remove your egg in a conscious, loving way.

● Laying Your Golden Egg

- Squat or lift one leg.
- Push out the egg with your muscles.
- Pull your string if you need to.

● Communing with Your Jade Egg

Feel the life pulse in your egg, the warmth coming from the core of your inner earth!

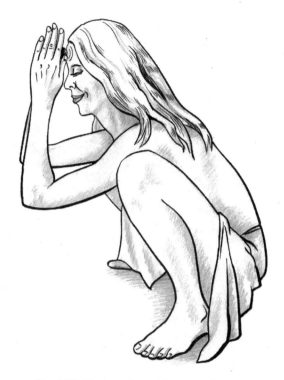

Fig. 6.13. Communing with your jade egg

Hold your egg close to your heart or third eye (fig. 6.13). Feel the alchemical connection between your yoni energy (yin) and your third eye (yang). Feel the warm, loving, golden vibration of your egg.

Say "thank you" and give your jade egg a kiss if you like!

Concluding Your Practice

Round up your Qi Weight Lifting practice by including a few shamanic sexual practices from chapters 7 and 8: Kali Stretches Her Tongue, Durga Rides the Tiger, Phoenix Washes Her Feathers, and/or Flying Crane (chapter 7), followed by Bone Toning, Tapping, and/or Wu Wei Qigong (chapter 8). To complete your workout, always circulate the energy in the Microcosmic Orbit, collect the qi that you have generated, and cool down with the triple warmer sound.

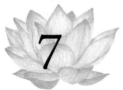

7

Tao Tantric Qigong
Shamanic Empowerment

If you ignore the dragon, it will eat you.
If you confront the dragon, it will overpower you.
If you ride the dragon, you will take advantage of its might and power.

CHINESE PROVERB

In this chapter we will bring alive through movement and sound Taoism's roots in Wu Yi shamanism, with its deep connection to nature, animal powers, and the pursuit of long life. Remember that Mother Nature has been with you from the beginning; you can always return to the nature spirits for healing, renewal, and transformation. This work is essential in accessing the sexual power from your inner animal's raw sexual nature.

✳ Sexual Vitality Warm-ups

Try the simple yet profound Qigong practices below to revitalize your qi, loosen up, and get your sexual energy flowing.

● Ocean Breathing

Feel an ocean of qi in your belly as you breathe in and out with the rhythm of the waves, rippling an ocean of breath throughout your body. Inhale for 6 seconds and exhale for 6 seconds—the average length of an ocean's "breath." Breathe into your toes, and as you exhale, sink into your sacrum and heels. Fill yourself with life force and relax into your core. Allow the breath to lift your arms to shoulder height and lower them as you exhale to hold on to a qi ball, an ocean of qi in the belly. Whole-body breathing will help you naturally spread orgasmic waves during whole-body orgasm.

● Qi Shaking

"Shaking medicine" is an effective way to toss out stagnation and freshen up! Let go of stress or something you are holding on to, shake it loose, and toss it into the ground. When your joints are open the qi will flow well.

- Bounce on your heels or the shock absorbers in your knees.
- Shake from the earth up through the joints and/or organs and glands.
- Let your sacrum bounce like a kangaroo tail!
- Loosen your joints.
- Relax your jaw. Make a sound between a sigh and a giggle.
- Lift your arms up and shake like you are at an uplifting concert! Allow the ecstasy to rise!
- Bring down the lightness of being. Shower golden cosmic light as a blessing upon yourself and the earth.
- Rotate your wrists down to your sides like falling leaves.
- Allow your body to shake spontaneously.

After shaking, feel the buoyancy of your qi—like champagne bubbles sparkling through your body!

● Bouncing Boobies

Support your breasts, cupping them with your hands as you bounce. Feel like your breasts are bouncing upward! "Up, up, up. I feel good, good, good. Happy boobies!"

● Yin and Yang Pelvic Rocks

Yin: Swing your hips back slowly as you inhale "ha-a-a-a-a-w" in a receptive, relaxed way. Breathe in and out with your mouth. Feel like ocean waves are moving through your hips.

Yang: Thrust your hips forward as you sound "ha-a-a-a-a-w" in a fiery, aggressive way. Your movement tends to speed up like a train going uphill. Then slow down again and keep the momentum going as you run the energy inside.

● Sacral Screwing

- Put one hand over your pubic bone and one hand over your sacrum. Spiral the sacrum as if it were floating. Imagine a pendulum is dangling and turning from your tailbone. Allow the cranial pump to spiral with it.
- Spiral serpent energy up the spine as it winds up the tree of life.

● Snake Goddess

- Spiral qi in and around your joints. Qi loves to move in spirals!
- Let your body-mind unwind. Dance like a snake goddess with many snake arms.
- Put half of your awareness on your yoni, source of creativity, and half of your awareness on moving the energy throughout your body. Notice how this makes your movement more sensual, spontaneous, and authentic.
- Peel off the old skin and mask and cast it into the earth. Caress your body. Bow to the serpent power within.

● Free Form

- Liberate creative Kundalini currents. Flow like a liquid flame or steam. Free up your body-mind to heightened states.

EMPOWERING YOUR SEXUAL VITALITY

When you begin to connect with the many sources of vitality in heaven, earth, and your own body, you'll find that even the simpler exercises are more exciting and more energizing. Use the following solo exercises to help prepare you for alchemical lovemaking with your partner (for more on that, see chapter 9). Remember that when you pull qi up to higher centers it is vital to counterbalance this with grounding practices. The more open and transparent we become, the more we need to root in the body for protection and safety.

✳ Rising Tide

Circulate sexual energy in progressively rising, expanding orbits up your body. The qi cuts through the chakras from back to front as if you were flossing and clearing them. The qi ball picks up on higher and higher frequencies of each chakra. Allow your pelvis to rock and your spine to undulate. Spread and refine the sexual waters with the rising tide.

- Hold a qi ball in your hands in front of your dantian. Move the ball down to the perineum, absorbing earth and sexual energy. Scoop energy across the PC pump to the sacrum. Lift the back of the qi ball up your spine to the sacrum, sweep it through to the Sexual Palace, and come back down the front to the perineum.
- Ripple up your spine to Mingmen, then sweep through to the navel and

soften down the front in a circular wave. Continue to move around and through the adrenal pump to the solar plexus, through the Wing point to the heart center, through the dorsal pump to the throat, and through the cranial pump to the third eye, over the crown, and back to the perineum.

- Make the "ha-a-a-a-a-w" sound as you offer love through your heart.
- Clear your creative voice as you sound "a-a-ah" through your throat.
- Clear your mind as you sound "he-e-e-e-e" through the third eye.
- Keep your tongue on the roof of your mouth to bring down the energy from the crown to the belly.
- Imagine the phases of the moon—from new moon at the perineum to full moon at the crown. The moon pulls the tides. "High tide" is orgasm!
- Return with smaller and smaller orbits and collect the energy at your navel.

✸ Drinking Jungle Juice

Replenish your savings account in the kidneys and build cash flow in the sexual organs. Imagine you are in a luscious jungle. Drink up life force from the earth to nourish the kidneys, ovaries, and uterus.

● Lotus Bud Breathing.

- Sip juicy Earth Qi into your tailbone like sipping nectar with a straw. As you inhale, tuck your sacrum and chin. Squeeze your yoni.
- Create "beaks" with your fingertips together and pointing down, like lotus buds, in front of your ovaries.
- Exhale and rock your sacrum backward. Release and open your hands.
- Repeat these steps nine times. This form of Yoni Breathing is quite quick and refreshing.

● Qi Balls Grounding

- Breathe Earth Qi up to the perineum and hold your breath as your hands hold a ball of qi.
- Split the qi ball into two separate balls and roll them down your legs to the Bubbling Springs points. Let your arms flow downward at the same time.
- Repeat Lotus Bud Breathing nine times.

● Kidney Qi Fills the Yoni

- Scoop up Earth Qi with your hands pointing to the kidneys. Pack qi into the kidneys and fill out their energy field.

- Blow with the "choo-oo-oo-oo" sound, sending the juicy essences down to the ovaries and uterus.

● Small Ocean Breathing

- Embrace the aura of your ovaries with your palms a few inches from your body. Feel your ovaries breathing and their warm, pink glow pulsating into your palms.

❋ Four-Leaf Clover

Pull up the "push-button controls" around the PC pump to shoot energy up the body to the brain. Subtle movements stir more qi movement than most big physical movements.

- Front: Squeeze and pulse the clitoral ligament.
- Back: Squeeze and pulse the anus/qi muscles.
- Sides: Press your left foot into the ground and tighten the left side of the perineum. Repeat on the right side.
- Figure eight: Swing an eight around the front and back, left and right, all four corners, and then center. See fig. 5.5 for an illustration of the figure eight.

❋ Ovarian Palace Compression

Pull up the pelvic floor as you bear down, compressing the qi ball from both ends.

- Squeeze the vagina lips and the cervix toward each other as you inhale. Your belly will draw in.
- Expand on the exhalation, noticing your belly pushing out. This is reverse or dantian breathing.
- Hold a qi ball with your hands above and below the Ovarian Palace. Hold out the exhalation to create empty force. Show this internal compression by pulsating a qi ball between your hands. See Qi ball compression in fig. 8.8.
- Place one hand on your pubic bone and the other on your sacrum. Squeeze the qi ball from front and back. Squeeze the mound of Venus and sacrum toward each other as you inhale. Bear down below the navel as you exhale.

SHAMANIC SEXUAL PRACTICES

In the following exercises, we embody shamanic animals, guardians of our sacred temple, who protect us with virtue and call it toward us. Celebrate our inter-being! We are one family, one creative force with all the animals who fly in the air, swim the sea, and roam the mighty grasslands.

Explore how the nature of the five elements is captured by these animal powers: metal/tiger; water/turtle; wood/dragon; fire/crane; earth/phoenix. We will bring to balance the physical strength of the tiger with the mysterious, spiritual qualities of the dragon. We will also play with soul archetypes of deities and mythological beings to expand our soul's expression. Virtue has the spiritual power to sublimate sexual energy in an effortless way.

✳ Turtle and Buffalo

The Turtle and Buffalo Qigong is done in a low, wide posture that opens the hips and strengthens grounding through the legs. The bent-over posture opens the groin for deep breathing, which builds digestive fire and clears excess coldness from the uterus. It also builds qi in the lower dantian, spine, and brain. The turtle goes into the water, then the buffalo charges out of the water. This is a great way of getting down and expressing your sexual power!

Note: Do not practice deep groin breathing in these postures while menstruating, as it will increase the blood flow.

● Golden Turtle

- Practice Six-Gate Breathing (see chapter 8) 9 times in a wide, deep Horse Stance.
- Lift your arms above your head and pull down the heavenly force with your fists facing you.
- Widen your hips internally like a big smile to make space for your back to hinge down. Your fists are facing your chest and your chin should be slightly tucked in.
- Exhale, slowly hinging yourself down until your back is parallel to the ground and your elbows are inside your knees, but not touching them.
- Stay bent over and sip sexual energy up the pumps along the spine (sacral, adrenal, and cranial) and up to the crown (see fig. 7.1 on page 266).
- Hook up to the stars by connecting your crown energetically to the Pole Star and your sacrum to the Southern Cross. Feel them pull in opposite directions to effortlessly suspend your spine. Energize your whole body and smile.

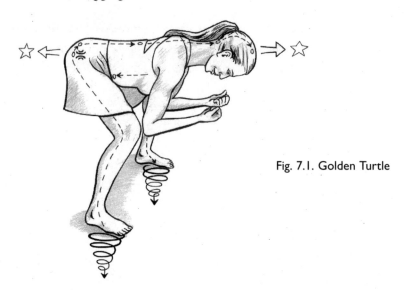

Fig. 7.1. Golden Turtle

- Bearing down through the dantian, exhale down the legs and screw the life force into the ground.
- Repeat for 3 sets.

● Water Buffalo

The deep groin breathing in this exercise tones the digestive and sexual organs. The charging ahead builds natural self-confidence.

- Remaining in the hinged-over posture, drop your sacrum a touch and lift your shoulders slightly. Hold on to a qi ball below your groin (fig. 7.2).
- Breathe deeply into your groin like a bellows: your belly expands on the inhalation and sucks in on the exhalation, lifting the urogenital muscles. Let air jet out of your wide nostrils; imagine you have a nose ring!
- Press your feet into the earth. Breathe in fully from the groin to the shoulders as if the water buffalo is charging out of the water. Pack qi into the shoulders. In between charging/packing, pump your belly with deep groin breathing in sets of 9 quick breaths.
- Repeat for 3 sets.

● Wash the Spine in the River

- After the Water Buffalo exercise, drop your torso in a forward bend and swing your spine sideways.
- Let your head and arms hang down, and let go of the base of your skull.

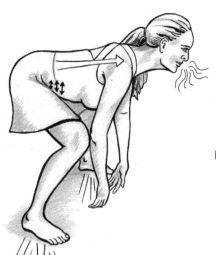

Fig. 7.2. Water Buffalo

Lunge from side to side, leading the movement with your hips. Sweep a figure eight on the ground with your arms.

- Roll up slowly. As you stand, enjoy the rising sensation like mist rising up and clearing your head. Absorb the warmth you have generated into your bones.

❊ Water Wheels with Three Archetypes

This practice mobilizes your sexual energy and refines it in the Microcosmic Orbit, activating the pumps along the spine to pump sexual waters up to the higher centers.

The practice helps make your soul responsive and flexible: at any appropriate moment you can shift to being a warrior, lover, or sovereign. In this way you become a full-spectrum lover who meets life and relationships with courage, love, and wisdom.

● Little Water Wheels

- Stand in Horse Stance with knees slightly bent.
- Imagine being near an ocean. Scoop the ocean power into your ovaries. Make rolling motions in front of your ovaries with your hands to help get it going (see fig. 7.3a on page 269). Roll qi around the ovaries—back, up, forward, and down, like little water wheels. Make a purring sound, "rrrrrr," by trilling your tongue. Rev up your motors! Everyone has their own signature rhythm.

- Inhale, suck up your PC pump, and notice how your sacrum tucks under. Exhale, rocking your sacrum back. Keep up the sacral rocking as you breathe.

● Three Archetypes: Warrior, Lover, and Sovereign

Roll the circular wave 6 times quickly around your ovaries. Roll the circular wave 3 times around each dantian: belly, chest, and head. Allow the whole body to wave rhythmically. Notice the different qualities of each dantian: power, warmth, and light.

O Warrior Archetype—"I Protect You"

- Scoop up to your kidneys, inhaling, and move the qi in a circle to the navel and down the front (fig. 7.3b). Pump up the power of the ocean to nourish the kidneys. Make a full, deep "waaaah" sound, as in "water."

O Lover Archetype—"I Love You"

- Scoop up the back and circle the qi around your heart and lungs (fig. 7.3c). Make a circle from your adrenals to your throat. Open your creative voice. Rock your chest forward and back in sync with the sacrum rocking. Offer love with the heart's warm sound, "ha-a-a-a-a-w."

O Sovereign Archetype—"I Understand You"

- Press your feet into the floor. Scoop up your back to your head and circle the qi around your brain (fig. 7.3d). Make a circle from your throat to above the crown. Pulse your tongue on the roof of your mouth. Your chin will rock, opening the Mouth-of-God point in the base of the skull and activating the cranial pump.
- Nourish your mental power. We say "m-hmm" and nod when we understand someone. Make a light sound of humming bees, "m-m-m-m," similar to the droning sound "Naad," the cosmic sound current of enlightenment.

This practice can also be done without the sounds. The etheric movements can naturally roll through you during an orgasmic experience. They generate tremendous energy on the dance floor too!

● Turning the Wheel of Life

- Hold a qi ball, scooping sexual water up the spine, over the crown, and down the front.

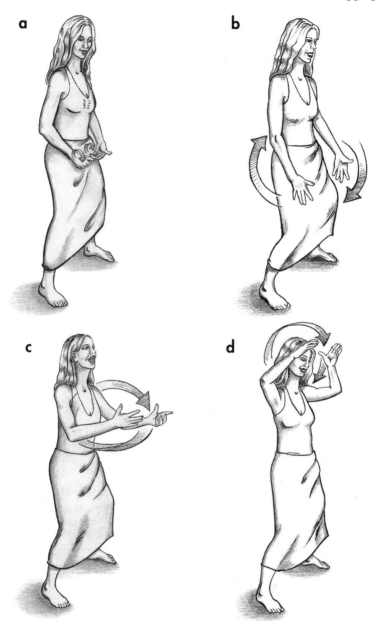

Fig. 7.3. Water wheels and three archetypes

- Inhale up the back and exhale down the front. Pulse your tongue on the roof of your mouth so the energy circulates down the body. Make a "mmmm" sound rising up the scale and down the scale as the movement rises and falls. Induce the Microcosmic Orbit.

● Ferris Wheel

- Circulate the Microcosmic Orbit as your hands move quickly around a Ferris wheel, faster than your breathing (fig. 7.4). Rotate your arms in front of you as if the yang hand were chasing after the yin hand! The faster it moves, the more light you generate!
- Stand with your hands over your navel and let the energy move by itself.

● Conclusion

Collect the energy at the navel and feel yourself as one with the ocean. Thank the ocean goddess for her healing power.

✺ Swimming Dragon

This curvy, sensual practice weaves sexual energy around the three dantians to integrate and evenly balance their soul fields of thinking, feeling, and willing. It circulates qi in the three Thrusting Channels, balances hormones, increases flexibility, and enhances your youthful body. You are as young as your spine!

The two dragons you create intertwine around the Central Channel like human DNA, forming the caduceus that is sometimes used as the symbol of medicine (fig. 7.5). The yin and yang dragons play with a golden pearl and take it on a cosmic journey through the central star, central sun, and central moon.

● Swimming Dragon Principles

- Move your spine like a snake (see fig. 7.6a on page 273).
- Keep your elbows in close to your body.
- Move from your spine, the "dragon bone."
- Let your head move with your hips.
- Stretch your eyes to look at your "dragon tail" trailing behind you.
- Keep your feet together.
- Going down, lead with your pinkies; going up, lead with your thumbs. Flip your hands on the out curve.
- Breathe like a serpent: make a snakelike sound, "sssss," as you descend; breathe in from the earth as you sweep across the bottom curve. Make the sound "sssss," as you ascend; breathe in from the heavens as you rise up on your toes.

● Hormonal Balancing

Smile to your glands as you move past them. The sideways stretching energizes the thyroid, thymus, pancreas, adrenals, and ovaries. The upward stretch

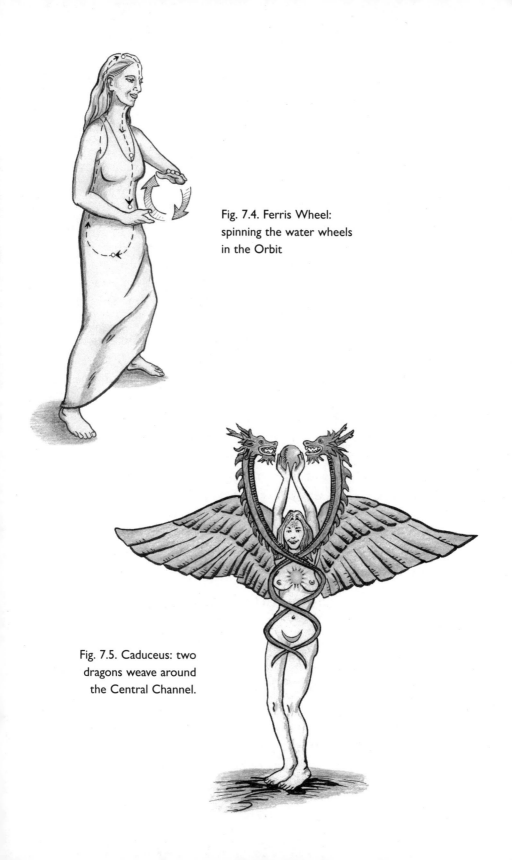

Fig. 7.4. Ferris Wheel: spinning the water wheels in the Orbit

Fig. 7.5. Caduceus: two dragons weave around the Central Channel.

energizes the pituitary and pineal glands. Thank your glands for all that they do for your health.

- Stand in heavenly posture with your feet together and your hands in prayer position at your heart.
- Sweep your arms outward, palms down, as the dragon gathers from the earth. At shoulder height, turn your palms up to gather from the heavens. Let your inner dragon spread its wings! Rise up on to your toes. Bring your hands into prayer position above your crown, holding on to a golden pearl (fig. 7.6a).
- Bring your hands and the pearl down the *left side* of your head like a sleeping dragon (fig. 7.6b).
- Sweep across your throat. This stretches the thyroid and parathyroid glands.
- Curve around the *right side* of your chest (fig. 7.6c). This stretches the thymus gland.
- Sweep across your solar plexus. The sideways pull stretches the pancreas and adrenals.
- Curve around the *left side* of your lower abdomen and across your perineum (fig. 7.6d). This gives a stretch to the ovaries. Breathe in from the earth.
- Ascend by swinging *right,* then *left,* then up the *right side* of your head (fig. 7.6e). Breathe in from the heavens. When your hands reach above your head, rise up onto your toes. Let the two snakes, yin and yang, kiss above your crown! This surges sexual energy up to the pituitary and pineal glands.
- Go down the same way you came up: *right, left, right.* Breathe in from the earth. The dragon takes the pearl on a journey around the Pole Star in the head, the sun in the heart, and the earth and moon in the lower abdomen.
- Ascend *left, right, left.* When your hands reach above your head, rise up onto your toes.

Repeat as many times as you like. You can add a soul flavor like an innocent, playful dragon or a dark, sexy dragon. Hold back on any judgments of what is saintly or sinful! The creative energy is pure and natural.

- At the end, bring the elixir that you have gathered in the pearl straight down your Core Channel. Drink the nectar like a drop of heavenly dew into each chakra flower. Bring your hands down in prayer position. Point your fingers downward below the solar plexus, then place your hands in Yoni Mudra (a V shape with the thumbs together) over the Sexual Palace (fig. 7.6f)
- Give thanks for this resource of creativity, vitality, and beauty. Smile and bow to the mystical magical dragon within you.

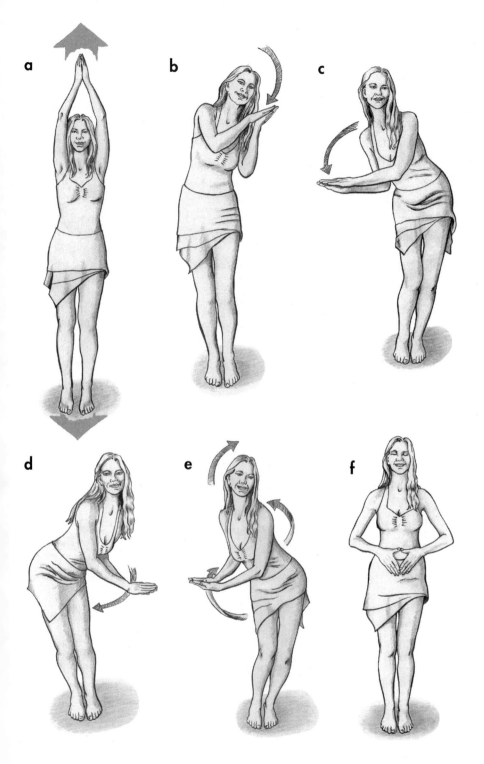

Fig. 7.6. Swimming Dragon, down to earth and up to heaven

❋ Belt Channels

Are you thin-skinned, finding that the moods of those around you affect your mood? By being aware of the spinning Belt Channels, you can develop a thicker, radiant, protective Wei Qi field.

These channels are the only channels that run horizontally in the body. They protect the front and back chakras with high-frequency energy and help you pull yourself together when you feel dispersed and all over the place.

As you spin in energy from the earth and the heavens, you'll develop healthy boundaries and bundle up with energetic protection.

- Spin rings of light around your roots, feet, knees, hips, waist, chest, throat, mid-eyebrow, crown, and halo.
- Spin counterclockwise up from the earth, front to the left (fig. 7.7a).
- Spin clockwise down from the heavens, front to the right (fig. 7.7b).
- Move both channels simultaneously, silver light spiraling close to the body and golden light coming down—yang protecting and containing the yin.
- Feel the whirling vibration inside of your yoni and Core Channel.

Qi Tree

Qi moves 'round
Spiraling from the ground
Up the tree of life
Whirling in the sky.

Qi moves 'round
Spiraling from the stars
Down the tree of life
Rooting in the Gaia.

❋ Qi Fountains

When you have an abundance of energy that overflows your body, you can channel it through your auric field, circulating it in a torus ring—a revolving doughnut shape of universal qi. In this practice, you can build healthy boundaries by employing the Fountain of Yin and Shower of Yang to wash and protect your auric field. You can circulate the energy in meditation or induce the flow through Qigong. Your qi will feel fresh like the air after a rain!

● Fountain of Yin: Pulling Up Divine Bliss

Scoop Earth Qi up the insides of your legs, up the Core Channel, and out your crown like a fountain (see fig. 7.8 on page 276). The qi cascades down your auric field and comes back into your feet. You can show this flow by lifting your hands up the front of your body as you inhale and lowering your arms down the sides of your body as you exhale. Sense that you are taking it all in—sky, mountain, forest, and ocean—with one big embrace.

Whole-body orgasm can feel like your body becomes one Jade Fountain! Squeeze your thighs together and then your buttocks, undulating qi up your spine and sending a rippling wave of ecstasy up your body, filling your aura with bliss. Show this fountain of bliss with your arms.

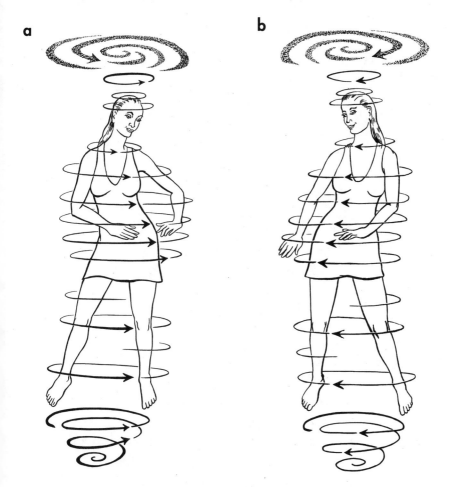

Fig. 7.7. Belt Channels spiraling energy from earth and heaven

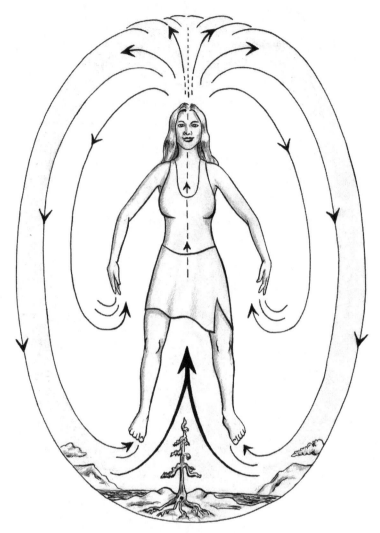

Fig. 7.8. Fountain of Yin

● Shower of Yang: Pulling Down Divine Light

Reach your hands up the sides and scoop Heaven Qi down through your crown, down the Core Channel, and through your feet (fig. 7.9). Then draw the qi up and around through your aura. Imagine that you are drawing qi from the stars and planets—the moon on your right and the sun on your left. Bring heaven down to earth. You can show this flow with your arms rising up the sides of your body as you inhale. Then bring your hands down the front of your body as you exhale.

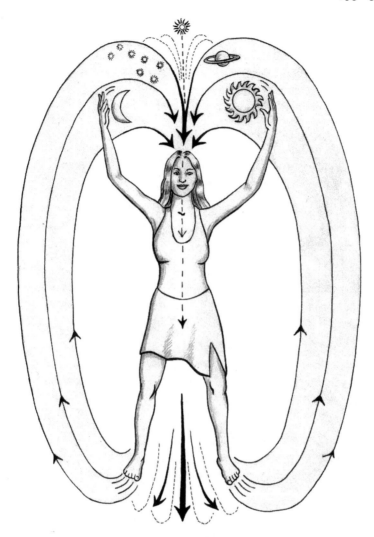

Fig. 7.9. Shower of Yang

Shower the clear light of the heavens down your Core Channel. Tuck in your auric field with a bubble of moving light. Gather refined light frequencies and bring them down to earth. Gather from nature: from the oceans, forests, mountains, and sky as you raise your arms. Bring the energy into your crown and down your Core Channel—a cascading waterfall of light to nourish your higher destiny. Feel yourself sustained, protected, and guided by divine light. Let the bubble of light attract positive events toward you.

● Torus Fountain

Run the Fountain of Yin inside the Fountain of Yang, so that they are both circulating simultaneously. Torus is a doughnut shape—apparently the shape of the universe and the magnetic field of the heart.

✺ Fountain of Sound

Lift the rejuvenating sexual waters up through the Inner Flute or Core Channel, from the perineum to the crown to water the lotus flowers.

- Standing in Horse Stance, inhale and scoop up Earth Qi with your hands. Channel juice from your Jade Fountain into your voice. Draw a fountain up to each chakra or energy center. Fluidly wash up through each center with the rising scale, seven tones for the seven chakras. Squeeze with your buttocks to shoot energy through your open throat and sound "la, la, la" up the scale. Squeeze the thighs and buttocks and send a wave of qi up through your core. Scoop with your hands and lift your palms up your midline. Open your hands out like the top of a fountain and lower your hands down your sides, palms down.
- Spray out through the crown to tone the eighth sacred chakra and shower down all around the body, washing your auric field.
- Reverse the flow. Turn your Palms up and scoop up the outside. Funnel energy back into the crown by pointing your fingertips together down your midline. Scoop up and point down to each chakra: halo, crown, third eye, throat, heart, solar plexus, Sexual Palace, and root. Resonate one chakra at a time sounding "tu, tu, tu" down the scale, vibrating into your roots.

✺ Kali Stretches Her Tongue

This dramatic exercise surges sexual energy through the tendon meridian lines and moves the sexual energy up to the higher centers, particularly the crown. It can be done with or without a jade egg.

This practice embodies the energy of Kali, fierce and wrathful, slaying egotistic delusion in your life. It removes stale qi from the body, making room for fresh, new impulses. Kali clears all that does not serve us—like a storm clears old leaves.

To ravish and be ravished with passionate energy!

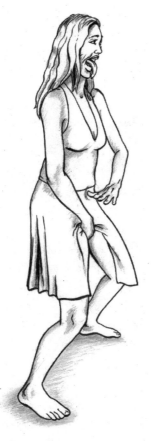

Fig. 7.10. Kali Stretches
Her Tongue

- Stand in a strong Horse Stance.
- Press your left thumb on the Sea of Qi point, two finger-widths below the navel. If you are using a jade egg, pull the string downward with your right hand as you sound the liver sound, "sh-h-h-h-h-h," three times, while thrusting the energy up the three dantians, through the sacral, adrenal, and cranial pumps. Lift the back of your neck. Without an egg, you can still pull an imaginary string.
- Exhale strongly as you stretch out your tongue, look up to your crown, and stretch the tendons of your fingers and toes (fig. 7.10). If you are using a jade egg, tug the string nine times while squeezing the jade egg, pumping the qi upward, and emptying out all the air. This opens the back of your throat and increases the empty force power (vacuum suction), which sucks energy up the spine to your crown.
- Inhale and pop your belly open to expand it with qi and breath. Let your arms lift above your head as you inhale and make the dragon's sound—a high-pitched surprised "a-a-a-a-a-ah."

- Pull down the heavens by bringing your arms down, sounding "s-s-s-s-s," to bring down excess heat from the head and heart to the lower dantian.

● Bone Breathing

Draw the sexual waters up your trunk like juicy sap rising up a tree, inhaling. Spread the juice into your branches and roots, exhaling.

✸ Durga Rides the Tiger

Durga, Goddess of Power, rides a tiger (fig. 7.11). She is a protector of what is precious to us. *Durga* means "inaccessible fortress," and thus this goddess represents protection power. She is seen as the power to overcome demonic forces.

The white tiger is the shamanic animal of the Taoists, the embodiment of courage and strength. Imagine that you are riding a white tiger, holding a white shield of protection and a sword, which cuts through to the truth with integrity.

This exercise tones the pelvic floor and builds potent energy in the left and right ovaries. It also builds compression in the womb, which can be used in childbirth for bearing down with inner strength.

The practice surges energy up through the spine and neck to build a confident and sovereign posture. It brings out the wild-woman instincts and protects our sexual energy by sounding like a growling tiger. When inner strength is present, no fight is necessary; naturally healthy boundaries declare, when needed, "Don't mess with me!" This inner power is of particular importance to women with a history of sexual abuse, who need to remember that they are masters of their own sexual energy.

- From a standing posture, inhale and pull up the earth force by squeezing up through your legs and buttocks. Grip the tiger with your thighs. Grip your fists in front of your groin, at the Rushing Gates. This pulls up sexual energy from your yoni to the core.
- Moving from your core, turn to the left and bear down the left leg, pulling up on the left side of the anus. Punch down with the right fist while making a growling tiger sound—a deep, guttural "hu-u-u-u-m." An equal force of energy rises up the spine and stretches open the cranial pump. From your core, project a pure white light outward into your second skin—the first Wei Qi field of your aura.
- Come back through the center, inhaling and pulling up the reins of your tiger energy.
- Repeat on the right side.

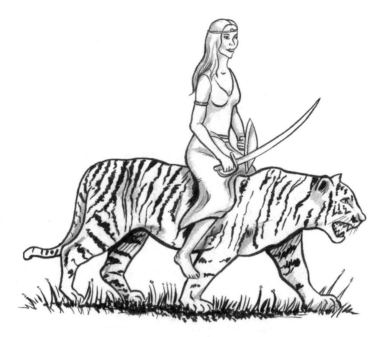

Fig. 7.11. Durga Rides the Tiger

✳ Phoenix Washes Her Feathers

The phoenix, the bird that rises out of the ashes, is a symbol of renewal and rejuvenation. This time-efficient, effective exercise cleans and nourishes all the vital organs and glands and spreads the Sexual Qi to all your meridians. It can be done with or without a jade egg in your yoni. In a more advanced version of the exercise you can hang some weight from the jade egg.

To do the "washing," we warm up the water (Yoni Breathing), add a cleansing agent (sexual energy), agitate (wrapping), rinse (healing sound), and dry (fan out). Sexual energy cleanses the qi back to its original blueprint. It is your best detergent! It also is a primal source of nourishment, which we absorb into the organs and glands like a superfood.

• Inhale and widen your upper back to open the Wing point behind your heart, making a little space for a small "qi egg" under your armpits, where the first point of the Heart meridian is located. Imagine you are a bird fluffing its feathers. Practice Six-Gate Breathing (see chapter 8) nine times, sucking fertile Earth Qi into your yoni, palms, and soles. Allow the tendons of your fingers and toes to respond by subtly stretching and releasing. Lift up an imaginary weight and then a real weight with your genitals, organs, glands, and tendons.

- Inhale (sip) one-third of your air. Gently squeeze up your yoni, perineum, and anus, and direct sexual energy to the kidneys. Scoop up energy with your hands, pointing and spiraling to the kidneys. Pack and hold the breath. Spiral the energy in and around the kidneys six times. Smile to your organs. Be gentle and calm, without strain (fig. 7.12a).
- Without exhaling in between, inhale and sip up to the liver and spleen, expanding the fascia in the side ribs. Spiral around the liver and spleen six times.
- Sip up the last third of air while raising the energy and arms to your chest. Spiral six times around and through your heart and lungs.
- Rotate your hands away from your center, palms up, leading with your thumbs. Push your palms forward, sinking the chest and tucking back your chin. Make the lung healing sound, "ss-s-s-s-s-s," as you extend your arms (fig. 7.12b).
- Make "beaks" with your hands, pulling all the fingertips together, as you inhale and draw up sexual energy to the master glands (pineal and pituitary) in the head (fig. 7.12c). Feel the power of these glands hooking up the sexual energy like an elevator is hooked from above. Smile up, clench your teeth, press up your tongue, and pull in your eyes. Spin a mini-tornado counterclockwise (front to the right) six times to spiral up Earth Qi and Sexual Qi from below.
- Inhale again, bending your elbows slightly. Pull up the energy with your thymus gland in your chest, and spin the mini-tornado.
- Sip again, pulling in the beaks slightly closer. Pull up the qi with your pancreas and solar plexus, and spin the mini-tornado.
- Exhale with the kidney healing sound, "choo-oo-oo-oo," pressing down your hands (fig. 7.12d). Compress the qi ball in your lower dantian.
- Pull up and pack the Ovarian Palace, twisting your hands inward, thumbs touching the ovaries.
- Exhale, stretching the tendons in your hands and feet, pinkies twisting back. Open your wings. Stretch out your tongue, which will tilt your sacrum back, fanning the long tail of the phoenix (fig. 7.12e). Look at your nose tip—the beak of the phoenix. Spread the sexual energy through all the tendon meridian lines, ending in the fingers and toes.
- Repeat packing and wrapping the organs and exhale the liver sound, "sh-h-h-h-h-h."

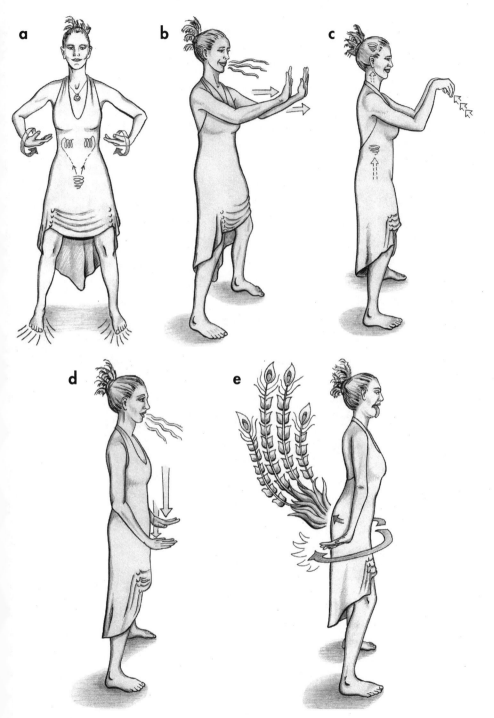

Fig. 7.12. Phoenix Washes Her Feathers

- Pack and wrap the glands and exhale the heart sound, "ha-a-a-a-a-w."
- Repeat packing and wrapping the organs and exhale the guttural spleen sound, "who-o-o-o-o-o."
- Pack and wrap the glands and exhale the triple warmer sound, "he-e-e-e-e."
- Twist the inner and outer tendon lines, bringing your feet gradually together like a Taoist Charleston dance. Twist your hands and feet: thumbs and big toes inward, then pinkies and pinkie toes outward. Toes touch, then heels touch.

✸ Flying Crane

The crane is the shamanic animal for the heart. The heart with wings beats throughout our whole life! In ancient China, the crane was symbolic of longevity and wisdom. It was believed that souls of the deceased were carried on the backs of cranes to the sky. In mythology, Taoist immortals would magically transform into cranes for astral journeys. It was said the mother of the Taoist priestess and Immortal Sun Bu'er dreamt that a crane entered

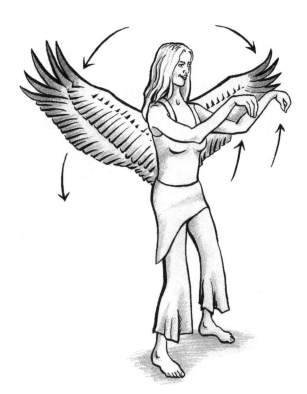

Fig. 7.13. Flying Crane uplifts sexual energy.

through her breast and she knew she would give birth to a divine being.

In this exercise, we lift earth energy and sexual energy up the Left and Right Thrusting Channels by activating the left and right sides of the anus. This exercise can be done with or without a jade egg. In a more advanced form of the exercise you can attach a weight to the egg.

- Standing in a wide stance, bend your knees slightly as you inhale and sink into the earth. Lift your arms forward to head height, with hands in beak positions (fig. 7.13). Lift golden-pink fish from the sea!
- Exhale as you spread your wings out to the side, palms pressing down. Press your feet into the floor, growing tall. Compress the qi ball by squeezing up the jade egg and lifting a real or imaginary weight. The force that compresses your qi ball is equal to the force projected into your powerful wings! Energize your fingers like the spread feathers of a flying crane.

8
Cultivating Your Qi
Exploring Sources of Vitality

A tree grows high when it has deep roots.

Whether you are beginning or refining your sexual energy practice, it is important to remember that the energy you seek exists all around you in the universe. Your body serves as a conduit of that energy and can also become an amplifier of it with regular Qigong practice.

This chapter explores how to deeply ground yourself in the pure life-force energy of nature—how to draw it in, store it, and channel it where it's needed so that it is ready when you are! As you cultivate energy, you become sensitive to the qi in the world around you and the qi moving inside your body. Tap into an abundance of sexual vitality in nature to be creative in your life. This approach to Qigong consciously cultivates sexual vitality to put fuel in your lamp to light up your world.

Create opportunities to bring spirit into matter. We celebrate life as sacred when we bring ritual into our lives, like full moon circles and blessing our holy water.

CONNECTING WITH NATURE

The Tao is the path of living in harmony with nature. Spend time in nature so that you can learn to feel the vitality all around you. While nature nourishes us all, we receive the fullness of the life force when we are conscious of our connection with it.

Beauty Without and Within

Allow the beauty of nature to caress and nurture your senses. Smile to nature with gratitude and it will "smile back" generously, filling you with natural energy. When we give our gratitude and delight to nature we boost the immune system of the earth, and she needs it! When we smile, our pelvic floor lifts effortlessly and uplifts our creative forces.

> *Before me beauty, behind me beauty,*
> *above me beauty, below me beauty,*
> *all about me beauty!*
> NAVAJO TRADITIONAL PRAYER

✳ Walking in Beauty

Smiling inwardly embraces your body with loving acceptance. Appreciate your unique beauty, and it will glow and grow from within. Coming to emotional, mental, and spiritual peace with yourself is the key for preventing illness and enhancing health. This natural self-confidence will reverberate into more harmonious relationships with the world around you.

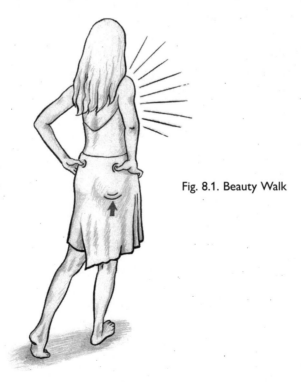

Fig. 8.1. Beauty Walk

● **Beauty Walk**

Press the "sex points"—the dimples beside your upper sacrum (see fig. 8.1 on page 287). This will open your chest and express confidence.

As you walk, squeeze the buttock on the side where you are stepping. This will bounce sexual energy upward and give you awareness of your beautiful behind! Feel the trail of conscious beauty you are leaving behind you.

● **Sensual Walk**

Feel your sensual curves and the natural sway of your hips and shoulders. Walk as if moving through liquid honey. Sigh and relax. Imagine that you are carrying a vase on your head as you walk with graceful poise. Caress the earth with your bare feet. Feel the breeze on your skin, smell the fragrances, and delight in all the colors around you. Breathe it all in!

Nature Qigong

Make a point of stepping outdoors to directly experience nature's vitality. Learn to feel and interact with the qi all around you and you will find your own energy resources expanding. Find a tree that attracts you. Step into its aura with reverence. Hugging trees is comforting and stabilizing.

❊ Tree Qigong

Release excess negative emotions with the healing sounds and channel them down from the tree's leaves and branches through the trunk and roots into the earth. Negativity will be composted and neutralized by the earth. Human emotions, like the carbon dioxide we breathe out, serve as food for the trees, just as their fresh oxygen is necessary to us.

Qi moves Love
Love moves Qi

When Qi moves, I sing
When Qi moves, I dance
When Qi moves, I smile

Breath moves through me
Breezes blow through trees
Community flows as one

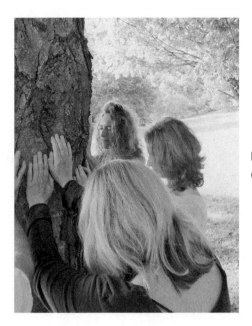

Fig. 8.2. Women hugging a tree
(Photo by Minke de Vos)

Return home to the source.
Listen to the sound current.

The trees tell me
to love, just love.

Lungs: Energetically sweep down the bark of the tree and let go of sadness with the lung sound, "ss-s-s-s-s-s." Breathe in the strength of the tree.

Kidneys: Bow to the tree and wash any fear into the roots as you make the "choo-oo-oo-oo" sound. Breathe in the peace and wisdom of the tree.

Liver: Lift your hands with open palms to the green leaves. Release anger and frustration with the "sh-h-h-h-h-h" sound. Breathe in the kindness and generosity of the tree.

Heart: Lift your hands with open palms to the aura of the tree. Release feelings of impatience, chaos, and selfishness with the "ha-a-a-a-a-w" sound. Breathe in the unconditional love of the tree.

Spleen: Curl down over your ribs and blow your worries down through the core of the tree as you make the "who-o-o-o-o-o" sound. Breathe in balance and stability. Trust that the rain and sun will come as needed.

Triple warmer: Sweep up the tree with your hands rising. As you bring your hands down, shower neutral, balanced tree energy down your Core Channel and sound "tree-e-e-e-e."

● Circulate Qi with a Tree

- Hug a tree and imagine that it is your lover in this moment. Sense unconditional love and acceptance in the tree.
- Circulate qi in the Microcosmic Orbit—inhale up your spine to the top of the tree, exhale down the tree to its roots, and inhale up your spine again, breathing in a continuous loop. Reverse direction, running the qi up the tree and exhaling down your Front Channel to the roots before looping back up again.
- Still hugging the tree, circulate qi in your horizontal Belt Channels from your feet to your crown and back down. At the same time, wrap energy up the tree counterclockwise and down the tree clockwise. Sense the rings of growth in the tree.
- Lean on the tree and breathe tree qi into your bones.
- Listen to the tree for any message or gift it may have for you.
- Bow with gratitude to the tree.

Cosmic Nourishment

Our life-body is like a plant that needs all the cosmic forces to flourish. Nature nourishes all beings; in Qigong we make this process more conscious so we receive from each natural energy source more fully. The moon is a cosmic source of divine feminine frequencies and the sun is a source of divine masculine frequencies.

❀ Moon Qigong

These practices are wonderful to do outside when the moon is full, though you can also absorb her qualities at other times. The waxing moon (from new to full) is a time of expansion, potency, regeneration, and rejuvenation. The waning moon (full to new) is a time of cleansing, completion, and reorientation.

The moon is the eye of the night
Seeing through the darkness,
Seeing through my life.
Give me inner sight,
Give me inner light.

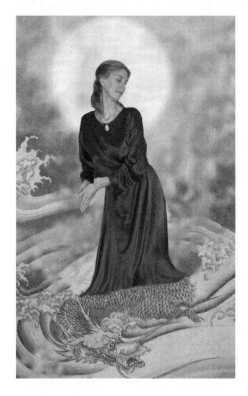

Fig. 8.3. Dancing with Luna
(Photo art by David Gyurkovics)

Moon Mirror: See the moon as a cosmic mirror. Bring Luna's light into your third eye. Imagine the full moon inside your head as a mirror reflecting light down into your body-mind, lighting up the dark areas in your life. Reflect on your life, seeing the perfection in the lessons and events.

Moon Bath: Let the moonlight's yin energy nourish you internally and emotionally. Lean back with open legs and allow the moonlight to bathe your yoni.

Pulling Moon Silk: Make a triangle or prism with your hands to focus moonlight into your Crystal Palace (center of the head). Let your Crystal Palace reflect the light into your body (see fig. 8.4 on page 292). Exhale and reach with your "qi fingers" to touch the moon. Inhale and pull the energy like silver silken threads toward your third eye. When you feel complete, wash it down your Front Channel and store it in your yoni.

Moonlight Shower: Bathe yourself in real or imaginary moonlight. Connect with the Divine Mother in the moon. Reach up and scoop some moonlight and then shower it down the front, back, and middle of your body.

Drinking Moon Milk: Make a cup with your hands and receive the "milk" of the moon (see fig. 8.5 on page 292). Drink and mix it with your saliva and swallow it down to your belly.

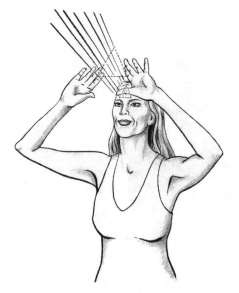

Fig. 8.4. Catching moonlight with Pulling Moon Silk

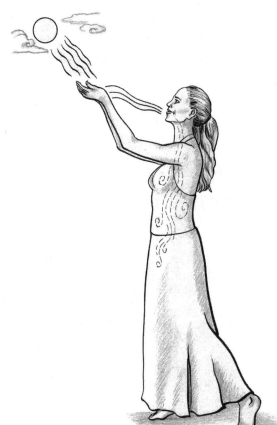

Fig. 8.5. Drinking Moon Milk

Moon Cream: Gather some "moon cream" in your hands. Massage the healing, nourishing balm into your body. Soak an extra dosage of moonlight medicine into any parts of your body calling for healing. Feel with all your senses that this part of you is already healthy, innocent, and glowing.

Moon Recharge: Breathe moonlight into your sexual organs and kidneys to recharge your "batteries." Store this energy in your bone marrow.

Moon Orbit: Circulate moon qi in the water cycle. Feel the phases of the moon within your Microcosmic Orbit, the dark new moon at your perineum getting brighter as it reaches the full moon at your crown.

Collect the moonlight in your center. Bow in gratitude to the moon.

Luna's Kiss

Luna, Luna	*rides the tides*
Luna, Luna	*goddess of the night*
Luna, Luna	*heaving, swelling*
Luna, Luna	*of ocean's passion*
Luna, Luna	*carry me high*
Luna, Luna	*to touch the sky*
Luna, Luna	*reflect sun's kiss*
Luna, Luna	*cradle divine bliss.*

❀ Sunlight Qigong

The bright warm sun nourishes our physical body with yang energy.

● Sun Bath

Find a private place to expose your yoni to the warm (not too strong) sunlight. Open your labia like a flower. Breathe in the light to purify and recharge your sexual organs (see fig. 8.6 on page 294).

Expose your kidneys to the late afternoon sun. Let them soak in the warmth.

● Sun Shower

- Gather sun qi, filtered through the trees in thousands of rainbow rays. Reach out to touch the rays and pull them into your third eye.
- Shower the light down your spine to fill the Governing Vessel. Replenish

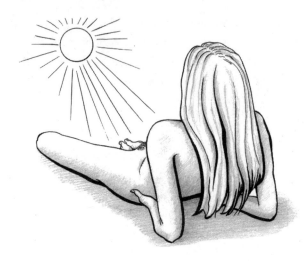

Fig. 8.6. Yoni sunbathing

the yang qi in the adrenals. Fill your sacrum with warmth so it can nourish your nervous system.

• Circulate sun qi in the fire cycle to energize the whole body.
• Collect the sunlight in your center.

In this moment the Sun is your Lover.
Allow Him to penetrate you with enlivening warm rays!

✺ Earth Bath

An earth bath nourishes your center, resetting your body's vibration to the earth's frequency of 7.8 herz. This frequency is the same energy you feel when you are happy or orgasmic!

Lie down on the earth and absorb the stable, supportive energy into your cells.

✺ Water Prayer

Bless your water in the morning, in a special ritual, or on celebratory occasions. Water changes into beautiful patterns like snow crystals when we send positive intentions into it. Water has memories of our feelings and thoughts, as many researchers have discovered.*

---

*See, for example, the book *Messages from Water and the Universe* by Masaru Emoto (New York: Hay House, 2010).

Hold up your glass of water and say this prayer:

> *Divine Palace of the Six Directions,*
> *infinitely flying Heavenly Gods*
> *and abundant Earthy Goddesses,*
> *quickly bring down vital qi into my water and cells,*
> *please, in accordance with Divine Law.*
> *Thank you, thank you, thank you.*

Take your time to drink and absorb the blessed healing water.

SUPPORTING THE KIDNEYS
Treasure House of Jing

In Taoist practice, the kidneys store the essential energy that powers all of the other organs. This energy is a combination of your Original Qi (formed at conception) and the Postnatal Qi that you acquire through the digestion and refinement of food and water. This combined energy acts as your core energy reserve, supporting all bodily functions throughout your life.

In addition to storing essential sexual energy for your survival and for emergencies, the kidneys govern the sexual organs, sexual energy, the bladder, the bones, and the brain. They are associated with hearing and balance and also govern the qi of absorption and storage.

When the orb of the kidneys is in balance and full of life force, we feel energized, calm with the strength of inner peace, and supported by Mother Earth. We have a healthy sex drive and feel passionate, sensual, gentle, and creative. Strong willpower creates the magnetism and charisma to manifest our dreams. We are able to surrender through our faith in our bodily wisdom. We feel safe to open and breathe in life deeply.

Kidney Energy

Kidneys are the "trunk where the gathered treasure takes root." This saying describes how the kidneys store jing—the inheritance or treasures you were given from your ancestors at birth. This jing, also called Prenatal Qi, cannot be replenished and is gradually spent during our lives. This is why it is vitally important to conserve it through Qigong practice, and to supplement it with Postnatal Qi—the types of qi we can acquire through food, drink, and respiration.

A positive attitude toward life is another source of Postnatal Qi. Spiritually we are nourished by inspiration of the highest good that supports us in our lives. By realizing the divine intention in all our experiences, we reap the potential energy to manifest our destiny, which we received at conception.

Yin and Yang Kidneys

The kidneys are the root of yin and yang energies in the body's organs and tissues. The left yin kidney is considered the "water of life"; it is the fundamental substance of all yin the body, moistening and nourishing the tissues. It rules the cycles of birth, growth, maturation, and reproduction. It is the foundation of yin energy in the body.

The right yang kidney is the foundation of all yang energies in the body. It is the primary motivator and is considered the "fire of life." Kidney yang provides warmth to the organs and tissues.

Mingmen, the Gate of Destiny, is the moving qi between the kidneys, which pulsates with the influence of ancestral qi.

❊ Kidney Balancing

Visualize the left kidney as deep blue and the right kidney as bright blue. Become aware of which kidney feels tighter or harder to breathe into. Take extra sips into the weaker kidney to internally balance the yin and yang kidneys.

Breathe into Mingmen to connect with a portal to Yuan or Source Qi, the foundation of all the yin and yang energies of the body and the spark of change. Thank your ancestors for supporting you in living to your highest destiny.

Your Kidneys Are Your Batteries: The Importance of Preventing Burnout

The kidneys are the bio-batteries of the body. If there is no charge on your battery, there is no connection! That means it's hard to connect to yourself and others and to listen to divine guidance. It takes a certain amount of charge in the kidneys to pull cosmic qi deeper into the body.

If your fire burns too hot and you don't turn down the flame, your water will boil away and the pot will be burnt or broken. Women tend to be big spenders who love shopping and pleasing others. This is all good if we balance this overgiving tendency by giving back to our bodies and topping up our energetic bank account.

When we are overgiving we crave stimulants like sugar and coffee; we stay up late and try to rev ourselves up with loud music or push ourselves into exercise. This is called "false yang"—a superficial energy without the real substance behind it. This will eventually burn up the adrenals and kidneys, the central source of willpower in our body. Taoist yoga offers ways of conscious resting that will allow our natural reserves to be replenished.

The signs of kidney energy depletion can be fatigue, weak knees, back pain, poor short-term memory, low libido, incontinence, stiff or achy joints, poor hearing, hypersensitivity to noises, fear, and lack of initiative or creativity. More signs are hormonal imbalance, especially after menopause, night sweats, dizziness, osteoporosis, and accelerated aging. As you can see by this list, it is very important to consciously replenish your kidney energy!

✳ Test Your Batteries

To test how much charge you have in your kidneys, you can intuit a number between 1 and 10, visualizing your energy like the green bars on a charger. There might be a different number for each kidney. Practice Packing the Kidneys (see page 300) for five minutes, gently holding the breath in the kidneys. Then take another reading. After decades of doing this test with groups, I've found that people consistently get about two more bars!

Building Your Core Reserves

Replenishing Yourself—Replenishing Your Kidneys

Women tend to be great givers. It is vital for us to replenish ourselves on a regular basis through energetic self-care. In order to build kidney energy, we need to balance movement with stillness, and doing with being. What are the ways we can replenish ourselves? Let's look at what women already do: soak in the bath, rest in nature, receive a massage, go to the spa, get pedicures, meditate, practice Qigong and yoga. We can enhance these activities by being quiet, being aware of bodily sensations, receiving pleasure, and conscious deep breathing. Simply by closing our eyes and basking in the dark yin, we can begin to restore our vital energy. Going to bed early (before midnight) and listening to soft music, to nature sounds like running water, or to silence replenishes our kidneys.

Building the core reserves is essential for women who would like to empower themselves. The following kidney practices will give you effective ways to get charged and stay charged up.

Kidney Neigong

Neigong is inner work, mainly focusing on breathing. Kidney Neigong fills the kidneys with nourishing earth energy. This increases stamina and helps prevent adrenal burnout. It can also help to regulate blood pressure. Any overflow of kidney energy will flow into the bones, which are ruled by the kidneys.

Kidney Neigong has been an essential daily practice of mine for decades. The kidneys are nourished by receiving the yin energy of the earth, like a geyser bubbling up from underground waters. There is an abundant wellspring of life force to be tapped. Kidney Breathing is nourishing before, during, and after menstruation, or whenever you feel tired. It feels supportive and eases lower back discomfort during menstruation. It prevents drying up after menopause.

✺ Basic Kidney Breathing

To initially access Kidney Breathing, hold your hands at your waist, with your thumbs on your back. As you exhale, hug/squeeze your floating ribs and gently press your thumbs into your kidneys (fig. 8.7).

Inhale and push out against your hands and thumbs. Breathe into the kidneys and feel them widen.

● Drawing from Deep Wells

- Rub your hands until they're warm, then tap the Bubbling Springs points in the soles of your feet. Tap into deep underground waters and draw from a healthy, energetic pipeline of earth's creative energy to nourish your kidneys.
- Claw your feet like suction cups. Suck qi in through the Bubbling Springs points, up the insides of your legs, through your perineum, and into the kidneys. Keep your perineum firm to enhance the suction power.
- Exhale into your kidneys.

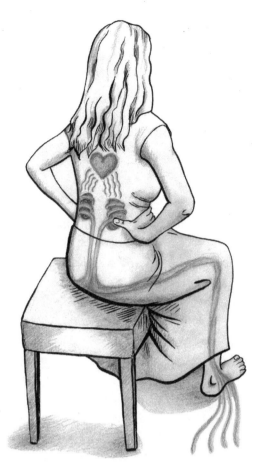

Fig. 8.7. Kidney Breathing,
melting the ice

❀ Kidney Packing

This practice can be done lying down, sitting against a wall or chair, or standing in Horse Stance against a wall or a tree.

• If lying down, press your kidneys gently into the floor or bed and feel them widen.
• In a sitting position, press the kidneys gently against the back of the chair.
• Standing in Horse Stance against a wall or tree, fill out your kidneys and lengthen your middle back into the support behind you.

Other postures that expand the kidneys are Child Pose (kneeling with head down), sitting and leaning forward over your bent legs, or lying flat with knees to your chest.

● Inward Mudra

This hand position helps focus energy in the kidneys.

- Tuck your thumbs into palms, with the thumbs touching the base of the ring fingers.
- Curl your fingers around your thumbs into a loose fist. Place your hands on your belly in front of the kidneys. This will draw your mind inward to build qi in your kidneys.

● Packing the Kidneys

- Sit or stand with your hands over your kidneys.
- Pack qi into the kidneys, filling them with calm, blue, luminous mist. Smile to the kidneys, making them soft, receptive, and comfortable.
- Hold and spiral earth energy nine times in and around the kidneys to absorb the energy.
    Say inside the words of internal power, "Peace" or "Shanti," three times.
- Exhale slowly into the kidneys.

● Packing the Qi Belt

- Place your thumbs over the kidneys, below the floating ribs.
- Feel the breath push against your thumbs as you inhale.
- Keep up the breath pressure against your thumbs as you exhale.
- Keep your "tire" pumped up around your waist as you continue to inhale and exhale.
- Do not strain, and smile into the power you are building in your abdomen.

● Turtle Drinks from Deep Pools

- Take sips into the kidneys and spiral the energy in them.
- Breathe in earth qi through your left Bubbling Spring. Pull up the left side of the anus to pack the left kidney. Make a fist with the left hand in front of the left ovary.
- Breathe in Earth Qi through your right Bubbling Spring. Pull up the right side of the anus to pack the right kidney. Make a fist with the right hand in front of the right ovary.
- Sip to both sides at the same time, then exhale deeply into the kidneys, blowing down warm qi from the heart with the "ha-a-a-a-w" sound. This is known as "melting the ice": love melts icy cold fear, which is a major

obstacle to liberating sexual energy. Melting the ice will relax and lengthen the psoas muscles—the "muscles of the soul."

❋ Filling Deep Yin Pools

In this version of Kidney Neigong we practice Empty Force Breathing. Imagine that you dig a hole in the sand and allow the water to fill it: the more you empty, the more you can fill.

This feels wonderfully relaxing lying down with your knees up.

- Place your fingers on the B spot ("b" for "breath") just above the pubic bone, and gently press in as you exhale. Exhale very long and pull up your perineum and urogenital muscles. Hold out the exhalation as you deeply relax into the emptiness. Feel the life pulse in your ovaries.
- Inhale and feel your kidneys magnetically drawing cosmic forces deeper into the body. Allow the water of life to fill the pelvic basin from below upward, widening your kidneys and filling them with yin energy. Your lower belly will push your fingers outward.
- Feel the peaceful grace and blue light of the water element. Relax. Breathe rhythmically and count by your heartbeat: 6 beats exhaling, 6 counts suspending the emptiness in the kidneys, 6 counts inhaling, and 6 counts suspending the fullness.

● Descending Yang, Ascending Yin

As you exhale, stroke down the yang meridians, down the back of the legs. Pick up some earth energy with your fingers, stroking around the toes. Stroke up the yin meridians, up the insides of the legs, as you inhale. Stroke around the waistline (Qi Belt).

Rub the kidneys warm.

Reverse Breathing

Reverse breathing is also called "tortoise breathing" for its longevity qualities, as the tortoise lives a long time. It is a natural breathing pattern that occurs with laughter, yawning, and shouting and during exertions of power. Express "HA!" as if you were doing a punch in martial arts, and notice how your belly moves outward or gets firm on the exhalation. This is the reverse of relaxed breathing, in which the belly moves inward on exhalation and outward on inhalation.

The belly comes in on the inhalation as the kidneys expand in the back, and it goes out a bit on the exhalation as the qi pressure builds in the dantian. Applying Newton's law of counter forces (for every action there is an equal and opposite reaction): the more qi pressure goes down and in, the more force is projected into the limbs, voice, mind, or wherever you direct it. This is why reverse breathing is practiced extensively in Qigong, Taiji, and other martial arts, as well as in some Zen circles to penetrate the riddles of life.

This breath pattern is also known as power breathing, dantian breathing, or paradoxical breathing. It is called "paradoxical breathing" because you cannot see from outside if someone is inhaling or exhaling. A striking samurai warrior would watch carefully because the opponent is more vulnerable on the receptive inhale.

The following exercises are reverse breathing practices that help build qi pressure in the dantian.

❀ Resilient Qi Ball

Use reverse breathing to compress the qi ball in your dantian. Use this breath to counter any deflation that happens in your Qi Belt when you are stressed. When you are stressed out, you have dropped the ball.

In this exercise, your perineum will bounce like a yo-yo as you pull up on the inhalation and pull up even more on the exhalation.

- As you inhale, fill up your dantian like a beach ball, expanding on all sides. Draw qi into the perineum.
- As you exhale, blow down into your core like blowing up a balloon in your belly, building qi pressure. Pull up the pelvic floor and squeeze the ball from above and below, noticing how the sides of the qi ball widen. This sends qi down the legs to root (fig. 8.8).
- Once the qi ball is pumped up (like a tire), do not deflate it.

Sounding the Six Healing Sounds or other vocal expressions can strengthen the compression of the qi ball and thus the projection of power in or out of the body. Lifting a yoni weight by bearing down on exhalation as you simultaneously lift the pelvic floor further compresses the qi ball.

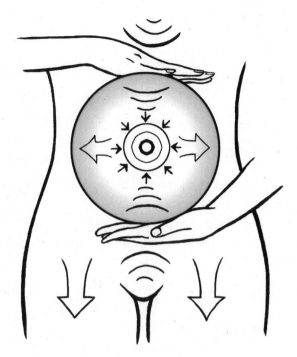

Fig. 8.8. Compressing the qi ball

Playing with Qi Ball

Breathing rewards you in the moment.
It is the expression of your Divinity.
Practice with joyfulness!

✳ Spinning Wheel

According to Chinese myth, the weaving goddess floated down on a shaft of moonlight. Her robe was seamless, for it was woven on a loom without the use of needle and thread. Thus the phrase "a goddess's robe is seamless" expresses perfect workmanship.

In this exercise, we apply reverse breathing to circulate the vital breath in a small Microcosmic Orbit around the lower dantian. With each turn of the wheel, weave golden silk threads (refined qi) into your center. This is very effective for building reserve energy in your core. It is a good practice for those who are low in sexual vitality.

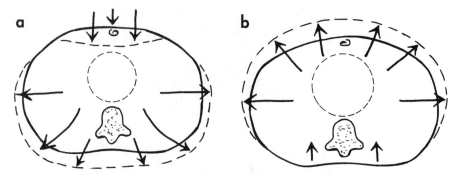

Fig. 8.9. Reverse breathing: inhale into the back, exhale into the front.

Rotate a spinning wheel with clasped hands in front of your lower abdomen, ascending close to your body and descending farther away from your body:

• Clasp your hands together and hold them close to your body in front of your navel. Exhale down to the navel, lowering your hands.
• Inhale and scoop golden Earth Qi from the perineum up the back to Mingmen (fig. 8.9a and 8.10a) Your hands rise to waist height, close to your body.
• Hold your breath in the kidneys to absorb the qi. Then exhale the qi forward to the navel and down to the cauldron just below the navel (fig. 8.9b and 8.10b). Bring your hands slowly down, away from the body, thus completing the wheel with your hands. Feel how your core starts to fill up. Scoop up more qi by sucking up your perineum and anus and draw up the back again.

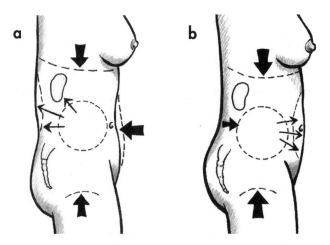

Fig. 8.10. Reverse breathing, side view: inhale and exhale.

❋ Deep Sea Turtle Breathing

Kuan Yin, goddess of compassion, is seen riding a sea turtle, rising from the sea (fig. 8.11). She is the embodiment of the yin principle and the turtle is the shamanic animal for the water element. In Chinese mythology, the turtle supports the world on the back of its shell.

- Stand or sit and practice Spinal Cord Breathing (see page 66) with reverse breathing. Imagine you are a turtle swimming slowly and steadily in the sea.
- Inhale, curl your back like a turtle's shell, and widen your kidneys. Fill your kidneys with blue nourishing mist and wrap them with qi nine times. You can internally say "Peace" or "Shanti" three times.
- As you exhale, arch your back and feel your dantian pushing forward (reverse breathing).

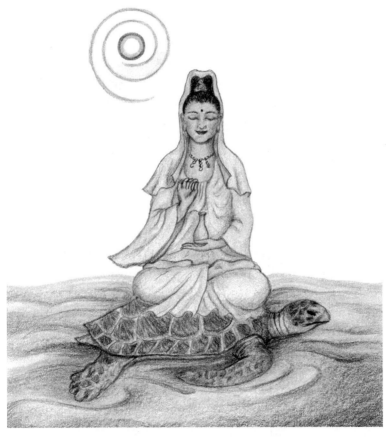

Fig. 8.11. Kuan Yin riding a sea turtle

CHANNELING
YOUR VITAL ENERGY

When you have become familiar with building your energy, you can begin to direct it with awareness. Understand yourself as an energy being!

✳ Embracing the Tree

Embracing the Tree starts with standing like a tree—standing up for yourself and what you believe in. As you align yourself with the heaven, earth, and human planes you become strong, yet receptive. At home in your body, you learn to balance form and internal flow, spreading sexual energy through your whole being.

● Standing in Horse Stance

A proper Horse Stance posture will drop your center of gravity as though you are sitting on a three-legged stool.

- Stand with your feet hip-width apart, with the outsides of your feet parallel to each other. Bend your knees in a comfortable quarter squat, being sure not to extend them farther out than the toes. Feel your weight going down through the backs of your knees and through the ankle bones and Bubbling Springs points (fig. 8.12).
- Tilt your sacrum downward, as if pulled by a weight toward the earth. Imagine you have a long, heavy dragon tail extending from your sacrum into the deep earth.
- Open your hips wide so the knees are over your ankles. Hug a horse with your thighs. This tones your inner tendon lines and yin meridians.
- Keep your joints relaxed and open, allowing internal qi pressure to hold them up.
- Widen your adrenal pump (T11) by filling it out with your breath.
- Soften your chest slightly, as if receiving a hug. Fan your scapulae to open the dorsal pump (C7).
- Keep your spine straight and your crown suspended by a star. Tuck your chin slightly to stretch open the base of the skull (occiput). Smiling gives you a natural uplift and strength!

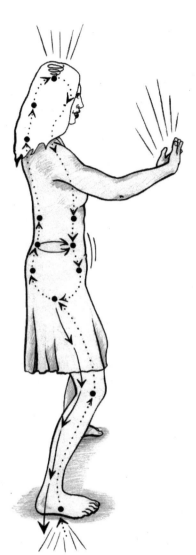

Fig. 8.12. I stand steady
on my own two feet.
I am ready to evolve!

Standing Tree

Standing like a tree
Head in the sky

Standing like a tree
Roots in the ground

Standing like a tree
Firmly in the wind

Standing like a tree
Stable and kind

Standing like a tree
Leaves spread wide

Standing like a tree
Still and wise

Tree, tree, tree
Standing free.

● Creating the Embrace

- Let your arms embrace a tree with relaxed shoulders. Drop your elbows with gravity—like rain falling down a steep roof into the ground. Face your palms toward your chest and feel your fingers connected by a magnetic force. Wrap chi from inside around the outsides of the arms.
- Twist your forearm tendons outward so that your thumbs are slightly out and your pinkies are slightly in. Say yes to life!
- Connect an iron bar between your palms and the Lung 1 points below your collarbone. Circulate energy in a clockwise circle around your arms from the right hand to the left hand.
- Jump a few times and fill your body with readiness and aliveness. Be engaged in life! Get ready to catch a ball that might come from any direction.

✱ Packing the Tree

The kidneys magnetically draw qi deeper into the body. We put some money into our savings account (kidneys) before spending all our cash. Packing is like a good handshake: if it is too loose the hand drops out; too tight and the qi is squeezed out. When it's just right, there is a good connection. This exercise packs qi (inhale and hold) into multiple areas of the body.

● Six-Gate Breathing

Standing in Horse Stance, breathe in and out from the six gates: Huiyin (perineum), Laogong points on your two palms, Yongquan (Bubbling Springs) points on the soles of your feet, and the Baihui point at your crown. Suck up with your perineum as you inhale to create suction power in your palms and soles. Suck up your yoni to activate the sexual energy. Breathe quickly 9 times.

Practice Six-Gate Breathing before each of the packing steps below.

● Packing the Qi Belt (Dantian)

- Inhale, squeezing up the yoni, perineum, and anus to draw energy up from the earth and sexual organs. Pack this energy into your kidneys. Inhale around the Qi Belt to pack your navel. Sip and pack the Sexual Palace. Pull up the perineum and hold your power in the dantian.

- Exhale down your legs. Screw out from the hips and wrap qi from inside around the outsides of your knees and ankles. Spiral giant screws into the ground.
- Practice Six-Gate Breathing.

● Packing the Qi Bottoms (Legs)

- Sip earth energy into the Bubbling Springs points, the backs of your knees, and your perineum. Feel the fullness of your legs. Exhale, spiraling down the legs, screwing into the ground.
- Practice Six-Gate Breathing.

● Packing the Qi Top (Microcosmic Orbit)

- Pull up the perineum and draw sexual energy in sips to the sacral, adrenal (T11), dorsal (C7), and cranial pumps (C1), then up to the crown. Spiral outward 6 times, then spiral inward 6 times, drawing in heavenly energy. Move your eyes to the left, then to the right to direct the qi in a vortex (like the Power Lock).
- Exhale a bit, releasing pressure in chest.
- Pack your solar plexus and your navel.

● Embryonic Breathing

Hold your breath while pumping your belly in and out 9 times. This increases the qi pressure and massages your organs with the packed qi.

● Bone Breathing

Suck qi into your bones like you are a sponge soaking up warm water. Exhale, spreading the qi to your whole skeleton. Practice 3 of these breaths, holding your form with fullness.

● Brush Down

Brush down your chest to your belly as you walk. Keep tall and feel the ground with your feet. Become aware of the majesty of your posture.

❋ Wei Qi Field Breathing

Light attracts light: the pure colored light that you breathe into your aura will attract high-frequency virtue energy from the universal energy field.

Stand in Embracing the Tree posture. Radiate the colored light from your core channel and breathe it into the three Wei Qi fields:

- Breathe out white light into the first Wei Qi field, which radiates about one to three inches from your body. Breathe in truth and integrity from the universe. Affirm: "I am true to myself."
- Breathe out blue light into the second Wei Qi field, which radiates about 12 to 18 inches. Breathe in self-understanding and wisdom from the universe. Affirm: "I understand myself."
- Breathe out pink and violet light into the third Wei Qi field, radiating about 24 inches. Breathe in love and compassion from the universe. Affirm: "I love myself."
- Pull down divine light to download and embody compassion, wisdom, and truth. "May the pure lights of virtue carry me on my life journey."

BONE TONING
Bone Marrow Neigong

Emerge from primordial roots into new life!

Bone Toning is simultaneously a way of strengthening and a way of sounding by sending vibrations through the bones. Our bones are transpersonal instruments for channeling the energy of the earth and the heavens. They are reservoirs of the deep ancestral, primordial, creative, sexual energy that create the bone marrow, red and white blood cells, stem cells, and the bones themselves.

Traditionally these practices are called "Bone Marrow Neigong" (bone marrow internal work), as the focus is on the mind's intention to move the qi in a meditative way. The intention is to penetrate qi deep into the marrow at the core of the bones, to support their fundamental functions and to help you find stability and security in your bone structure.

It is essential to fill the kidneys, which rule the bones. Their overflow qi pours into the bones and bone marrow. Practices include Warm-Ups, Bone Venting, Bone Breathing, Bone Packing, Bone Compression, and Tapping.

Bones are like crystal transmitters that tune in to celestial sound. Consciously breathing in sound vibrations deeply cleanses the bone marrow, activates the production of red and white blood cells, and awakens our DNA's potential to create new life.

Bone Toning can be practiced in many positions—lying down, sitting, or standing. Explore the different positions, which facilitate the channeling of cosmic forces into the bones in different ways. Standing, for instance, allows for channeling gravity through the bones to strengthen bone mass.

After a self-love ritual, rest on your back with your palms up and absorb the warm, steamy energy into your bones. Feel the pulsations of your yoni spread and pulse in the bone marrow. Breathe in light, and mix it with your internal warmth. Soak it into the bone marrow, where your blood is grown. Store excess sexual energy in your bones.

❋ Bone Breathing Warm-Ups

Use these practices to prepare your body for the Bone Breathing exercises below.

● Bone Rocking

- Extend a long tail into the deep earth from your spine—the "dragon bone." Rock your spine like a snake from side to side.
- Ripple your spine forward and backward with the Turtle Neck and Crane Neck, moving from below as you press and rock your feet.
- Rotate your head, ribs, hips, and knees, loosening the joints.

● Trembling Horse

After a fight, animals release their traumas right away by trembling. What do humans do? Sometimes they hold on to resentments even into the next life! When the inner thighs and hips tremble, quickly opening and closing, it loosens any constriction in the psoas muscles, part of our instinctive fear response. This can release sexual trauma that may be stored as emotional residue in the body. This is a great way to let it go!

Vibrate all the bones from side to side to release stress. Inhale, shaking your wrists and arms and shimmying your shoulders. Exhale, shaking down your hips and knees (moving them in and out) and tumbling the stress down and out your feet. Vibrate your lips like a horse.

● Bone Shaking

Shake your bones to loosen the joints. Bounce up and down on your heels. Keep a lift in the pelvic floor so your bladder does not overshake. Relax your jaw and let the teeth chatter.

Flick out your hands and feet as you blow out your mouth. Toss sick winds out of your bones into the earth. Tell the stress, "Don't come back!"

✸ Bone Venting

Bone Venting is an effective way to cleanse the bone marrow and blood. The practice begins with Earth Qigong, a simple standing Qigong that is the foundation of many Bone Toning exercises.

● Earth Qigong

Breathe in: Sink into the earth like it is soft sand or moss. Relax and open your joints. Smile and be receptive. Soften your whole being with feminine qualities. Allow your arms to float to solar plexus height.

Breathe out: Press your feet into the earth. Root down and stand tall like a tree. Your arms will press down. Feel qi strengthen the bones. Stand your ground to activate your masculine qualities.

● Venting the Bones

• Practice the Earth Qigong above. As you inhale, breathe in infrared light; sunny, warm, golden qi; and clean, fresh oxygen through the skin, joints, fingertips, and toes.
• Melt excess toxins and fat in the bone marrow and breathe it out like gray, cloudy smoke or exhaust. You can use the "ha-a-a-a-w" sound to purge with heat. As your arms come down on the exhalation, press your feet into the ground and send toxic qi out your toes into the earth.
• The bones expand like sponges on the inhalations and squeeze out dirty water on the exhalations. A jet of sexual energy, our best detergent, helps push out congestion. Purge toxins out of areas and joints that feel stiff. Release shock, fear, and trauma from the bones.
• Rinse with cool blue vapors. Blow out from the bones with a descending "yoo-oo-oo-oo" sound (as in "you"). Your bones can feel like silver flutes.

Bone Breathing

Bone Breathing involves drawing in earth and heaven energy as well as sexual energy into the bones. If Healing Love practice gets you too energized to fall asleep, Bone Breathing will settle you down; simply store the excess sexual energy in the bones and build a reserve of energy.

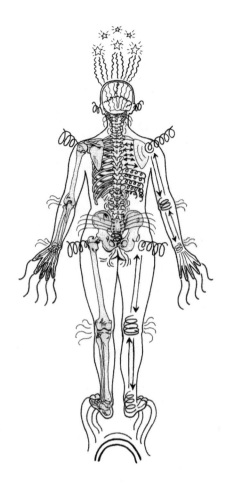

Fig. 8.13. Bone Breathing

❁ Bone Breathing Practice

This Qigong is a meditative journey into the depth of your body.

• Draw earth, heaven, and sexual energy into your body using one of the three methods below. Hold it there for a moment to absorb the qi into the bone marrow (fig. 8.13).

Straw method: Breathe through your fingertips and toes along the bones as though they were straws. This is a nice method to start with, as you gradually work qi from the extremities deeper into the body.

Spiral method: Spiral, coil, wrap, or drill the qi in and around your bones and joints. This method is good for protecting the body—like a qi bandage—and also good for penetrating qi deeply into the joints, spine, ribs, facial bones, and ear bones.

Piercing method: Visualize light coming from all directions and piercing through the skin, joints, or protrusions into the bone marrow. This method is particularly effective for penetrating light into the flat bones. It is a nice way to complete the practice, sensing your whole body being penetrated at once.

- Let the qi penetrate and spread along all the bones. Exhale into the body rather than out your skin. The action of Jing Qi (sexual essence) in the marrow stimulates the production of red and white blood cells.

✳ Restorative Bone Breathing

Filling the bones with qi is a great way to restore depleted energy.

- Lying down on your back, loosen and rock the spine with the Spinal Pelvic Rock (see chapter 6).
- Loosen your joints with the Laughing Baby practice—arms and legs shaking up in the air as you laugh.
- Hug your knees and pack the kidneys, wrapping the qi and holding your breath.
- Lean your legs against a wall. Embrace the tree with your arms, elbows resting on the ground.
- Breathe earth energy into the spine, around the ribs to the arms, and into the sacrum and legs.
- Turn your palms up. Feel your hands and feet like satellite dishes picking up light and sound frequencies. Listen to the sound current.
- Bring the soles of your feet together in Butterfly position and bend your arms above your head. Breathe into your hips and shoulders.
- Relax in a spinal twist, legs twisted to the right while your head looks left. Breathe into the open left side with smiling energy. Repeat on the other side.
- Roll over into Child Pose and bask your spine in the starlight.
- Lie flat and feel your whole skeleton breathing.
- Roll over to your right side to relax your heart.
- Sit up and rub the Bubbling Springs points on the soles of your feet.

Packing Qi into Your Bones

The following exercises will help you pack the qi you have absorbed deep into your marrow, until the bones become dense yet light, like diamonds.

🏵 Bone Packing

- Draw qi into your bones using one of the above methods. Feel your bones contract as the qi is sucked in. Let the suction power of your dantian draw sexual energy up, and let your smiling attention direct it into specific areas.
- Hold your breath for a moment, compressing the qi in the bone marrow. Keep your muscles soft, like cotton or silk wrapping around the diamond bones.
- Exhale and penetrate the energy deeply into the bone marrow. Dantian breathing will distribute the qi pressure from the dantian along the bones, like water pressure unkinking a hose. The qi pressure warms and softens the tissues and muscles around the bones. Blow along the bones against an imaginary counterforce, as though you are blowing up a balloon.
- Imagine someone pushing you from any direction and channel their force into the ground.
- Especially fill out the adrenal pump (T11) to link your upper and lower structure together.

🏵 Light-Filled Skeleton

In this exercise, you will use all three methods to gradually fill your bones with warm, liquid light. Fill up your arms and legs simultaneously, then fill up your torso and head.

- Breathe into your fingers and toes, filling the hands and feet with qi.
- Wrap your ankles and wrists from the inside around the outside, like protective bandages.
- Breathe up your lower leg and lower arm bones like straws until they are filled. Or you can breathe up the inner leg bones (tibias) and down the outer leg bones (fibulas), and up the radii of the arms (thumb side) and down the ulnae (pinkie side).
- Wrap the knees and elbows. Breathe up the upper leg and upper arm bones.
- Spiral qi into the ball-and-socket joints in your shoulders and hips to lubricate them.
- Breathe into your pelvis and penetrate the eight holes in your sacrum.
- Breathe sexual energy up into your spine in stages, wrapping counter-clockwise.

- Drill around every rib from the spine to the sternum, as if someone were hugging you from behind. Breathe with your shoulder blades like wings.
- Penetrate the light into the skull and face. Spiral into the ear bones.
- Clench your teeth lightly to strengthen the roots of your teeth.
- Breathe extra qi into weak, stiff, or injured areas.
- Breathe into your whole skeleton as one piece. If your mind is single, your whole body will be filled with light.

✸ Light Touches the Bones

Extend qi through your fingers like laser beams to "touch" the bone marrow. Let light spread into your whole bone structure.

- Channel cosmic light through your fingers. Touch your pubic bone. The marrow of the flat bones is where white blood cells are created. Imagine a white light there. Feel the dantian and Sexual Palace become warm.
- Touch the femur bone in your thighs. Long, round bones are where red blood cells are created. Imagine a red light like mercury in a thermometer.
- Touch behind your hip bones. Warm and lubricate the ball-and-socket joints in your hips.
- Touch your sacrum with your right (sending) hand and the cranial pump with your left (receiving) hand. Let the warm pink sexual energy rise up your spine into your skull.
- Feel your temples pulse. Fill the Sea of Marrow in your brain with white light. Continue with the next practice.

✸ Chalice for Celestial Qi

- Open and lift your arms like a funnel for receiving heavenly energy. You will receive what you are open to receiving. Let your fingers be held up by light strings from the stars. Drop your sacrum and ground. Your bones are simply frozen starlight!
- Ask the stars to give you the energy you need right now to live your life's purpose. Listen to the celestial sound. Your bones are like quartz crystals in radios, picking up light and sound frequencies.
- Reach up to the Pole Star and channel violet light into your skull. Bring your hands slowly down the front of your face and body. Feel light glowing from inside your face.

- Light up the tiny hyoid bone in your throat.
- Touch your sternum and smile to your thymus gland. Radiate white light to stimulate the growth of T cells.
- Giggle into your sternum and let laughter spread through all your bones until every bone is vibrating with orgasmic vibrations. This is great for your immune system!
- Spread your arms down like a mountain. Feel heavenly energy streaming down and earth energy streaming up, heaven and earth making love in your bones.

Bone Compression

Compress the qi into your bones with the following exercises.

❋ Internal Bone Compression

- Inhale and spiral qi into your bones. Hold your breath to absorb and condense the energy, warming the bones.
- Squeeze warmth into the bones as you exhale. Penetrate your bones with light until they glow inside like diamonds.

❋ External Bone Compression

Yoni Breathing will warm and activate the sexual energy in between the packing practices. Breathe with your yoni, 9 quick breaths, squeeze and release, then slowly exhale.

- Pull up the sexual energy and pack, wrap, and squeeze your muscles against the bones in your arms and legs.
- Hold the qi compression, then exhale and slowly release, allowing the qi to run between your muscles and your bones.
- Repeat the Yoni Breathing, then pack and squeeze the muscles around your spine, jaw, and teeth. Slowly exhale.
- Repeat this sequence for the rib cage.
- Repeat this sequence for all the bones simultaneously. When you release, let your arms float up.
- Feel the blood pulsing in your bones, fingers, toes, crown, and perineum. Feel the pulse of new blood and qi in your bone marrow: feel the qi that moves the blood, the blood that moves the muscles, and the muscles that move the body. Organically allow movements to arise out of your

spine and inner body. Let go and allow the qi to move you into the freely flowing state of Unwinding.

Tapping

The tapping practice comes from a long tradition of twist-and-tap doctors of ancient China who practiced preventive medicine. Toxins get trapped in the joints like dust that collects in the corners of the room; the stuck toxins can accumulate and cause arthritis. Tapping the body releases stagnation and toxins like dusting your bones, organs, and tissues. It increases lymph drainage, loosens old cells, invigorates new growth of the stem cells, and helps prevent cellulite buildup.

Vibrate sexual energy into the bones and organs. Bones heal through vibration!

❈ Tapping Practice

During this exercise, inhale and pull sexual energy up to an area, then pack it by holding the qi there. Exhale as you need to so as not to strain. With loose fists, palms, or bamboo hitters, tap well around the elbows, knees, and other joints as they are major detoxification points. You can bounce rhythmically with soft knees as you tap your body.

Avoid tapping on the spine.

- Tap clockwise around your belly (fig. 8.14a). Tap down the sides of the ribs in a zigzag (fig. 8.14b). Tap your chest and thymus gland as you smile (fig. 8.14c).
- Tap the back of your neck, without hitting the spine.
- Pull up sexual energy as you clench your teeth. Lightly tap your head with your fingertips, or gently tap around the hairline and jawline with a bamboo hitter (fig. 8.14d).
- Tap down the yin meridians on the inner part of your arms, and up the yang meridians along outsides of your arms (fig. 8.14e).
- Swing your arms and slap your shoulders. Cross your arms and slap between your shoulder blades or tap there with the bamboo hitter.
- Tap your kidneys, Mingmen, and your lower back (fig. 8.14f). It feels great to share tapping with a friend or lover: tap lightly in the kidney area and quite vigorously around the sacrum. Express how much you like it!
- Tap down the yang meridians of the legs, along the backs, sides, and front (fig 8.14g).

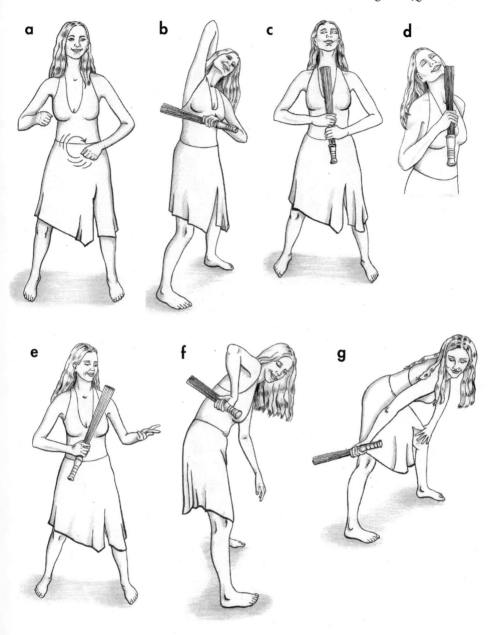

Fig. 8.14. Tapping vibrations

- Tap up the yin meridians on the insides of the legs.
- Tap the soles of feet and Bubbling Springs.
- Tap the Sea of Qi, 2 finger-widths below the navel (fig. 8.14a).

Wu Wei Qigong (Unwinding)

Allow yourself to be moved. Let it happen.

When the bones are full of qi, you can release it from inside into spontaneous movement. This Wu Wei Qigong is also called "Unwinding."

✸ Unwinding

Surrender to the wisdom of your spirit with Wu Wei—effortless effort. When you enter the state of Wu Wei, the path of effortless unfolding, you live in total surrender to divine will or the Tao. Living between heaven and earth, in complete alignment, we become a channel.

Through spontaneous, free-form movement we unwind old, conditioned energy patterns. Releasing trauma held in our structure, we allow harmonious sound and higher frequencies to vibrate into the core of our being. Filling the bones with qi, we liberate the flow from deep inside our bone marrow and cells. By letting go of control and surrendering to spirit, we allow ourselves to be moved by divine energy.

- Let go of all control areas such as the eyes, jaw, and solar plexus. Soften your eyes. You can touch your temples, cuing the brain to relax, or you can yawn into the back brain, signaling involuntary movement.
- Breathe deeply into your body, letting go with each exhalation. Trust the wisdom of the spirit to unwind your body-mind and be creative. Penetrate your deepest form with Bone Toning and then release into formless flow. The liberated energy moving through your body unleashes free and natural movement.
- Movements may unfold from different levels:
    Personal: releasing individual holding patterns, tensions, and memories, while allowing freedom from habitual movement
    Collective field: tapping into the space that originally created Qigong, yoga, and dance
    Divinely inspired: creative forms of movement
- Sense the pulsating, orgasmic, authentic movement arising from within. Simply go with the flow. It is not improvisation to music but a deep listening to the impulses of your spirit, which calls the qi inward, outward, or into movement. Allow free movement to clear the way so that you can be fully present in your practice.

• Smile inside to keep playful and spontaneous, like a child exploring movement for the first time. Smile with acceptance of any discomfort that may arise as part of the liberating process. Allow the energy to move you spontaneously. Your spirit is your best, personal bodyworker.

• Qi likes to move rhythmically: you may feel an urge to stretch, massage, shake, or dance. Allow internal knots to unravel and ripple out into whole-body movement. Allow the qi body to let loose. Surrender to the wisdom of the energy.

• Breathe consciously to keep the wind in your sails!

• Hum or sound into the places that want to open. The bones are like flutes and your qi is the breath that resonates in the body. Listen to the little whispers, "Free me—let me move!"

• When you feel complete, come into a symmetrical position to channel the free-flowing energies into the central river, the Microcosmic Orbit. Circulate qi up the Back Channel and down the Front Channel.

• Lie flat and place your hands over your navel. Collect the energy you have generated by spiraling counterclockwise and then clockwise into a pearl. Center yourself in the still, pivoting point amidst the inner dance. Come to peace.

• Bring down clear light with the triple warmer sound—"he-e-e-e-e"—to empty your mind. Enjoy the inner silence for a while.

✺ Partner Wu Wei Qigong

This is a great way for friends or lovers to sense and move each other's energy.

Start with your backs together, with no one leading and no goal. Both of you follow the qi. Allow your bodies to be moved like seaweed in ocean currents, carried by the force beyond personal urges. Allow your bodies to gracefully roll on and off each other, swimming in an ocean of qi.

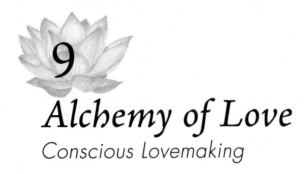

9
Alchemy of Love
Conscious Lovemaking

Are you aware?
Awareness is the continuum.

Are you present in every changing moment?
Presence is the giving of love.

Your experience of Tao Tantric Arts will grow more sublime as you continue to practice. Sexual alchemy is worthy of an in-depth education as well as reviving what feels natural.

The Taoist sexual arts will heighten your awareness of the energetic, emotional, and spiritual connection with your lover. They will help you develop ways to enhance healing and harmonious energy exchange with the men in your life and can be applied to same-sex partners as well.

SEXUAL ENERGY IS SACRED

Sexuality and spirituality are linked for Taoists: the passion and intimacy that you cultivate in your relationship can deepen your whole spiritual life. Body, soul, and spirit are one being and work together naturally if we do not separate them and judge them as sinful or taboo. When our raw passionate energy is refined and channeled upward to higher energy centers, it becomes the power behind love, creativity, and communion with Universal Love.

Compassion is a high state of consciousness, which ripples out into your relationships and the world around you. When partners are committed to supporting the highest in each other, they become portals for unconditional love. A couple might start with a physical attraction of sexual energy (jing), develop psychic flow between them (qi), and then raise their consciousness to perceive the most subtle spiritual presence (shen). Other couples might start with a strong heart connection and become more physically close. When we consciously cultivate the virtues of loving-kindness, our qi flows well and synchronicity happens easily.

The more we give pleasure, love, and compassion, the more we receive. We can heal each other and help each other expand our consciousness. We urgently need this powerful energy to heal this world and generate more love for generations to come. The whole universe is continually pulsating and vibrating. When we orgasm, we harmonize our own pulsations with those of our partner and nature. Becoming a multiorgasmic lover is realizing that you are one with the continuous, orgasmic, creative, and mysterious universal process!

GROWING MORE LOVE IN YOUR LIFE

How can we grow more love in our life? The ancients cultivated the intimate arts for centuries. They considered physical health the foundation of a vigorous, enduring, and fulfilling love life and vice versa.

Our essence is love; it is mainly our emotional and thought patterns that get in the way of our remembering that. Taoists believed that negative emotions are toxic to our bodies, health, and relationships. Instead of suppressing emotions or dumping them on others, we can recycle them into vitality. The Inner Smile is an easy way to do this and bring out the best in yourself and your partner. Listen to your partner with love, look into his eyes, hold hands, and honestly express how you feel. Keep "in touch" by communicating and touching with tenderness, even during troubled times. When the storms hit, be present for each other. Anger or harsh words can hurt our vulnerable insides and damage trust and responsiveness in lovemaking for a long time. Practicing the Healing Sounds benefits our relationships.

Lovemaking and Enlightenment

Lovemaking brings our presence into focus with intense pleasure, multiplied energy, and loving connection. When both lovers unite in body, soul, and spirit, we are on the edge of enlightenment—the merging of Shakti /energy and Shiva/consciousness. When we surrender with expanded consciousness, we can potentially pass though the mysterious portal into oneness.

Stairway to Bliss

In conventional sex, arousal rises to a peak, followed by compression and explosion. (See fig. 9.1 showing two kinds of lovemaking in relation to pleasure and time.) With ejaculation, the man's arousal quickly dives down; perhaps he will roll over and fall asleep. Yet the woman's experience may be very different. Perhaps her water has not yet become warm, or it is still steaming and longing to move.

In contrast, the tantric orgasmic graph looks like a staircase to heaven: waves of orgasmic bliss keep rolling in. Each wave shows a rising of arousal and exchange of energy, shown as a figure eight. By consciously sublimating the energy and merging with the Tao, we allow these waves to ripple through the five-element cycle, where they can be expressed through the following natural urges. These expressions might pop up at any time and in any order. In the surprise is the art of spontaneity.

Fire: Connecting with your hearts and feeling the urge to kiss. The heart is pounding and the blood is pumping, expanding into a heart orgasm. Sensitive sex is expressed through devotion, adoration, and caresses, and through giving and receiving love.

Earth: Connecting through touch and taste and feeling the urge to massage, stroke, grab, and lick. Earthy sex is expressed as ravishing, pounding, grinding, and thrusting.

Metal: Connecting through breathing and the urge to smell; breathing each other in and being sensitive to the skin. Breathing speeds up into ecstatic sex.

Water: Connecting through the bones and the urge to bite. Vibration expands into spine and brain orgasms. Sensual sex is expressed as undulating, erotic movement.

Wood: Connecting with the eyes and the urge to move, surge, and change positions. Passionate sex is expressed as playful, vocal, sweaty, and emotionally intense.

Lovemaking may weave through the various qualities of the elements. If you are predominantly more of one element, or your lover is, you might pace with familiar qualities as well as surprise your partner with expressions of the other elements. Lovers can play with the alchemy of the ele-

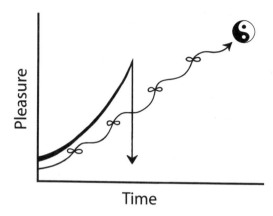

Fig. 9.1. Short-lived sex vs. tantric orgasm

ments. A "spiritual" lover might crave "earthy" sex for balance. All flavors can be expressions of love and are powerful medicine for the body, soul, and spirit.

Sexual Kung Fu

Men can have whole-body orgasms without ejaculating. Instead of exploding through the genitals, the vibrations rise through the organs, heart, and head and penetrate through the woman's channels as it circulates through the man. This circuit multiplies the energy. Sexual Kung Fu is learning the art of seminal retention: how to pull up and circulate the sexual energy with breathing, mindfulness, and muscle control so that the semen is recirculated instead of ejaculated. It is essential that the man minimizes and eventually withholds from ejaculating or he will lose much of his energy.

Use the word *circulate* instead of *stop coming,* which could stop the flow of energy. If a man circulates the orgasmic energy, then he will lose less essential qi even if he does come, as he has distributed it inside his body and his lover's. The woman also learns how to expand her experience of a genital orgasm into a whole-body orgasm. She will feel full and good for days!

Soul Orgasm

Soul orgasm is possible when you feel orgasmic energy circulating and waving through the body. Circulating energy in the Microcosmic Orbit balances warm yang energy and cool yin energy. It becomes a way to receive and give energy and also to generate love and light.

Once this pathway is open, you and your partner can exchange energy, linking your Orbits into figure eights, connecting through your genitals, tongues, foreheads, or hearts. The yin energy of the woman flows into the man and the yang energy of the man flows into the woman, creating a harmonious field of united energy. This exchange of energy can be felt even without touching. When a soul orgasm overflows beyond the physical, it can feel like a fountain rising out the crown. In bliss, souls can unite above the body. This energetic bonding deepens the potential of long-term relationships. Together you can cultivate a perennial garden of love, joy, trust, and respect.

Soul Mating

Have you ever longed for your soulmate? A soulmate is someone with whom you feel a mind-heart-spirit connection, which could have been cultivated in past lifetimes. This connection is cultivated by sharing in all three aspects of your being: thinking (views on life), feeling (what you care for), and willing (your lifestyle). Soul mating is a profoundly intimate experience of union and oneness. It can be felt at a distance. You can experience orgasmic lovemaking on the other side of the world from your partner! Like remote viewing or remote healing, remote soul union is a vivid reality.

Shakti dances, Shiva plays

Shakti swirls inside my body
Rising, rippling, rushing,
in upward waterfalls.

Bobbing golden bubbles
Shimmer through silk
Shakti emerges for air.

No mind, open throat, Ahhh
Hair extending into rainbow fields
wind blowing, allowing.

Shiva's musical fountains
Wash her with bliss
As she lies spread open
On endless shores of love.

Keys to Energetic Lovemaking

While lovemaking is instinctive, the refinements of the sexual arts are not always obvious. Keep in mind the following tantric concepts as you explore the deeper aspects of sexual alchemy.

Invitation. Your openness is very seductive. Enjoy following as well as leading. Tune in to your partner's signals, like subtle expressions and breathing changes.

Subtle communication. Lovemaking is like a conversation. Your vagina will become more alive and subtle. Feel your vagina from within. Allow natural sounds of pleasure to arise freely.

Active-Receptive. Touch with tenderness and presence. Receive your partner's gift of love through his or her penetration. Give your gift of love through your breasts. If you are too passive, your energy is too heavy and your mind sinks. If you are too tense and uptight, your body is more rigid and the energy does not flow well. Being active-receptive is a co-creative, flowing dance.

Breath. Let your breathing be free and wild. Breathe in and let in the cosmic orgasm, channeled through you and your partner. Allow yourself to soar in the vast ocean of bliss! Breathe out and let go.

Sound. Breathe with an open mouth and allow sound to naturally arise. The sounds may range from deep moaning to heart-opening "aaaaahs" to high-pitched blissful sounds. Be willing to feel emotion and pleasure and to express them.

Relaxation. Relax your jaw and throat. Your jaw reflects how open your hips are. If you are tight above, you will be tight below.

Touch your partner with the impulse arising from your whole body. Feel your touch sinking in beyond the surface of the skin or stroke the energy field of your partner.

Kiss with your yoni and heart, not just your mouth or from your head. Become aware of your yoni gently squeezing when you kiss.

Dance with your inner body. Flexing your yoni muscles during intercourse heightens pleasurable sensations for you and your lover. Gently contract your muscles to grip on your man's penis. Rhythmically squeeze and relax. Explore different sensations of prolonged gentle contractions, firm squeezes, or a series of quick pulsations. Be aware of building energy together.

Riding movements. While riding on top of your lover, you can play with the Crane Neck (fire cycle) and Turtle Neck (water cycle) while you brush his body with your hair or breasts. Sacral Screwing (Belt Channels) sets the energy spiraling up through your bodies.

Playing the Jade Stalk. While sucking your partner's "Jade Stalk" (also called "playing the flute"), open the back of your throat. Allow passionate energy to surge through you and play up and down your Core Channel. Send energy up through his Core Channel with your intention.

Love paint. If your partner ejaculates in your mouth, feel the photons as bursts of liquid light essence! Drink the love potion and paint your face with nature's rejuvenating lotion with gratitude.

Channeling orgasmic energy. As you are making love, smile to your kidneys, liver, spleen, lungs, heart, and brain. Smile into your lover's organs with the intention of growing virtues with the orgasmic energy. Orgasmic energy amplifies our feelings and makes the cells multiply in the right way.

Intuitive movement. Move your body intuitively so your partner's Jade Stalk stimulates the reflexology zones inside your yoni that are calling for healing. The penis is the best acupuncture needle in the world!

Spontaneous postures. Be aware of where the orgasmic energy is moving. Back bends open the heart to orgasmic energy; forward bending postures expand the kidneys to receive orgasmic vibrations; side bends allow the liver or spleen to fill with orgasmic energy.

Hands-on healing. Allow your hands to touch or hold organs that are calling for extra healing energy. Orgasmic energy is potent medicine!

Guiding the energy. Help each other open the channels and circulate the sexual energy by stroking your hands up the spine or down the Front Channel of your partner.

Timing. If you or your partner is tired after a long day or week or after a big meal, rest to replenish your qi; when you are well rested you will have more to offer each other. Morning is a time of uprising energy. Making love in the morning is energizing and gives us the openness and joy to greet the day as well as any stresses that may occur. Each organ has an optimal time when it receives healing energy. The ancient doctors would give prescriptions of when and in which postures to make love to heal specific organs.

Energy exchange. Smile with loving attention to the energy in yourself and your partner. Feel your movements extending into each other. Connect your tongues or sexual centers and feel your energy weaving through each other. Allow your excess yin qi to stream into your partner and your partner's excess yang to stream into you, making harmony.

Third eye connection. Connect at your third eyes and feel one circle of energy that moves through them and your sexual centers. The woman's third eye is a masculine sexual organ (yang within the yin) and the man's is feminine (yin within the yang).

Heart connection. Connect your hearts and let the energy overflow like a fountain of love.

Belly connection. Place your warm hands on your lover's belly to center. Lie belly-to-belly and breathe deeply into the dantian to ground.

Multiorgasmic energy is stimulated by breathing aroused energy upward and letting it expand from your heart to your body, your loved ones, the earth, and the vast universe. Affirm: "Create wisdom, compassion, and vitality in us all."

Being in the moment. Be totally present and caress like you may die the next day. Each moment with this being is precious!

Nesting. Take the time to lie together and breathe the orgasmic energies into your bones. Circulate the rejuvenating energy into your Microcosmic Orbit and collect it. When you spoon together and connect your feet, the qi in your meridians—which end in your toes—will harmonize.

🔥 Seamless Play

My partner's full presence allows me to open my heart and body in trust so we can both surrender to the bliss of union. He takes me on a journey and I

*respond with energy in motion. Cascading sounds express my pleasure. En-
ergy spirals in and around us. We are channels of the universal orgasmic life
force weaving through us, for the sake of all beings. Deep peace soaks into
our bones as we nest.*

*Our joyful play and touch throughout the day is a continual, seamless
foreplay. We meditate together and experience alchemical bliss just sitting
still in the same room. When I travel far away I still feel his presence cuddling
and comforting me and I do not feel alone. I am so grateful to have our warm
and loving connection in my life.*

MINKE DE VOS

Sapphic Lovemaking

Jade egg practices can enhance polarity in lesbian relationships. The woman
with a stronger yang core can chose to practice more standing, empowering Qigong, while the woman who has a more yin core can choose to practice more
yin. Cuddling is so relaxing and nourishing. It relieves depression and anxiety
and strengthens our immune system.

The jade egg practices are a natural form of penetration that will prevent
weakening or atrophy of the vagina muscles, which can occur if there is no
penetration for a long time. "If you don't use it you lose it!"

Whether you choose to make love with a woman or man, these playful
ways to weave the jade egg into your lovemaking add another dimension to
your love life. These movements can be a tantric massage to help a woman
open up to her deep yoni and whole-body bliss.

❋ Pulling the String to Bliss

Making love, one lover can pull the string of her lover's egg as she squeezes her
yoni and channels the energy internally. Here are some playful variations . . .

- The lover who pulls the string can stroke the awakened qi upward through
  the body to induce various forms of orgasm.
- The couple can have each a jade egg inside and can alternate pulling each other's
  strings like a seesaw. Connected at the hips, with legs draped over each other
  and heads away from each other, they can run their Orbits like an infinity symbol!
- One lover can rub the jade egg and imprint her loving intentions into it, then
  massage with the jade egg around her lover's belly and mound of Venus (pubic
  bone).

- One lover lies on top of the other, both facing up. The lover on the bottom can pull the string and massage the breasts of the lover on top or touch her heart with one hand.

- One lover rides on top of the other, facing each other. The lover on the bottom holds the rider's kidneys and pulls the string rhythmically as they breathe together. Another posture is holding behind the heart at the Wing point.

- Lying on their sides in a spooning position, the lover who is behind can pull the string as both partners both rock rhythmically together.

- As the active lover pulls the string, the "active-receptive" lover squeezes inwardly as she inhales or exhales. Entrain your breathing and become one as you ride the waves of ecstasy!

SEXUAL MASSAGE PRACTICES

The following sexual massage practices are a great way to get the sexual energy flowing in both partners.

❇ Energy Massage for Your Lover

This energy massage spreads awakened sexual energy to the three dantians, supporting personal power and will in the lower dantian, growing love and compassion in the heart dantian, and expanding the ability to grow mental and spiritual energy, thinking, insight, and intuition in the upper dantian.

The massage accelerates the frequency of energy in your partner and clears the passages for multiorgasmic experience by facilitating communication between the three centers.

● Quality of Touch

Slow, sensual, warm, smooth, continuous, flowing, penetrating touch will move energy through the density of the physical body and awaken the sexual energy on a cellular level.

Light feathery touch with the fingertips will awaken the sensitivity and move energy in the first Wei Qi field, which is like a second skin.

Stroking the qi about a foot or more away from the body in the subtle energy fields will help move the soul and spiritual levels of your partner's being. Become aware of the layers of auric field with the intention of harmonizing and integrating these layers.

Creating sacred space. Start by connecting with the golden smiling light washing down the front, back, and center of your body. Feel it flow into your roots, grounding in the unconditional support of the earth. Draw energy from the earth up into your body during the massage.

Connect with the heavens, stars, sun, moon, and planets and with the vast healing energy of the great eternal Tao. Connect with your guides, guardians, and beings of light, and those of your partner. Call on the Divine to create a safe and sacred space for this healing in accordance with divine will.

Warming the stove. Sitting beside your lover, place one hand on the Sexual Palace/organs and the other on the dantian/navel. Start massaging in a breast-stroke away from you, moving your hands apart and together again in circles. This direction expands the qi. You can also reverse this direction, moving your hands away on the outside and toward you in the middle. This direction gathers qi between the centers.

By connecting the sexual organs with the navel center dantian, you build core power and "warm the stove" below the navel. This helps build sexual fire and digestive fire. For women this is very important for evaporating excess dampness and bloating.

Warming the heart. Move your upper hand over your partner's heart, keeping your bottom hand over the Sexual Palace. Massage with the same circular movements as above, while making the heart sound, "ha-a-a-a-a-w."

Lighting up the third eye. Keep one hand on the Sexual Palace and move the other to the third eye. Massage in circles as above. You can also do some light tapping with your middle finger on the third eye. Move the sexual waters up to fuel the inner light in the third eye.

Figure eights. Sweep with both hands in a figure-eight movement from the Sexual Palace across the solar plexus, around the heart, and over the throat, crossing again over the solar plexus and back down to the Sexual Palace. Make continuous eights, moving with your whole body. You can also reverse the direction.

String of pearls. With the same weaving, you will now add another loop to your eight, making three loops that integrate the lower, middle, and upper dantians. Start at the Sexual Palace, cross the solar plexus around the heart, cross at the throat, and circle around the third eye and crown. Cross back down over the throat and solar plexus to return to the Sexual Palace. This can also be done in the reverse direction. Use your intuition to feel which way the qi wants to flow.

Collecting energy. Help your partner collect the energy by spiraling your hands outward counterclockwise nine times, then inward clockwise nine times. Press gently inward, sending your loving blessing into your partner's pearl.

❈ Reflexology Massage

Connect the reflexology zones along the Jade Stalk (penis) with the associated organs. See the sexual reflexology organ correspondences in fig. 5.2 (page 181).

If you are helping to raise the energy, follow the arousal and what makes your partner hard. If you are sublimating the energy, massage from the kidney zone toward the head. If you are cooling down and settling into peace, massage from the head down to the kidney zone.

- Touch the heart zone on the head of the penis with your left hand and touch your partner's heart with your right hand. Imagine a pink sunrise lifting up to your partner's heart.
- Touch the lung zone on the sides of the head of the penis and sweep an infinity symbol around each lung with white light.
- Touch the spleen zone just below the head of the penis with your left hand and hold or gently rock the spleen and stomach with your right hand. Imagine a yellow light of openness filling the earth organs.
- Touch the liver zone in the middle of his Jade Stalk and hold or gently rock his liver. Imagine the green light of kindness filling his liver.
- Touch the kidney zone at the base of the penis and hold one kidney at a time, filling the organs with a peaceful blue light.
- Hold his Jade Stalk in one hand, and with the other hand collect the energy at his navel.
- Bow with gratitude and honor of the great mystery.

● Fountains of Bliss

Sit between your lover's legs. Make a breaststroke with your arms, spreading his aroused qi in three expanding fountains up through his body.

- Stroke the sides of your partner's Jade Stalk, then up to the navel, down the belly, and inside his hips.

- Stroke up his Jade Stalk and make a fountain in the solar plexus, stroking around the ribs to hug his kidneys and down the folds in the hips, following the grooves of the body.
- Stroke the sides of his Jade Stalk and up to the heart, down the side ribs, and inside his hips, making a big heart shape!

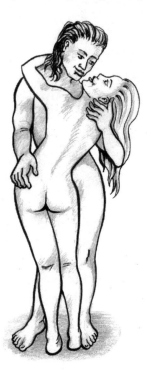

Fig. 9.2. Sexy, romantic lovers

Sexy Lover

I've got a whole lot of lov'n
My fountain is boil'n over
Stroking down my skin
Sending my lover in a spin
I'm a sexy lover!

I've got a whole lot of lov'n
Rolling with my baby in bed
Sliding in sweaty heat
Pulsing to heart's beat
I'm a sexy lover!

You've got a oooo lot of lov'n
Present in every move
With eyes of a hawk
And muscles of a rock
You sexy lover!

You've got a oooo lot of lov'n
Tasting every inch of my body
Creamy and fully baked
Lick the icing off my cake
You sexy lover!

We've got a whole lot of lov'n
Flowing with the steam of life
Alive in every cell
Glowing in love's spell
We're sexy lovers!

HARMONIOUS EXCHANGE

Qi flows between us continuously. By consciously exchanging energy, we can harmonize our relationships and develop deeper, more sensitive friendships (see fig. 9.3 on page 336). Practice with your partner or a close friend to bring subtler dimensions to your friendship. Some of the exchanges can be practiced by yourself, by imagining your inner man or inner woman in front of you.

✻ Partner Breathing

Allow your breath to carry masculine and feminine essences between you and your partner.

● Sacred Kiss

The partner with feminine essence channels the beauty of nature into her mouth and lips: sunrises, sunsets, forests, oceans. . . . She implants all this beauty onto her partner's lips, forehead, cheek, or hand. He breathes in the essence.

The partner with masculine essence channels the vastness of the heavens, stars, sun, moon, planets, sacred geometry . . . and fuses it in his mouth.

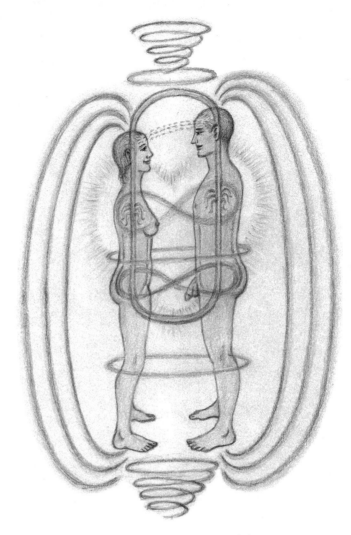

Fig. 9.3. Weaving of energy through lovers

He implants through his lips the universal presence onto his partner's lips, forehead, cheek, or hand. She breathes in the essence.

● Humming Hugs

Hug your partner heart-to-heart with your left ears together.

Both partners hum "mmmmm" warmly from your hearts and feel yourselves merging into the oneness of resonance.

● Channeling Cosmic Polarity

In this dynamic breathing practice, two people channel cosmic masculine and feminine energy to increase polarity. Sit with your partner with your eyes closed. The man—or the partner who wants to increase masculine essence—sits tall with palms facing upward to the heavens. He channels the sun and stars into his crown, down the Core Channel, and into his "wand of light" (penis).

The woman—or the partner who wants to increase feminine essence—sits tall with palms facing downward to the earth. She channels the moon and earth into her perineum and yoni, up the Core Channel, and into her heart and breasts.

Both partners breathe together from opposite polarities. Allow the qi to gather in the heart and sexual organs with each exhalation. Then open your eyes and give the gift of light and warmth over to your partner, letting it pour over into a circular flow. Follow with the next practice, Heart to Sexual Palace Circular Breathing.

● Heart to Sexual Palace Circular Breathing

In electrical circuitry, a positive pole flows into a negative pole. On our bodies, what protrudes is positive and what recedes is negative. So there is a natural energy attraction between a woman's breasts and the flat chest of a man, and between a man's Jade Stalk and a woman's yoni (fig. 9.4).

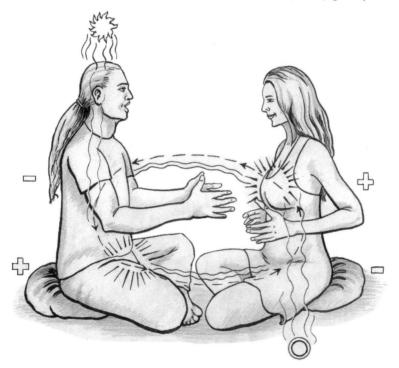

Fig. 9.4. Channeling cosmic polarity through the heart and Sexual Palace

Partners sit facing each other. The woman exhales with the heart sound ("ha-a-a-a-a-w"), overflowing her love from her breasts to the man's heart. Her partner inhales and receives it. He then brings the energy down to his Jade Stalk and sends his love over to her yoni as he makes the heart sound. She inhales and receives it. Both their arms can follow the same circle.

● Embracing Fire and Water

In a standing position, both partners hug each other and place their right hands over the back of the partner's heart (fire) and their left hands over the back of the partner's kidneys (water). Breathe together with love and peace.

● Linking Orbits

Embrace your partner with your foreheads touching, becoming aware of your Orbit and the Orbit of your partner (fig. 9.5). Your tongues can be kissing or resting on your own palates, tasting the sweet nectar of the Heavenly Pool. Sense the Orbits linking up through any of the chakras or all of them. You may feel the life pulse coursing through both of you like one heartbeat.

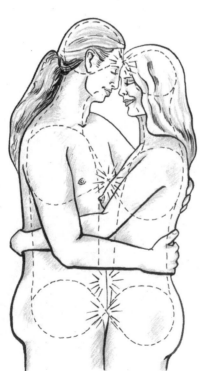

Fig. 9.5. Linking orbits, dantians, and chakras

If your Orbits are both running in the fire cycle, the qi dives and penetrates into both partners, tying you together like a bow!

If your Orbits are both running in the water cycle, the front doors of your hearts can open together and waterfalls of blissful qi run down your backs! Once your Orbits are flowing the possibilities are endless.

● Back-to-Back Orbit Breathing

Sit back-to-back with your partner. Entrain with your partner's breathing until you are breathing as one. Your kidneys will become warm and feel supported. Feel the current of qi in your partner's spine.

One partner initiates inverted breathing and rocks forward slightly while exhaling. The other will rock backward while inhaling. Allow your bodies to gently rock forward and backward together with the qi flow.

● Fire and Water Breathing

Sit back-to-back with legs wide and elbows interlaced (fig. 9.6).

One partner bends forward, making the kidney sound, "choo-oo-oo-oo." This opens the kidneys and stretches the Urinary Bladder channels on the backs of the legs.

The other partner rides on top in a back bend, making the heart sound, "ha-a-a-a-a-w." This opens the heart and stretches the Heart channels in the arms.

Both partners inhale together and suspend for a moment in the upright position before rocking in the opposite direction.

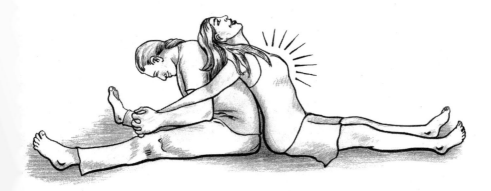

Fig. 9.6. Fire and Water Breathing, back-to-back

● Double Eagle

Sit back-to-back, legs wide. Keep your elbows interlaced with one another and your arms extended, forming two wings together. Feel the Wing points at the back of your hearts connected and warm.

Sway sideways, with one wing down and the other up. Circle the upper wing forward while the lower wing circles backward, so that you soar like eagles catching the wind. Imagine you are soaring up over the trees, over the clouds, past the moon and sun. Then return through the clouds, over the forests, and back to your nest.

Say "thank you" to your partner with a gentle wiggle in your back. Slowly peel off and turn to each other. Bow and say, "I set you free!"

✸ Exchanging Energies

> *I am opening up to sweet surrender*
> *of the luminous love-light of the One.*
> ANONYMOUS

For the moving exercises, stand in Taiji stance with one foot back at a forty-five-degree angle. Shift your weight forward by pushing your back foot and shift your weight back by pushing your front foot. Change legs after each exercise.

Between exercises, stand and get in touch with your "pillar of light."

● Pillars of Light

Stand in an open gesture with your palms facing each other. Connect your personal stars. Ask permission to share subtle communication and communion. Become a conduit for unconditional love.

Mostly we meet on the horizontal human plane; here you can support each other's path by meeting in the vertical plane. Feel like two pillars that uphold the temple of goodness, truth, and beauty. Support the highest in each other. Feel your spines and Core Channels aligning and entraining in parallel tones like tuning forks.

● Soul Gazing

Look deeply into your friend's eyes and third eye, creating an even triangle. See into his/her inner goodness and mystery. Express the depth of your love with your smiling eyes. Become calm and empty your mind. Breathe deeply. Keep your eyes open, soft, and panoramic, embracing each other's whole body and aura.

Two primal human needs are to love and be loved and to live in freedom. Ordinarily possessive attachment creeps in as we want to get closer, the opposite to freedom. The more we let go, the closer we get. As the limitations of the personality fall away, the celestial beauty of the soul attracts us naturally. We can experience our essential unity as our consciousness becomes inclusive. Melt feelings of separation. We are different but not separate. Feel merged yet individual. Let your hearts relax and become vast and all-embracing.

Affirm: "We are one. I honor you as an aspect of my universal self."

Practice Bone Breathing together. The bones are transpersonal channels for light frequencies. Come to peace by simply doing nothing—a practice called Silent Tantra. By just being together, we can heal relationships and make space for issues to shift on their own.

● Waves of Qi

Stand in a Taiji stance with one foot forward. Shift your weight forward by pushing your back foot and shift your weight back by pushing your front foot.

Allow a tidal wave of unconditional love to flow from behind you and wash toward your partner. Practice inverted breathing: as you exhale, your partner inhales.

Send the wave as you exhale. Receive the wave from your partner as you inhale. As you move forward your partner moves backward and vice versa. Let the qi breathe back and forth between you. Balance the giving and receiving aspects of your relationship. Touch into the naked energy of the primordial void and become fresh as a sea breeze.

- Send waves through your lower dantians. Clear any blockages that limit your passion and enjoyment of life. Sweep away any desires and attachments, which may obstruct the embodiment of compassionate action. Sound "sh-h-h-h-h-h" as you exhale. Generate the fullness of vitality and kindness.

- Send waves through your middle dantians. Clear any blockages that limit love from growing. Dissolve the ego's delusion of separation. Open to the oneness of compassion. Sound "ha-a-a-a-a-w" as you exhale. Generate the warmth of love.

- Send waves through your upper dantians. Let the wind of grace clear your

third eye of any limiting thoughts that may obstruct your inner vision. Sound "he-e-e-e-e" as you exhale. Generate the light of consciousness.
• Then return to the middle and lower dantians.

● Seesaw

As you exhale, swing a wave up the Core Channel of your partner to his crown. Receive the wave up to your crown as you inhale. Indicate this seesaw motion with your arms, making a U-shaped vessel between you. Breathe back and forth. As you exhale, sound "choo-oo-oo-oo."

● Wheel of Light

Taking turns, one partner stands in a receptive gesture as the other partner showers blessings of rainbow light, love, and adoration. Inhale up your Core Channel and send a rainbow from your crown into your partner's crown. Shower rainbow light down your partner's Core Channel, with a descending "he-e-e-e-e" (for him) or "she-e-e-e-e" (for her).

Become a hollow bamboo for the light to shine through. Become vast and empty, full of creative potential to grow your relationship. Yang light fills the yin vessel. Yin water fills yang's protective vessel. Yin water balances yang fire, within and between you. Bless each other with harmony. Feel the wheel generate light.

● Infinity Orbits

Connect your Microcosmic Orbits like an infinity sign between you (fig. 9.7). As you exhale, swing the energy over to your partner and follow it up the back and down the front of his or her Orbit. As you inhale, swing the energy over to yourself and follow it up and down your Orbit.

Alternate back and forth. Build a momentum that wants to go on infinitely, in a silken continuum. Indicate this flow with your arms, offering and scooping toward you. Extend your fingers of light to move the qi in this uniting flow. You can make this infinity flow around each of the dantians as follows:

Lower dantian. Weave Sexual Qi in a figure eight. The crossing point is a central Sexual Palace between you. Exhale and toss a qi ball over to your partner, who catches it and moves it in a loop around the core—from the root to Mingmen, to the navel, and back to the root—generating life force.

Middle dantian. Weave qi in a figure eight. The crossing point is a central heart

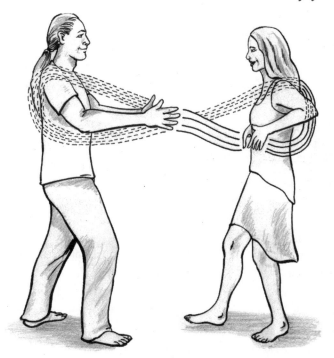

Fig. 9.7. Infinity Orbits exchanging qi at the heart

between you. Exhale and toss the qi ball over to your partner's solar plexus, circulating it up his spine, forward through his throat, and around his heart center, generating love.

Upper dantian. Weave light qi in a figure eight. The crossing point is a central third eye between you. Exhale the qi ball to your partner's throat and up the back of his or her head, circling it over the crown, generating light

Follow your intuition to generate qi in any center, wherever you would like to grow more power, love, or consciousness. This can shift from moment to moment. You can also weave small loops through the throat or solar plexus, wherever you feel more energetic clearing or connection is needed. Breathe together and embrace both Orbits in your awareness simultaneously. Feel your auric fields overlapping and glowing.

● Ocean of Compassion

Swim in fluid golden light with a breaststroke. Scoop energy into your Wing point, receiving compassionate energy from the universe through the back door to the front of the heart center. Exhale, sounding "ha-a-a-a-a-w," and let compassion flow from your heart forward to your partner in a freely giving gesture.

Your partner, the receiver, inhales "ha-a-a-a-w" with an open mouth into his heart center. Then he exhales and opens his wings from the Wing point, making a big embrace with his arms. Let your bodies be moved by the power of love.

After the heart chakra you can repeat this process for each of the seven chakras. Finish by repeating the heart chakra exercise again. Change roles and repeat the sequence. To close, cross your arms over your heart center. Generate reverence and respect for each other.

● Fountain of Life

Tap into a bottomless well of unconditional love and joy. Both partners inhale "oo-oo-oo" like sucking up a straw, pulling up a fountain of energy between you. Make a descending sound "la-a-a-a-a-w" as you let it shower down your backs. Follow the fountain movement with your arms and your whole body, rocking forward and backward.

Play in the spray! Frolic in the light of ecstasy! Shed karmic heaviness and conditioning off your back so you can be spontaneous in the moment. Lift lusty desires into the light of love. Let the overflow of love infuse every cell of your being. Soak in the warm mist.

✳ Ball of Joy

Create a collection ball between you to grow joy and love. Create a sacred space. Embrace with one arm up and the other arm down. Embrace like angels without ruffling each other's feathers. Feel embraced by a soft pink cloud.

Draw in warm, loving energy from the universe. Feel the ball pulsating magnetically between you. Smell the fragrances of the flower of friendship. Pack and condense the qi ball between your hands like a pink snowball. Hold it close to your heart, embracing your blessings for cultivating harmony in your relationships.

● Free Form

Open your heart and stretch the qi ball into two balls. Mirror dance, holding on to your common balls. Let the balls stretch and play between you. Let the qi move you, with no leader and no follower. Enjoy the buoyant currents of co-creative flow!

The Zen poet, Ryokan, describes this playful exchange of love between people as:

. . . playing ball,
Together in the fields—
*Two people, one Heart.**

● Rings of Light

Send protective rings of light around each other. Toss a qi ball or comet around. Starting and ending at the waist, spiral the qi counterclockwise up the chakras and clockwise down the chakras. Indicate that the ball goes behind your back. Let it spin like a cocoon of light. Bundle up in warm qi.

You can also do Push Hands in Taiji stance with your right foot and right wrist forward. Put the left palm in the right palm. Touch your right wrists together and circle them, like you are stirring the same cauldron, front to the left. A circuit of energy connects your "hugging points," C7. Switch arms, legs, and the direction of stirring. This helps resolve competition and overcontrolling issues in a relationship.

● Heart Salutation

Stand with your hands in prayer position at your heart. Be still and come to peace with your true nature. Give thanks for the gift of love and harmony you receive from the universe.

Bow to your partner, saying with your eyes, "The Divine in me bows to the Divine in you." Say to your partner, "I love you. I bless you. I set you free."

● Closing

Practice the triple warmer sound, "he-e-e-e-e," to sweep out any energies you may have picked up that do not feel right in your personal energy field. Smile down to balance your emotional body. Center yourself in your sovereign space.

Divine Marriage

I love the way you move,
The way your passion rises,
Pulsing, waving, spiraling

---

*Translation by John Stevens in *One Robe, One Bowl: The Zen Poetry of Ryokan* (Boston: Shambhala/Weatherhill, 2006).

Born into life
I bow to you, dear sex, and say I do.

I love the way you radiate
Shining light on my mystery
Pulsing, understanding, embracing
Born into consciousness
I bow to you, dear heart, and say I do.

We are the marriage
Of fire and water
Our child plays in the steam of creation
Born into humanity
We bow to you, dear Divine, and say we do.

MULTIORGASMIC POTENTIAL
Taoist Sexual Alchemy

Tantric sexuality contains three basic levels of progression, referred to as "lower tantra," "middle tantra," and "highest tantra." All three levels of practice mutually support one another.

Lower tantra emphasizes prolonged sex through the holding back of climaxing and the creation of valley orgasms. Many techniques also develop increased pleasure. The danger, if lust and pleasure are the only goals, is that the benefits are only temporary.

Middle tantra has spiritual overtones, working with healing, growing virtues, opening channels, and developing the chakras. Through consciously exchanging energy, more harmonious relationships can be encouraged. The Taoist practices for cultivating sexual energy are effective for this.

Highest tantra is the sublimation of aroused or unaroused energy into divine union. In Taoist practice, this is accomplished in the alchemical process of Kan and Li, meaning water and fire. By reversing fire and water, a steaming process refines sexual essence and uplifts it to higher centers.

The Metamorphosis of Inner Alchemy

Through sexual energy we got here.
Through its transmutation we return to our spiritual home.

Inner Alchemy is a spiritual practice of returning to the source, the Tao. When we incarnate, spirit (shen) generates energy (qi), and energy generates essence (jing). Essence then generates the body. In alchemy, we reverse this process to return to our original nature, returning body to jing to qi to spirit. In the metamorphosis of a cocoon into a butterfly, we can sense the power of the transmutation of matter into spirit.

As part of the reversal process, the fire of the heart descends and the sexual waters of the kidneys ascend, making an alchemical kitchen in your Core Channel. Imagine a fire under a cauldron filled with sexual essence: the fire brings the water to a boil. The cooking of raw substance creates steam, which is intensely healing and can dissolve old, stubborn patterns and blockages in the meridians and vital organs, as well as in the nervous, lymphatic, bone marrow, and blood circulatory systems.

Sexual alchemy couples the inner male and female essences within the body; our yin and yang energies literally make love inside and produce a blissful field of Yuan Qi, or unconditional love. Yuan Qi is a conductor for spirit to infuse the body. As we practice Inner Alchemy, we become sensitive to the collective spirit as a vast ocean in and around us. Body, energy, and spirit fuse into a single elixir field. The universe is no longer perceived as separate or outside but coexists inside of our beingness.

Sexual Alchemy Practices

The Kan and Li practices unite the masculine and feminine forces within, allowing the immortal body to be "impregnated." To lay the ground for the growth of the immortal seed, the energy body, qi, and channels need to be purified through awareness and deep, coherent breathing. Through responsible caring attention, the soul and spirit bodies mature.

Vital elements of the alchemical union of sun and moon are concentration/metal/sun and the internal cultivation of life force/wood/moon. If the body is still, the generative force is strong enough to turn the five elements back to their source, into one whole. In dual cultivation the arousal is maintained in still penetration of the sexual organs. Through one-pointed concentration of mind for over twenty-eight minutes, profound absorption is possible. The heart, seat of Original Spirit, becomes serene. Cosmic orgasm can be experienced as energy melting in the heart chakra into radiance and immense bliss.

The indiscriminate loss of sexual essence from the lower gates prevents the sublimation of this divine ecstasy. One doesn't "let down" but "let rise" into higher consciousness. The signs of a beautiful "Aha!" moment are the temporary effortless cessation of heartbeat and breathing, as when we say, "It took my breath away."

Wisdom, love, and compassion naturally arise out of the "reborn" soul body. This body can be still yin and illusory, like a doll. When this translucent, holographic, dreamlike body is investigated, we can apprehend only emptiness. Its lack of separate existence is like a rose, which cannot exist without heaven and earth. Through the realization of emptiness, interdependence, and oneness, an adept can attain enlightenment in the form of the primordial spirit body. Now this "holy body" is immortal, a constant experience of spontaneous great bliss fused with emptiness.

❀ Water Wheels Meditation

This is a solo meditative practice that refines sexual energy and balances the feminine and masculine energies in the deep Thrusting Channels.

● Thrusting Channels

- Visualize your Thrusting Channels by looking down inside your body to your ovaries. Your eyes guide energy and are openings to the Thrusting Channels. The Left Thrusting Channel (yang) goes through the warm heart. This yang channel is on the yin receptive side, where the stomach is receiving nourishment.
- The Right Thrusting Channel (yin) is on the yang, active side, where the liver is actively in charge of movement. Yin within yang creates an alchemical dynamic.

● Golden Boy and Silver Girl

- Imagine smiling energy as a golden boy coming into your left eye and a silver girl coming into your right eye. These children are representatives of the sun and moon. They invoke the pure, innocent, playful qualities of sexual energy.
- Let the children slide down your Thrusting Channels like firemen's poles and land on your ovaries. Imagine your ovaries are water wheels; as the cosmic children run toward your spine, water wheels roll up the back and down the front, like mini Microcosmic Orbits.

- Let your eyes roll in the same direction as your ovaries, drawing energy up the spine to your head. Continue to use the spinning qi in your eyes to pump, circulate, and refine qi in the Microcosmic Orbit.

● Refining the Energy

- Breathe deeply down into the water wheels like blowing into a fan or windmill. Feel the liveliness this generates! Traditionally, the energy generated by a windmill has been used to grind grain into flour; so, too, the jing or essence is refined into Jing Qi/sexual energy and then into shen/spiritual energy. Inhale and pull sexual waters up the spine. Exhale and bring the refined energy back down. Distribute the refined energy around the body and collect the balanced qi in your cauldron.

✸ Divine Union Meditation

This sensualization balances the universal yin and yang aspects of your Self. Marry your inner woman and inner man together to give birth to your inner sage.

- Sense a beautiful deity of the opposite sex smiling into your eyes with unconditional love. The warm light illuminates your Crystal Palace and flows down your Front Channel to the tip of your clitoris. Couple the energy there with a deity of the same sex as you are. These deities represent the primal power in male and female sexuality. Allow their exchange of energy to pulsate in your yoni and ripple pleasurable excitement up through your body.
- Their quickened qi rises up your Core Channel to your lower dantian. The blue water goddess and red fire god make love in your cauldron with the goddess on top. Imagine a volcano under the ocean. Practice Breath of Fire—a long deep breath in followed by short forceful exhalations through the nose—like a bellows fanning your inner fire. The fire gets the water to boil and generates steam. Steam rises and purifies the heart. Enjoy their "steamy" affair! Feel the steam infuse your body with vitality. Let it circulate freely. Cultivate pleasurable energetic satisfaction.
- The steam pressure lifts the god and goddess higher to your heart center, the Palace of the Spirit. Movement becomes internalized as the two deities sit in open lotus with the moon goddess on the sun god's lap (Yab Yum posture). Feel their hearts beating together and merging in loving embrace. Let warm vibrations pulsate through your bloodstream. Steam rises and

purifies your head. Cultivate radiance and serene spiritual surrender.

- The power of love lifts the two deities up to your Crystal Palace. The heaven god and earth goddess join in blissful, still penetration. The yang pineal gland penetrates the yin hypothalamus gland above it. Become attuned to celestial sound, overtones, and pure light vibration. Steam rises out from your crown and purifies your halo. Let your awareness brighten as their communion generates light.

- Open your crown like a flower. Let the divine couple launch up to the personal star above you. Surrender to your higher presence. Their light raises the sexual energy effortlessly.

- These representatives of male and female sexuality call the majestic creative forces of the universe toward you. Their light attracts high-quality yin and yang energy. The yin and yang aspects of yourself unite in harmony. Merge these cosmic forces—emptiness and bliss—into one light of Divine Oneness, Source, or the pregnant void.

- Bring a pearl of clear light down to your crown and Crystal Palace. Illuminate wisdom and imagination. Consecrated, sacred sexual energy produces nectar that drips down, clearing the passageway to your heart center. The pearl descends down to your heart and kindles love, joy, and inspiration. The nectar drips down, clearing the passageway to the navel center. The pearl descends down to the cauldron and empowers compassionate will and intuition.

- Circulate the high-quality energy in qi fountains and the Microcosmic Orbit.

- Collect the energy into a pearl in your center. Sense in your pearl an inner sage smiling.

✺ Kan and Li Meditation

Kan and *li* mean "water" and "fire." This Taoist Inner Alchemy practice brings the fire of the heart energy under the creative essence of water, like a volcano under the ocean. Your loving smile is the sunshine glistening on the water. The steam is Jing Qi, refined sexual energy.

Your alchemical kitchen takes place in the Core Channel, where the fire will cause the water to boil and create steam. With this steam we open up and purify our energy body. It has the potential to dissolve ancestral knots and deeply rooted patterns. The steam rises up and fuels our spiritual development.

● Steaming Sexual Energy

- Blow fire down your Front Thrusting Channel (within the Core Channel) to below the navel with the "ha-a-a-a-a-w" sound.
- Suck up water from your perineum by inhaling the cool "choo-oo-oo-oo" sound. Bring the sexual waters up the Back Thrusting Channel (within the Core Channel) like a pipeline with a faucet that pours water into your cauldron.
- Connect with the warm core of the earth as you would with a heartbeat. Fan the fire with Breath of Fire. Look down with crystal wands of light from your eyes and stir the steam. Caress the inside of your body with pink, luscious steam. Spread and soak it into the body, into any dry, stiff, closed parts of yourself. Steam open any old glue or residues from this earthwalk.
- Steam up the chakras, organs, and glands, opening them like flowers. Steam up your Core Channel and overflow out your crown into a fountain, cascading through your aura. Then reverse and bring the energy down the chakras, drinking in the heavenly dew and restfully closing the petals into potent buds.
- Let the pulsing, orgasmic energy generate bliss. Place your right sending hand over your Sexual Palace and your left receptive hand over a part of your body needing extra healing energy. Absorb the healing steam into your body.

● Self-Intercourse

The ability to have a spiritual orgasm is within us; stimulation from outside is not required. One universe does not go hump another universe! Couple the fire god in your pineal gland (cosmic love) with the water goddess in your Sexual Palace (cosmic creative energy). Join the cosmic couple in the neutral force of your center with loving, smiling energy. In other words, in your Core Channel, join Shakti/power—in the base of your body—with Shiva/consciousness—in your crown.

Feel the center of your brain and your uterus pulsating together. Then bring them together like long-lost lovers in your navel center. Let their energies make love, blue female on top of the red male. They can be in penetrating, sitting meditation posture with erect spines. Allow their orgasmic pulsations to spread everywhere in your body.

● Inner Eye

Let the divine union give birth to an animated pearl with awakened, heightened inner senses. Move this pearl through the chakras and channels, checking them out and clearing them. Check out your inner world like a child, for the first time.

Let the pearl settle back into the nest/cauldron/core and be nourished by steam. Sense your inner being smiling with contentment, wholeness, and the harmony of yin and yang.

Taste the nectar that drips down from the Heavenly Pool in your mouth and swallow it down to your navel.

● Immortal Child

- Let the steam grow your inner child—your highest potential—within the pearl. Let the pearl rise up a column of steam to the transpersonal point above you. See your life in a broad view. Bring the pearl down to the center of your brain, illuminating your mind.
- Incarnate your vision down to your feet to take your next step. Feel the essence of the universe within the pearl in your dantian. See the pearl as a miniature of your being like a smiling Buddha or Kuan Yin, content just to be.
- Absorb the steam into your bones. Rest like after a steam bath.
- Circulate the steam in the Microcosmic Orbit and collect the elixir into a pearl.
- Cool down excess heat with the triple warmer sound, "he-e-e-e-e."

EVOLUTION OF DIVINE HUMAN TREASURES

The Taoists saw the human body as a microcosm of the natural world, as illustrated in fig. 9.8. Our inner world is portrayed in this image as a landscape with mountains, rivers, streams, lakes, pools, forests, fires, and stars.

The nine sacred mountain peaks are like funnels that draw down universal energy. The boy and girl represent the testicles and the ovaries connected to the kidneys and eyes. They are stepping on the water wheel to pump the sexual waters upward.

In the center is the seed of long life and wisdom (the immortal fetus or the golden pearl). Below this golden pearl are the cow herder and the

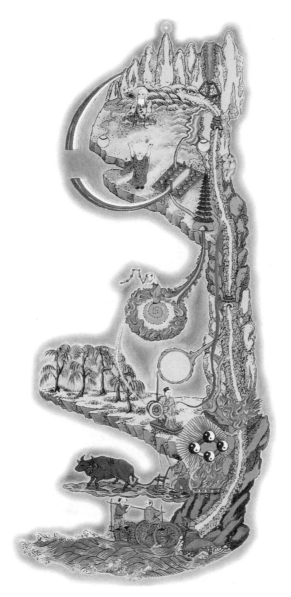

Fig. 9.8. Ancient image of Inner Alchemy
(Illustration courtesy of *The Taoist Soul Body* by Mantak Chia)

weaving maid, who have the ability to store energy and to go inward to instill quietude. The maid weaves silk out of moonlight with her mind, using gentle, soft, long, and deep breaths like spinning or pulling silk, drawing in the cosmic forces and weaving an internal web of qi.

The meaning of life is finding your gift,
and the purpose of life is to give it away.

ANONYMOUS

We are so fortunate to be freely exposed to once-secret tantric teachings from various spiritual traditions. Does the vast perspective of the Tao seem "beyond you" or do you dare to venture "beyond"? Allow yourself to be touched by the intangible, caressed by the sun's warmth, the wind's breath, and the ocean's flow. Awareness of our loving, creative nature lays the path for multipossibilities of orgasmic experiences. May our cultivation of potent sexual energy fuel greater love, light, and goodwill in our lives.

Sexual energy is the primal power of evolution. Evolving our limitless potential is possible with the masterful transformation of sex, love, and spirit. What I most want is to inspire women to cherish the magnificent, divine treasures that we are and to remind them how to cultivate the pure sexual life-force energy within us. We can create our lives consciously and commune with all beings with loving-kindness and compassion. I would love to see us playing with these arts, making them our own, and sharing them with our loved ones. The ripple effect multiplies the love and bliss!

The Divine Feminine is emerging and calls the Divine Masculine to walk hand in hand on this path of love. We walk together and make love together, merging heaven and earth through our oneness. Out of this harmony the new earth evolves with respect and reverence for all life.

May your feminine treasures be abundant,
making this world a more beautiful place.

SHARED WITH LOVE,

MINKE DE VOS

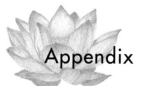

Appendix

Inspiring Your Daily Practice

Luscious Ladies

Ladies in love with themselves
Lure the lusciousness of life
Through their bodies and inner eyes
Gushing, the jade fountain flows
Into a river of opalescent nectar
And condenses into a golden pearl,
Each a unique gem of beauty.

DAILY PRACTICE

Even if you don't finish a complete practice, always end by circulating energy in the Orbit and collecting the energy in your navel center.

✹ Morning: Wake-Up Practice

When you first wake up, lie flat in bed, taking the pillow from your head, and lift your knees.

Inner Smile. Put your hands on your heart. Smile to your heart and fill it with love, joy, and gratitude. Radiate love to every gland and organ. Melt down from head to toes with the relaxation response. Smile down a waterfall of golden light, telling every cell, "I love you. Thank you for supporting my life."

Belly Massage. Brush down to your navel. Massage the wind gates around the navel and expand clockwise to massage the small intestine and colon.

Deer Breast Massage. Place one hand on your mound of Venus as the other hand massages your breast 6, 12, 24, or 36 times. By the time you reach 6 you will most likely be smiling! Repeat on the other side.

Kidney Packing. Restores and builds energy.
- Round your back to open the kidneys: lie down, hugging your knees up and crossing your ankles in the air; or lie down with your knees bent and feet on the floor; or kneel bent over your legs in Child Pose.
- Place your hands on your kidneys, widening the sides of your rib cage as you fill it with breath and qi.
- Hold your breath and spiral earth energy in and around the kidneys to absorb the qi.
- Exhale warmth from the heart down the lower back to "melt the ice" and comfort the kidneys.

Microcosmic Orbit. Place your hands over your navel. Run energy up the spine and down the Front Channel to balance and generate energy. Collect the energy, spiraling out and in to condense and store it.

✺ Daytime Practices

The following practices can be performed anytime during the day, as often as you like.

● Spinal Cord Breathing

Inhale, arching your back and opening wide your heart and pelvis.
　　Exhale, curling forward, arms in front of your chest, relaxing.

● Shaking the Tree

Shake your body like shaking old leaves off a tree. Make deep sighing sounds that come from your bones and ancestors.

● Swinging Bear

- Swing your arms around your hips, twisting from the lower back and pushing off with your feet. Tap the front and back of the body with both hands. Breathe in life-force energy and breathe out stress.
- Tap below the navel, releasing stagnation.
- Tap the kidneys, liver, spleen, lungs, and heart, knocking out toxins or tiredness in the belly and sexual organs.
- Tap the sacrum and shoulders.
- Push off with your big toes. Let your arms ride on currents around you. Send out smiling energy, rippling it out into the universe and letting it come back to you. What goes around, comes around!

● Full Vase Breath

Include conscious breathing throughout the day. It relaxes the organs, expands lung capacity, and balances the emotions.

It is more comfortable to wait a while after you eat to practice deep vigorous breathing.

- Breathe from the groin to the tip of the lungs like filling a vase with water.
- Expand on all four sides like blowing up a balloon.
- Check what moves when you breathe, including the belly, diaphragm, and rib cage.
- Find more and more places to breathe into. Stretch the breath from inside.
- Relax. Place your hands over the navel. Take a centering breath and feel a ball of warm energy collecting there.
- Come to peace.

❋ Evening Practice

Bone Breathing. Feel like a sponge in warm water, absorbing qi into your bone marrow. Plug yourself into the universe to charge yourself up!

Wu Wei Qigong. Lift your arms like a chalice and fill your body with universal energy. Allow the qi to move you spontaneously. Relax your jaw and allow the body to unwind. Lie down, surrender, and feel the support of the earth. Lie on your right side and "spoon" yourself. Let your heart relax.

Foot massage. Rub the Bubbling Springs points on the soles of your feet until they become warm. This will relax your body-mind and prepare you for a peaceful sleep, which replenishes deep yin reserves.

Triple Warmer Sound. Lie down and press your hands down the length of your body as you make the "he-e-e-e-e" sound. Feel like a rolling pin is rolling down your body, clearing away mental tension. This promotes good sleep as it cools the head and warms the feet.

Jade Fountain

My hands wash up your back,
Tossing luscious curls,
A waterfall cascades over my breasts,
My Jade Fountain rises again.

Summary of a Self-Love Ritual

In addition to the daily practices described above, you can devote time to a self-love ritual once, twice, or several times a week.

Inner Smile
Breast Massage
Massage ovaries, uterus, and kidneys
Jade egg practices/Tao Yoni Yoga
Bone Breathing
Microcosmic Orbit and Collect Energy
Triple Warmer Sound
Bow

For a more vigorous sexual energy workout add: Qi Weight Lifting, Tapping, or Wu Wei Qigong

---

Pracice with love, gratitude, and joy!

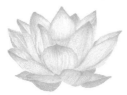

Resources

Recommended Reading

The Emergence of the Sensual Woman by Saida Desilets. Kihei, Hawaii: Jade Goddess Publishing, 2006.

Exploring the Hidden Power of Female Sexuality by Maitreyi Pointek. York Beach, Me.: Weiser Books, 2001.

Healing Love through the Tao by Mantak Chia. Rochester, Vt.: Destiny Books, 2005.

The Multi-Orgasmic Woman by Rachel Abrams and Mantak Chia. New York: HarperOne, 2010.

Women's Anatomy of Arousal by Sheri Winston. Kingston, N.Y.: Mango Garden Press, 2009.

Tao Alchemy Products

CDs: *Bells of Love* and *Tao Basics*

DVDs: *Move with Flow* and *Heart Qigong*

For these and more CDs, DVDs, jade eggs, and other related products, see the author's website: **femininetreasures.com.**

Workshops, Retreats, and Trainings

For listings of workshops, retreats, and trainings see:

silentground.com ◆ taotantricarts.com

Teacher trainings and workshops in Sacred Femininity, Taoist Priestess, and Divine Alchemy are available through Tao Tantric Arts. Seasonal retreats and certification programs are also available. Please see **silentground.com** for more information.

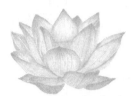

Bibliography

Camphausen, Rufus. *The Yoni*. Rochester, Vt.: Inner Traditions, 1996.

Deadman, Peter, and Mazin Al-Khafaji. *A Manual of Acupuncture*. Hove, UK: Journal of Chinese Medicine Publications, 1998.

Douglas, Nik, and Penny Slinger. *Sexual Secrets*. Rochester, Vt.: Destiny Books, 1979.

Jarrett, Lonny S. *Nourishing Destiny*. Stockbridge, Mass.: Spirit Path Press, 1998.

Johnson, Professor Jerry Alan. *Chinese Medical Qigong Therapy*. Vol. 1. Pacific Grove, Calif.: The Institute of Medical Qigong, 2005.

Maman, Fabien. *The Tao of Sound*. Stockbridge, Mass.: Tama-Do, 2008.

Zhao, Xiaolan. *Reflections of the Moon on Water*. Toronto, Canada: Random House, 2006.

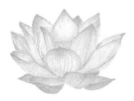

Index